Human Resource Management in Nursing

Dale Kayser Jernigan, R.N., M.S.N.
Consultant for Health Care Services
Gulf Shores, Alabama

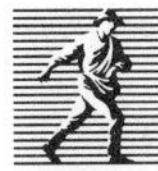

APPLETON & LANGE
Norwalk, Connecticut/San Mateo, California

0-8385-3952-1

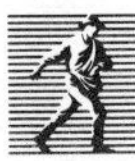

88 89 90 91 92 / 10 9 8 7 6 5 4 3 2 1

Prentice-Hall of Australia, Pty. Ltd., Sydney
Prentice-Hall Canada, Inc.
Prentice-Hall Hispanoamericana, S.A., Mexico
Prentice-Hall of India Private Limited, New Delhi
Prentice-Hall International (UK) Limited, London
Prentice-Hall of Japan, Inc., Tokyo
Prentice-Hall of Southeast Asia (Pte.) Ltd., Singapore
Whitehall Books Ltd., Wellington, New Zealand
Editora Prentice-Hall do Brasil Ltda., Rio de Janeiro

Library of Congress Cataloging-in-Publication Data
Jernigan, Dale Kayser.
Human resources management in nursing.

1. Nursing services—Personnel management. I. Title.
[DNLM: 1. Nursing Staff—organization & administration.
2. Personnel Management—methods. WY 30 J55h]
RT89.3.J47 1987 362.1'73'0683 87-14442
ISBN 0-8385-3952-1

Production Editor: Nancy C. Greenberg, Lynne Krupa
Designer: Steven M. Byrum

PRINTED IN THE UNITED STATES OF AMERICA

To the two people who enabled me to
seek truth,
learn compassion,
actualize potentialities,
and to face the forces of change:
My mother and father,
Jule Basch Kayser and
Sam Joseph Kayser, Jr.

I dedicate this book to you.

Contents

Preface

As a consultant in health care, I am continually asked similar questions by nurse administrators. Whether I'm in a hospital or home health setting, or providing a management seminar, questions are always raised regarding personnel problems and concerns such as "How do I attract and retain quality people?"; "How do I develop a productive and enthusiastic staff?"; and "How do I maintain good employer/employee relations?". When turning to health care literature, only bits and pieces of information can be found that address human resource concerns. Books on leadership, staffing, or organizational development may be found, but books that thoroughly review issues on and management of people in an organization do not exist. This book is devoted exclusively to the concept and practice of human resource management, and will hopefully fill that void.

In these difficult times it is all too easy to focus only on problem employees or performance deficiencies. As leaders, we must base our practices on a philosophy that views the human being as the answer, rather than the problem. We must value those who provide the care, and supply the structure and guidance to maximize their potentialities. The answers lie within the vast source of human talent and creativity that surrounds you every day. Your job is to tap and nurture these abilities. I hope this book will assist you in this endeavor.

Acknowledgments

I would like to express my special thanks and appreciation to Suzanne Smith Blancett, R.N., Ed.D., Editor-in-Chief of *The Journal of Nursing Administration* and *Nurse Educator*. Suzanne extended a hand to an unknown author, and offered friendship and guidance. My promise to you is to perpetuate the cycle of giving.

I would also like to thank the following nursing authors and leaders, who offered their insight, expertise, and time in reviewing selected chapters of my book:

Minerva Applegate, R.N., Ed.D.
Tampa, Florida

Majorie Beyers, R.N., Ph.D.
Evanston, Illinois

Dorothy J. del Bueono, R.N., Ed.D., C.N.N.A.
Philadelphia, Pennsylvania

Cecelia Golightly, R.N., B.S., M.P.H.
Minneapolis, Minnesota

Joellen Hawkins, R.N.C., Ph.D., F.A.A.N.
Chestnut Hill, Massachusetts

Margaret O. Jobes, R.N., M.S.N.
Phoenix, Arizona

Nellie Abbott, R.N., Ph.D.
University of Pennsylvania-Hospital
Philadephia, Pennsylvania

Jackie Dienemann, R.N., Ph.D.
George Mason University
Fairfax, Virginia

Sara J. Mapstone, R.N., M.S.N.
Charlottesville, Virginia

Gaye W. Poteet, R.N., Ed.D.
Galveston, Texas

Ingeborg Mauksch, R.N., Ph.D., F.A.A.N.
Ft. Myers, Florida

Belinda Puetz, R.N., Ph.D.
Indianapolis, Indiana

Mary Ann Rose, R.N., Ed.D.
Greenville, North Carolina

Julie Wine Schaffner, R.N., M.S.N.
Chicago, Illinois

Mary Yeager
University of Virginia-Hospital
Charlottesville, Virginia

SPECIAL ACKNOWLEDGMENTS

I would also like to give special thanks to *Leo Kemp Jernigan,* my husband—who believed in me, supported me, and understood. This book would never have been written without his devoted patience and love.

Introduction

The most important element in health care facilities today is the people who provide the care; the success or failure of an organization is determined by how its human resources are used. This book is different from many other management books in that it highlights personnel processes, rather than leadership style, communication theory, or organizational theories. These and other theories are interwoven throughout this book and applied to personnel practices.

The book is divided into two sections, the first of which presents some theoretical background for human resource management. Administrative functions, principles and patterns of change, effective planning, and fostering and developing creativity are explored to provide a foundation for Part II, The Personnel Process. This second section specifically examines the organization and effective implementation of each of the eight personnel processes: recruitment, selection, orientation, performance evaluation, counseling and coaching, retention and productivity, staff development, and labor relations. Together these personnel processes form the major aspects required for maximizing the human talents, potential, and resources within the health care organization.

This book was designed for both nursing graduate students and practicing nurse administrators, but its principles can be applied by managers and administrators in almost any field. Although it is health care oriented, this book will prove useful to anyone responsible for the management of human resources.

DEFINING TERMS

A few terms must be specifically defined for the purposes of this text.

The term *human resource* includes any individual employed by the institution. Although other human resources are often available on a consulting or contractual basis, or by referral to outside agencies or services, the focus of this book is upon the available human resources within the institution. The registered nurse is often used as the focus of the examples in the second section, but of course most examples are applicable to other personnel as well, e.g., aides, orderlies, unit secretaries, technicians, and licensed practical nurses.

The term *nurse administrator* is defined as anyone who is responsible for managing human resources, with the authority to hire, evaluate, fire, and promote. In some institutions, this will apply to first line managers, while in others it will apply to higher levels of management. The reader may discover that different parts of this text apply to different administrative levels in their institution. Because management roles and responsibilities are constantly changing and vary among institutions, the term "nurse administrator" is defined by actions rather than by titles.

Finally, the chief *frame of reference* throughout the text is that of the hospital. The principles and examples in this text may be applied in many other types of health care delivery systems, such as home health agencies and long-term care facilities, as well.

PART I
Concepts for Human Resource Management

Part I of this book provides concepts that are instrumental to effective human resource management. These concepts provide a framework for Part II, The Personnel Process, which focuses on the specifics and practice of human resource management. Chapter 1 provides an overview of four major functions of the nurse administrator. Each function is interdependent and linked to organizational success. Conceptualizing these functions as a whole is necessary to effectively implement the processes of human resource management.

Chapter 2 discusses some fundamental principles of change. This discussion provides a perspective of change that directs purposeful planning and intervention. Our response to change depends on our understanding of the process and workings of change, and determines our effectiveness as administrators in human resource management.

Chapter 3 presents the evolution of change in relation to the nurse administrator's function. Successful human resource management depends on a broad knowledge of trends, patterns and environmental conditions, to determine the effect of these conditions on the nature of work, the human resource and the organization. In order to adapt and control the forces of change, we must understand its direction. This chapter reviews dominate trends and changes effecting the health care system and provides a knowledge base of change.

Chapter 4 presents the planning function. The effects of change are continually assessed and analyzed, then put to use through deliberate planning. Planning is critical to all administrative actions and is necessary in order to effectively implement the processes of human resource management.

Chapter 5 explores creativity. All aspects of human resource management must involve analytical processes and practices blended with creative and innovative thinking. Creativity is essential for controlling the forces of change. It facilitates effective human resource management in a changing world. This chapter explores the creative process and ways to tap and foster the creative potential within the human resource.

Many skills and processes are critical to effective human resource management. The concepts presented in Part I will serve as a basis for operationalizing the skills and processes presented in Part II. With a broader perspective of the administrative functions, insight into principles and forces of change, and understanding of purposeful planning and creativity, we can be better prepared for the practice of human resource management.

1 Administrative Functions: An Overview

Human resource management is only one of the administrative functions of a nurse-administrator, albeit a critical one. In order to dispatch duties successfully, a nurse-administrator must implement several important functions. These include information synthesis, business management, planning and, of course, human resource management. What follows is a brief overview of these administrative functions.

INFORMATION SYNTHESIS

The first and most important of these functions is *information synthesis,* or the collecting, analyzing, and integrating of information. An *information system* can be department oriented or organization oriented; it is often both. Information synthesis is the deriving of meaning from facts, events, schedules, and data. The meaning derived from this synthesis is then used to evaluate a current departmental or organizational performance and to forecast future implications, trends, and needs.

The data used in information synthesis can be gathered from any number of sources, which range from conversations with patients and colleagues to the reading of newspapers and professional journals to the interpreting of computerized information printouts. Information synthesis first examines this collected information and breaks it down into basic elements for analysis. The information is then manipulated or processed into meaningful arrangements for problem solving and/or further analysis.

Last comes the synthesis process, in which the effects, meanings, implications, and usefulness of the information are derived. Computers, consultants, support networks, and decision-making models often aid in this final process.

It should be noted that effective information synthesis takes into account environmental and organizational conditions and changes. True information synthesis correlates past and present conditions and factors to provide future directions.

BUSINESS MANAGEMENT

With the recognition that health care is an industry, nursing has become more than just a service, it has become a business. Nurse-administrators have therefore become entrepreneurs, charged with running and managing a business. Indeed, *effective business management skills* are now necessary to exist successfully in today's health care system. Included in business management skills are financial planning and evaluation, marketing, public relations, cost-containment strategies, quality control, and risk management.

One of the most demanding business management skills is *quality control,* which is concerned primarily with patient satisfaction, enhanced health outcomes, prevention or management of complications, decreased lengths of stay, and cost efficiency. From a nursing standpoint these areas involve delineating nursing's independent functions and developing tools to evaluate their implementation, but from a business standpoint they involve improving efficiency, reducing costs, increasing market shares, and decreasing outliers. Viewed from this second standpoint, they become part of business management.

PLANNING

Planning is a process inherent in all administrative functions. In many organizations, planning is a separate department altogether, with employees devoted to the tasks of researching, developing, forecasting, and strategically planning. However, in recognition of the clinical expertise of professionals, planning is becoming more integrated within hospitals and organizations, with strong participation and input from operational as well as administrative levels in the organization.

Planning is intimately linked to information synthesis, as identification of environmental forces and potential conditions dictates the focus of planning. Planning is also a component of business management strategies, including cost-benefit analyses, projection of future financial needs and allocations, and establishment of a competitive edge while striving for excellence in service.

Human resource management planning is critical to matching employee competency to the organization. Plans must be made to develop current and potential staff to meet organizational goals.

HUMAN RESOURCE MANAGEMENT

Human resource management is the crossroads of all administrative functions: without employees, nothing gets done. The nurse-administrator must be able to manage human resources so that both the organization and the employee benefit. A nurse-administrator who can tap employee creativity and ability is not only providing the organization with creative benefits, but is also providing the employee with the opportunity directly to influence and *change* the environment for the better. Change is inevitable but, with proper human resource management, rather than feeling powerless, employees can take part in shaping their future.

2 Managing Change

The world is in a state of continual change—nothing stays the same. Our response to change determines our vitality and progress; consequently, the response and adaptation of our human resources determine the vitality and progress of the organization. Managing change to the best advantage is one of the hallmarks of an effective nurse-administrator. This chapter will discuss some basic workings of change.

WHAT IS CHANGE?

We can roughly define *change* by stating that it is the constant movement of energy from one source to another. This, of course, is an abstraction: for our purposes, change is more realistically defined as the movement and process of energy in transformation, through action and reaction. Change does not occur in isolation, but is interwoven in all the threads of our daily lives. How does the nurse-administrator harness the forces of change? The philosophy of *pragmatism* is useful in developing an approach to change.

WHAT IS PRAGMATISM?

Pragmatism is a philosophy that tests truth and knowledge through the results of practical application. It has its basis in the writings of the ancient Greek philosopher Heraclitus. It is a philosophy strongly influenced by modern science—Francis Bacon, Charles Darwin, and William James are only a few of the scientists who have contributed to the philosophy of pragmatism.

Generally speaking, pragmatism is concerned with making things work. Ideas have value only when they have social significance. Progress is not certain, but possible; one can face each situation with purpose and intelligence, and strive for progress. To the pragmatist, knowledge is organized facts or patterned hypotheses that have been validated by tested results. Pragmatism emphasizes problem solving and scientific methodology for a useful outcome. The value of knowledge is judged by its usefulness in practical applications. Thought and knowledge are weapons for controlling and improving the future.

THE DYNAMICS OF CHANGE

Change occurs within a pattern that can be interpreted and predicted. Certainly, radical changes do occur, but usually result from the lack of preceding smaller changes. The following *fundamental principles of change* reflect its dynamic processes and provide a guide for using change advantageously.

1. The world is a place of continual change in which all processes of nature are interconnected.
2. Perpetual change creates an order and regularity within nature.
3. Conflict and tension create an environment for adaptability and evolution; human survival depends upon the ability to adapt to change.
4. Creativity and innovation are tools for controlling change.

Continual Change

Change occurs to each of us every day. Our calendar and century systems are based on the fact that with every rising of the sun, a change occurs. Within the medical field, in the past 40 years, changes have occurred rapidly. There has been a knowledge explosion in both our understanding of disease processes and medical interventions. Disease is now seen as caused by multiple concurrent factors that are interdependent. Simultaneously, organizational science has expanded its understanding of organizational behavior to recognize that conflict and change are continuous, healthy processes. Each department within an organization is intimately connected to all others and to environmental influences. One small departmental change *can* have an impact on the entire organization.

Change Creates Order

Change has a stability and continuity of its own. We know that change will happen, and we can often predict what changes will occur. A simile for a change is that of a cloth with an intricate pattern being woven on a loom.

We can see how the cloth started out, see the present design, and perhaps guess at the final pattern. The weaver, like the nurse-administrator, chooses what threads to use, adapts the tension appropriately, and has a plan for what the cloth will look like when it is taken from the loom. The weaver, like the nurse-administrator, must pay attention to the individual threads, actions while using the loom, and the whole cloth. The nurse-administrator must fulfill *all* the administrative functions of the job in order to produce a tapestry.

Conflict Creates an Environment for Adaptability

Change is an infinite chain of cause and effect. One change can create a conflict, adapting to that conflict creates a second change. Because change is a constant factor, humans must adapt to change in order to survive. Conflicts also provide a means for improvement—rather than just adapt (or survive), we can also evolve (improve).

Creativity and Innovation Are Tools

Beyond adaptability and evolution is another level: control. Creativity and innovation are tools for controlling change and making it work for us. Although control is never complete or permanent, we can influence the chain of events within specific systems. Rather than allowing events to occur and then changing accordingly, we can initiate our own energy forces. By creating, we produce our own changes and affect the sequence of events, thereby controlling change.

CHANGE AND HUMAN RESOURCES

Change benefits both the employee and the manager. It provides the employee with the opportunity to use creative potential, while it provides the manager or administrator with the opportunity to tap into that potential. By the same token, the manager must provide the employees with tools—support, guidance, working conditions, resources, and reinforcement—to help them adapt to change. All aspects of the organization must continually help to maintain balance and equilibrium by learning, improving, and progressing one step ahead of change. Human resource management involves providing the right conditions and processes to foster innovative and expert human resources. An enlightened leadership team can attract, retain, and develop the human resources who will contribute to a vital, progressive, and successful organization.

SUGGESTED READING

Ames, R., & Siegleman, P. The age of Darwin. In *The Idea of Evolution.* Minneapolis, Minn.: Meyers, 1961.

Bakewell, C. M. *Source book in ancient philosophy.* New York: Scribner, 1907.

Browning, D. (Ed.) *Philosophers of process.* New York: Random House, 1965.

Butler, J. D. *Four philosophies and their practice in education and religion.* New York: Harper & Row, 1968.

Conklin, E. G. *The directions of human evolution.* New York: Scribner, 1922.

Dewey, J. *Democracy and education.* New York: Macmillan, 1944.

Durant, W. *The story of philosophy.* New York: Simon & Schuster, 1961, p. 2.

Eames, M. S. *Pragmatic naturalism—An introduction.* Carbondale, Ill.: Southern Illinois University Press, 1977.

Edel, A. *The theory and practice of philosophy.* New York: Harcourt, Brace and Co., 1946.

Huxley, T. H. The struggle for existence in human society. In R. Ames, & P. Siegleman (Eds.), *The Idea of Evolution.* Minneapolis, Minn.: Meyers, 1961.

James, W. Pragmatism: A new name for some old ways of thinking. In G. H. Knobs & R. K. Snyder (Eds.), *Readings in Western Civilization.* New York: Lippincott, 1960, pp. 716–718.

James, W. The stream of consciousness. In D. Browning (Ed.), *Philosophers of process.* New York: Random House, 1965, pp. 142, 143.

Johnson, O. A. *Man and his world: Introductory readings in philosophy.* New York: McKay, 1964.

Kirk, G. S. *Heraclitus: The cosmic fragments.* London: Cambridge University Press, 1962.

Kramer, M., & Schmalenberg, C. E. Conflict: The cutting edge of growth. *The Journal of Nursing Administration,* October 1976, p. 24.

Levenstein, A. Philosophy for nurses? *Nursing Management,* June 1982, p. 51.

Marcell, D. W. *Progress and pragmatism.* Westport, Conn.: Greenwood Press, 1974.

Maslow, A. H. *The farther reaches of human nature.* New York: Penguin Books, 1971.

May, R. *The courage to create.* New York: Bantam Books, 1975.

Partridge, G. W. *A reading book in modern philosophy.* New York: Sturgis and Walton, 1913.

Rodgers, J. A. Theoretical considerations in the process of change. *Nursing Forum, 12*(2), 162, 1973.

Rogers, M. E. *An introduction to the theoretical basis of nursing.* Philadelphia: Davis, 1970.

Russell, B. *The problems of philosophy.* New York: Oxford University Press, 1912.

Terreberry, S. The evolution of organizational environments. In W. G. Bennis, K. D. Benne, R. Chin, & K. E. Corey (Eds.), *The Planning of Change* (3rd ed.). New York: Holt, Rinehart & Winston, 1976, p. 179.

Thomas, H., & Thomas, D. L. *Living biographies of great scientists.* New York: Garden City, 1941.

Webster, H., & Wesley, E. B. *World civilization.* New York: Heath, 1940.

Whitehead, A. N. *Science and the modern world.* New York: The Free Press, 1953.

3 Changes in Health Care

Now that we have looked at some principles of change, let us turn to specific changes that have been occurring in the field of health care, and look at some implications and future challenges for nurse-administrators. First we will discuss some primary changes. These are forces that initiate further, major environmental change.

PRIMARY CHANGES

Demographic Trends and Changes

Demographics can provide important information about the birthrate, life expectancy, and health practices of a population. In 1982, only 5 percent of the population was 75 years of age or older. It is predicted that by 2030, 10 percent of the population will be in that age category. By 2050, those 85 years of age and older are projected to comprise 5 percent of the total population. With aging comes the need for more health care services. According to the American Hospital Association statistics of October 1984, older Americans represented 11 percent of the population, but consumed 20 percent of all personal health care expenditures. The "graying of America" is resulting in an increasingly elderly patient population and a requirement for greater access to hospital, nursing home, and home health care services to serve this population.[1]

With this growing elderly population, there has been a shift in epidemiological trends. With the aging population, there is a higher prevalence of people with multiple, chronic diseases associated with living longer and with poor health habits and practices. The incidence of chronic diseases associated with obesity, stress, and respiratory and cardiovascular disease has thus increased. This in turn has increased Americans' interest in prevention and fitness, and has also led to a fascination with health food, megadosing of vitamins, and other fads to "ensure" a long and healthy life.

The implications for nurse-administrators of this larger elderly population with multiple, chronic problems, requiring more complex nursing care, are that consumers will require increased education and counseling for health promotion, altering life-styles, stress reduction, and self-care. The "graying of America" will require an expansion in gerontology, long-term and home care services, and clinical staff competencies.

Advances in Technology

Advances in technology are currently sweeping the health care industry, and providers as well as consumers associate quality of care with the presence of the most modern technologies in a hospital. Health care facilities have invested in the most sophisticated diagnostic and treatment technology in an effort to increase market shares and attract physicians. However, the rate at which these extremely expensive investments become obsolete is increasing. For instance, nuclear magnetic resonance imaging now threatens to antiquate the CAT scanner after a relatively narrow time span. Small hospitals are also caught up in the technological race, so as not to lose patients and physicians to larger, city hospitals. These trends have contributed to escalating health care costs. In turn, escalating costs have led to government efforts to regulate the distribution of advanced technology instruments in hospitals. And the failure of hospitals to control costs has led to the current prospective payment plan and move to deregulate health care in the belief that market forces will lead to rationing of purchases.

The growth of technology has also brought an increase in the complexities of patient care. New treatment procedures keep patients with multiple health problems and illnesses alive, where previously they would have died. Larger aging patient populations and advanced technology have increased the acuity level of patients in hospitals. In order to keep up with rapid technological changes, nurses, like physicians, have begun to specialize and become more technically oriented.

Other technological trends include increased use of computers for invasive and noninvasive diagnosis and monitoring of patients' care and conditions. Computers are also increasingly being used to automate the management information systems in hospitals. This ranges from activities such as order entry to productivity reports. The impact of discovery and mass production of the microchip in computing has led to inexpensive, usable size and powerful hardware. Managers' emphasis is focused on software and training in computers to improve case management with record keeping; effective and efficient use of staff with patient classification tools, data base management, and electronic spreadsheets; and financial management of all resources with the automated management information systems.

Shifting of Payment from the Patient to Third Parties

The idea of insurance coverage against catastrophe began with marine insurance by shipowners in world trade. With the growth of cities and susceptibility to damage from fires came fire insurance for businesses. Insurance coverage for individuals began with burial insurance, and after the Depression, insurance payment became a negotiation by unions as a worker benefit. By 1945 benefits included life, health, and hospital insurance. Meanwhile, the government equivalent of health and hospital insurance for the elderly and disabled developed as Social Security. This began in 1935 as a joint federal and state plan for social assistance of the needy, aged, and disabled, and certain families with dependent children.

In 1965 the government began financing the health care of the elderly, disabled, and disadvantaged with the passage of the Social Security amendments Title XVIII (Medicare) and Title XIX (Medicaid). Medicare granted funds for medical insurance to the elderly, thus departing from the original welfare intent of the Social Security Act, and granted funds to all people 65 years of age or older, regardless of financial need. Medicare was intended as health care insurance for all elderly people, while Medicaid was established only for the needy.

As of 1984, there were 30.6 million people enrolled (12.7 percent of the population) in Medicare, with 61 billion dollars spent on coverage. The costs of both the Medicare and Medicaid programs have dramatically increased annually since inception, despite increases in copayments, caps on payment to physicians, and other attempts to control costs. Many factors have contributed to this increase: life expectancy has increased; there is a growing elderly population; use and intensity of medical services have increased; and health care costs have risen. Medicare coverage has also been expanded, adding to cost increases. Some expansions in coverage include the end-stage renal disease (ESRD) program covering kidney dialysis and transplants, and the Physician Peer Review Program (PSRO), instituted to monitor quality and utilization of services. Other added coverages included hospice, ambulatory surgical procedures, outpatient rehabilitation, and the pneumococcal and hepatitis vaccines.[2]

As a result of the continued rise in Medicare and Medicaid expenditures, the Social Security funds began to run out. The federal government could no longer afford to continue to finance health care for the elderly and the indigent in the existing system. Strong measures to cut spending have resulted.

Simultaneously, employee health care insurance benefits expanded to cover a higher percentage of costs and more services, such as new and better technologies, dental care, mental health care, and treatment of alcoholism and substance abuse. People came to expect all medical care to be paid by their insurance.

The third-party payer system is one whereby a third party pays for a service given to another person or subscriber. For example, an individual or employer pays insurance premiums to Blue Cross. When this individual is hospitalized, Blue Cross will pay a set percentage, such as 80 percent, of all the hospital costs. Blue Cross is then a third party, paying a hospital (second party) on behalf of an individual (first party). This third-party paying for health care has made patients insensitive to costs. This was another factor contributing to the increased percent of the gross national product devoted to health care.

Nationally, both the public and government have become concerned with the rise of health care costs. The media have made the public aware of the increasing cost of health care and its impact on the depleted Social Security system, shrinking natural resources, the growing federal deficit, and so on. In an attempt to hold down costs, cost ceilings, wage and price freezes, and various regulatory measures were instituted, along with the promotion of voluntary cost containment measures. None of these methods has worked. Economists realized that health care providers had no real incentives either to contain or decrease their costs despite these controls, due to the retrospective reimbursement system. Under this system, a hospital was reimbursed based on its cost in providing health care services. This "cost" included the diagnostic procedures and specialized services available through advanced technology. Cost versus effectiveness of each service was rarely considered. New technologies were purchased to increase revenues and prestige of hospitals. This reimbursement system actually encouraged hospitals to spend more so they could earn more.

The Consumer Movement

Another major force of change affecting health care is the consumer movement. Consumers want to know what services they are receiving, when, where, why, and how much these services cost. This consumer movement has evolved for a variety of reasons, including a general increase in both the average standard of living and educational level, as well as greater media exposure to health-related information. Information about medications, surgical procedures, birth control, and other health information can be found in women's magazines, newsmagazines, newspapers, and on television. In general, the public has higher expectations of quality and access to health care, and demands more information as well as reasonable costs.

Consumer special interest groups are another important force in health care. Lobbying by groups can help to change federal policy; the direction of change is influenced by those with the most power. Agencies and businesses can contract with law and public relations firms to influence court decisions and/or congressional action. Lobbying efforts can also influence resource allocation decisions. For example, federal funds allocated to nursing research in 1955 were $500,000; in 1987, due to lobbying campaigns by nurses, federal funds allocated were $19 million.[3]

The American Medical Association exerts a powerful influence on legislation, as does the American Hospital Association. But with increased competition within the health care industry, other interests are gaining the ear of Congress. Big industry, with its powerful lobbying influence, is complaining about exorbitant insurance premiums for health care benefits.

Health care providers other than physicians are lobbying for legislation to allow alternate entries into the health care system, rather than through physicians. Nursing is pitting itself against medicine in an effort to obtain third-party reimbursement for nursing services. Consumer movements for the elderly, such as the American Association of Retired People, are having an impact on health care legislation as well as gaining political clout. Women's rights as part of the consumer movement has become a special interest group affecting change. Women now comprise 49 percent of the work force, and politicians are taking notice.[4]

The consumer movement has had definite effects on patient care. Consumers want to know more and participate in their care; the client's right to negotiate and choose services among providers is now being recognized. Health contracting is one trend that has emerged as a direct result of this.

Health contracting is becoming increasingly popular with providers and clients. It involves the client and the provider agreeing to expected outcomes of health care, clarifying what care is to be provided. Based upon a philosophy of self-determination, health contracting hinges on the idea that patients are the experts on themselves, and so should provide input and be involved in their own care. The provider is the expert on health care technology and shares this expertise to help patients achieve the agreed-upon outcome. Health contracting emphasizes consumers as being responsible for their own health and participating in health care.

Health contracting often involves long-term relationships with clients and providers, in a primary setting. It is often effective with the chronically ill patient. The desired behavior is outlined in measurable terms, agreeable to both parties, and laid out in contract form. Health contracting is similar to nursing care planning, where the nurse and the patient set mutually agreeable goals. Health contracting takes this one step further and places part of the responsibility on clients for achievement of the expected outcome. Because consumers expect so much from health care providers, it is only just that the same expectations should be placed upon them.

SECONDARY CHANGES

Secondary changes are those changes that are efforts to adapt or respond to or are the effects of primary changes. It is important to remember that the changes in health care discussed below have occurred in relation to primary changes.

The Prospective Payment System

Prospective payment is a system whereby payment or reimbursement has been determined prior to the use of services. Rates for various health care services are preset, and payment is based on this, rather than according to the actual cost of the service provided. This is the latest approach by the federal government to attempt to contain the rapidly escalating health care costs in the United States.

The impact of prospective payment, first instituted in 1983 as the Social Security Amendment H.R. 1900 (P.L. 98-21), is far reaching. The amendment legislated that Medicare reimbursement would be based on prospective payment according to the DRG case mix method, and phased in over four years. The diagnosis-related group (DRG) method groups patients according to similar diagnoses that use similar amounts of services and treatments. This method identifies the hospital service as a product or output rendered to a patient mix; the hospital input is the cost put into providing that service. Each DRG uses similar resources or costs. Under this method, reimbursement is based upon costs allocated for each group of diagnoses; these costs are determined by averaging the cost for services per DRG, taking into consideration factors such as age, surgical procedures, and complications.

In an effort to stay within or under the DRG payments, hospitals are taking measures to increase productivity and decrease operating costs; these efforts include earlier patient discharges and shorter lengths of stay. Success requires adequate discharge planning, especially teaching of self-care and/or complications of illness as well as provisions for community-based follow-up care. Failure of adequate discharge planning increases readmissions of patients with more acute illness.

Physician Surplus

Another government attempt to decrease health care costs and increase equitable distribution of care was to support an increase in the number of physicians in the United States. Over the past decade there was a dramatic increase in the number of medical schools as well as rapid expansion of existing schools in the United States. To some degree, this attempt has been successful. A growing number of graduates began moving to rural communities, due to the oversupply of physicians in cities; they moved mainly for economic survival. Many hospitals, in response to the increased number of physicians seeking staff privileges, have tightened their credentialing processes. Peer recommendations are now required by the Joint

Commission on Accreditation of Hospitals, and evidence of professional liability insurance is also being required prior to granting hospital privileges.

There is increased competition among physicians, with generalists referring fewer cases to specialists. Physicians are performing more services in their offices, and are competing with hospitals for this income. The use of advertising has grown, as has the need for marketing consultants. Physicians are seeking new sources of revenue in physician-run emergency centers and clinics, and alcohol and drug abuse centers; this causes still more competition with hospitals. However, hospital-based physicians are becoming more prevalent, due to the secure, steady income that these jobs offer.

Many physicians have changed their approach as health care providers, to increase their market size. Office hours are more flexible for patient convenience, and medical and dental offices in shopping malls offer customers the convenience of shopping while waiting. Physicians are beginning to take more time to provide counseling, education, and emotional support. Consumer satisfaction and competitive pricing are the current focus, although physician salaries have not decreased to the degree the government predicted. Most physicians are charging more in order to maintain incomes at their previous levels.

Competition in Health Care

In an attempt to contain costs, the federal government has been reducing health care planning and regulation to increase competition. Consumer "shopping" and cost sharing are seen as two ways to increase competition among health care providers. Private insurers and Social Security have increased copayments and deductibles by the individual. Employees are being offered cafeteria-type benefits plans, and employers are limiting the amount they contribute. If employees want fuller coverage, they may have to pay larger portions of the insurance premium. This trend may discourage seeking health care when unnecessary, but it may also cause consumers to delay necessary treatment.

As consumers begin to share health costs and have choices in types of coverage, they are becoming more selective and are choosing more economical coverage. Therefore, a chief concern is the lack of public knowledge about health care and what various health care packages include. Efforts to require a minimum standard of coverage, types of catastrophic coverage, and public education are now being considered. By giving consumers a choice of health insurance plans and incentives for choosing a low-cost plan, a price and cost competition is hoped to be created among providers.

Disease Prevention and Health Promotion

The federal government has not only taken steps to contain health costs, but also to change the focus of health care from curing to prevention. It has recognized the need to prevent illness and promote health, and is advocating prevention and early detection; shifts toward coverage for prevention, screening, and health education are being seen in the rise of HMOs, ambulatory clinics, and prepaid group plans. Some insurance companies offer discounts to clients who exercise and who seek preventive services and screening. It is now recognized that prevention and health promotion is less costly than a cure-oriented approach.

Uncompensated Care

The problem of access to health care is a force that may affect the entire health industry. Poor access to health care is not new, but with cuts in Medicare and Medicaid, intense competition in health care, and unemployment, there are concerns that health care access for the poor could be still further limited. Hospitals can no longer afford to treat the nonpaying patient. The poor or those who cannot afford the initial deposit may be turned away from hospitals, unless there is a life-threatening emergency.

The urban poor, those in rural areas, and elderly nonwhites have the poorest access to health care. These populations often have no available physician and instead seek routine care at hospital emergency rooms. This increases the number of bad debts to hospitals, thus causing the cost of health care to rise. Because the poor are the most impeded in access to health care, they delay getting help and then develop multiple problems. Many who need care cannot afford private health insurance, and do not qualify for Medicare or Medicaid.

Legislation to address the issues of uncompensated care and the poor is being proposed. The Prospective Payment Assessment Commission (ProPAC) recommended Medicare adjustments to hospitals based on Medicaid volume, bad debt, and charity care.[5] In New Jersey, where all third-party payers operate under a prospective payment system, each payer contributes to the cost of indigent care. In some states, hospitals are developing financial pools to share the cost of indigent care, and physicians are teaming up to provide indigent care at no charge.

EMERGING TRENDS IN HEALTH CARE DELIVERY

Primary and secondary changes have led to recent trends in health care delivery. Hospitals have become increasingly business oriented, and are expanding and marketing their services. Let us look at some of these emerging trends.

Increased Business Orientation of Health Care

With cost containment, prospective payment, and intense competition, hospitals must operate as a business and effectively weigh the benefits or effectiveness of a service against its cost. Cost-benefit analysis has become the rule, as has provider participation in this analysis. In the past, hospital management decisions centered on costs, and physician decisions centered on care. These decisions must now be merged to involve admission procedures, diagnostic testing, length and course of treatment, and use of services and costs from a patient care and a business perspective. Nurse-administrators must analyze effectiveness of care in terms of achieving established plans, improvements in services, and increasing market shares. Cost-benefit decisions concerning hospital technology and services must involve medical and nursing participation along with hospital participation.

The nurse-administrator is a crucial link in effective cost-benefit analysis. With the largest number of employees in the hospital, nursing services provide patient care and coordinate all patient services. Its cooperation in cost-containment and cost-benefit decisions can determine the success of the entire organization. Nurse-administrators are more involved in executive-level decisions, in order to integrate nursing goals into the overall aims of the institution. Only by involvement in hospital planning strategies and policy formation can the nurse-administrator effectively manage human resources to help achieve the system's goals.

Marketing

Another direct response to competition is the health care industry's growing involvement in marketing research and strategy. Marketing is a powerful competitive weapon involving strategies such as a hospital promoting its doctors' expertise, and even the installation of video games and juice bars in waiting rooms.

Marketing involves assessing information about the service area and planning ways to respond to the needs of this area. Questions concerning the hospital's image, the effects of competition, low utilization of services, and the need for new services can be answered. This information is then analyzed and strategies planned.

In times of intense competition, marketing is geared toward increasing market shares (the number of consumers that would purchase a service). Decisions involving the classic four "P"s of marketing must be made: the product to be offered, the place it is to be offered, the price, and its promotion. A product can be a service, a building, or personnel: its value is proportional to the perceived benefits of the consumer.

Multihospital Systems

In October 1983, *Newsweek* did a feature story on the health care industry.[6] The business of health care was cited as being a larger industry than defense. According to *Newsweek*, this industry had consisted mainly of private physicians and nonprofit hospitals. Now group practices and profit-making hospitals have become the trend. With cost containment and competition, hospitals must now adopt the "for-profit" philosophy in order to survive. Many hospitals are selling out to investor-owned chains, and others are becoming part of nonprofit, multihospital systems. These systems can range from affiliated public facilities to religious hospital chains. The majority of the multihospital systems are investor-owned and profit-making.

The number of profit-oriented facilities grew as a result of money from Medicare and retrospective insurance reimbursement. Now the business tactics of these facilities have become a necessity for all hospitals. Thirty percent of the country's hospitals are members of multihospital chains, and by 1995, 80 percent will be part of a profit-making subsidiary. Independent hospitals are disappearing, while investor-owned chains are proliferating. Many independent hospitals are forming nonprofit trade associations and other alliances to increase their lobbying effectiveness, pool resources, and enhance purchasing of supplies and equipment. Some of these alliances and associations invest in separate businesses in order to make money to support their political functions.

PPOs, Prepaid Group Plans, and HMOs

These represent another major trend in health care delivery. *Preferred provider organizations* (PPOs) involve reaching an agreement to provide a specific service for a set price, in return for a guaranteed market. With PPOs the provider has incentive for cost-effectiveness and early discharge. Because prices are reduced, utilization review, claims screening, and monitoring measures are incorporated into the system to evaluate services and costs. Claims are paid quickly in this plan, offsetting discounted fees and bad debt costs.

The latest in selective contracting is the *prospective provider arrangement (PPA).* A separate organization (the O in PPO) is not required to be a preferred provider; all that is necessary is a contract covering payment, utilization, and claims, in an arrangement where consumers are channeled to certain providers. Under the PPA. as with many PPOs, the consumer is not locked into a specific provider, but has incentives such as more extensive health insurance coverage and benefits, or reductions in copayments, when a preferred provider is used.

Prepaid group plans are similar to the PPO, being offered to consumers by a group of physicians who offer services at reduced rates. Individual consumers or employers pay a set monthly rate to this group in return for discounted medical costs. Most of these plans include primary care and prevention services, with physicians sharing cost risks with employers or insurance companies. Members in these plans can select from several doctors, but their physician controls all of the care and any referrals to specialists. Any profits or deficits are usually shared among the physicians, employers, and employees.

Although discounts in physician and hospital services have increased, so has the consumer's role in payment for care. As mentioned earlier, the trend is moving toward increased cost sharing by providers, employers, *and* consumers.

Health Maintenance Organizations. Health maintenance organizations (HMOs) have filled a need for easier access, preventative services, comprehensive care, and cost containment. The Health Maintenance Act of 1973 helped support the formation of new HMOs with federal grants and loans. Certain services were required in order to meet federal guidelines and receive financial support. These requirements include physician consultation and referral, in-and outpatient hospital services, mental health, drug and alcohol abuse services, diagnostic and radiological services, home health, prevention, and well-child care. The HMO Act also required businesses with over 25 employees to offer employees the choice between regular insurance coverage and a community HMO.

The goals of an HMO are to decrease costs and inpatient care. They focus instead on outpatient services, preventative health care, peer review, and monitoring of quality of care.

Since 1983, HMOs could compete for Medicare business and contract with the Health Care Financing Administration for prospective payment. While HMOs aim at decreasing hospitalization, hospitals will contract with them because they need the business. Billing is simpler, there are no bad debts, and hospitals have guaranteed patients. More hospitals are participating in HMOs, due to the increase in surplus beds and the large market share of HMOs. In many cases, financial risks are shared by the HMO, the hospital, and the physician.

Consumers find HMOs attractive because there is a minimum of out-of-pocket expenses such as deductibles and copayments. Some hospitals are creating their own HMOs, offering yearly, renewable contracts with physicians, where selection into the HMO is based on quality care and cost-effectiveness. Hospitals are also networking to expand availability of an HMOs services: several hospitals and physician groups offer wider geographic accessibility. The networks of hospitals and physician groups usually consist of low-cost providers who are willing to discount, have minimum competition and overlap of services, have common objectives, and provide a broad range of services.

Expanded Hospital Services

Reimbursement changes and increased competition have resulted in a push to expand hospital services into areas that will increase revenues. One such area is hospital-based home health service: with the need for early discharge, communication systems from hospital to home can help effective discharge planning and increase the number of procedures and treatments performed at home.

With the popularity of HMOs and PPAs, it has become essential for hospitals to offer more comprehensive services, particularly for the elderly. Hospitals are now contracting with other agencies such as community home health agencies or home health management firms. These arrangements provide existing financial systems, expertise, and home health services currently developed and operating effectively. Skilled-care nursing services, private nursing duty, durable medical equipment, surgical supplies, high-tech services, home health pharmacy, self-care products, and exercise products are all being offered through hospital joint ventures with home health agencies and/or other affiliations.

Many hospitals are developing their own freestanding outpatient clinics in order to compete with other community clinics. New technological advances have contributed to the growth of ambulatory surgery centers: a procedure such as cataract removal used to require several days of hospitalization, but now can be performed in 30 minutes on an outpatient basis. Developments in anesthesia, lasers, and endoscopes have created an unlimited potential for outpatient surgery.

The use of *swing beds* in rural hospitals is another way to extend health care services, as well as respond to financial limitations imposed by PPS. The swing-bed system is when small hospitals of 50 beds or less use empty acute care beds for nursing home care, and are then reimbursed by Medicaid and Medicare. These hospitals must obtain a certificate of need and meet certain guidelines, and they can use up to 10 beds with patient stays of up to 30 days. The swing-bed system can help small hospitals with low occupancy increase revenues and provide a needed service.

IMPLICATIONS FOR NURSING ADMINISTRATORS

Primary and secondary changes and recent trends in health care delivery have produced many implications for nursing-administrators and nurses in general. Some of these will now be discussed.

While *high-tech* capabilities such as computerized monitoring and information systems serve to simplify, coordinate, and ease the work load in the long run, they also cause dramatic changes in how nurse-administrators accomplish their work. Intensive in-service training and orientation are required to keep staff abreast of rapid changes. Turnover costs for reorientation and training of nurses in high-technology procedures can be considerable. Nurses not only need to be computer literate, but also to be able to balance high-tech care with personalized high-touch care.

Prospective payment has increased the demands on nursing care in the hospital. The increased patient turnover has added to nursing demands for admitting assessments, patient teaching, and discharge planning; this is coupled with the increased complexity of care and a high level of acute illness. Despite these evident demands for increased nursing care, hospital administrators still desire to cut staff level in order to decrease costs. Benefits such as tuition reimbursement, continuing education workshops, and special programs such as internships and extensive orientation training are being cut back or even abolished to save money. In some areas salaries have been reduced or frozen and certain vacancies are not being filled.

Workers such as nurses' aides and L.P.N.s have been cut back, leaving more responsibility and work for fewer R.N.s. Personnel issues related to intensity of care will peak in response to pressure to contain salaries and to cut staff.

One of the greatest challenges the nurse-administrator will face is to provide high production at low cost while preventing nursing turnover and dissatisfaction. Nurses will find themselves concerned about patients' needs but realizing that there are limited resources for providing care. The philosophy of "optimum" care is being replaced with "minimum but safe" care. Nurses have traditionally been concerned with meeting patients' needs regardless of cost, and will have difficulty adapting to this change in philosophy.

The concern over cutting nursing staff is reinforced by the fact that few data are available to substantiate the type, amount, and cost of nursing care required for different types of patients. Without such data, nursing cannot be represented adequately in the preset reimbursement payments to hospitals. Many nurses believe that if third-party payers to hospitals itemized and included the costs of providing nursing services in their reimbursement, then nurses would have support to maintain appropriate staffing levels for patient care. The result is that nurse-administrators are beginning to separate the costs of nursing from the regular hospital charges, and listing nursing care as a separate item on the patient's bill. This way the patient knows what nursing care costs, and nursing is acknowledged as providing a specific service that has produced specific revenues.

Research is underway in many facilities to develop methods for determining the cost of nursing, and methods for *variable billing* based on these costs.[7] Nursing costs are being separated from room and food costs, and being based on the acuity level, or degree of illness, of the patient. Patients are classified according to degree of dependency, complications, and other factors contributing to the amount and type of nursing; each classification requires a specific skill level and type of nursing care. By determining the number of patients in each classification, the nursing staff needs can be determined. The costs for nursing salaries, benefits, and overhead are figured into the patient care costs per classification; this determines the cost of nursing service for each patient classification. Because classification levels of patients change daily, so do costs for nursing services. The daily cost of nursing is added to the patient's bill, along with room, food, and other charges. A concurrent monitoring of documentation and patient classification must be instituted to ensure accuracy.

Variable billing is also being calculated by nursing costs per time spent (such as in operating and emergency areas), and for one admission charge. This charge includes room charges, clinical charge per diagnosis and procedure, as well as acuity and ancillary charges. The patient pays for what he or she receives.[8]

Another method, presently being researched in New Jersey, is the relative intensity measure (RIM) for determining nursing costs.[9] Nursing personnel documented the number of minutes required to give direct and nondirect care to patients on all shifts. The use of nursing services was then calculated into RIMs, one RIM equaling one minute. The cost of one minute of nursing services was determined by the hospital's skill mix, overhead costs, and salaries. Thus one minute of nursing care, or one RIM, can vary from hospital to hospital. The number of RIMs used per case is determined according to patient classification or case mix. Patients were classified into nursing "clusters," or categories where the number of RIMs used are computed. Variables used in this computation were primary diagnosis, surgical procedures, length of stay, and admission and discharge status.

Once the number of RIMs per patient has been calculated, the patient is assigned to a DRG. This provides data concerning the average cost of nursing care per DRG. This RIM method for determining nursing costs per case mix was integrated into the New Jersey PPS in January 1984, for a group of voluntary hospitals.

Under prospective payment, efficient and accurate record keeping, cost analysis, budgeting, and planning are imperative. Any uneconomical or unnecessary services will be cut. Because business management and financial planning are integral to the nurse-administrator's work, it is necessary to have current information available in a useful form. Computers are playing a more important role not only in analyzing patient classifications against costs and services, but in linking clinical departments and increasing employee productivity. Appropriate and progressive *management information systems* (MIS) must be in place to maximize operations.

Extensive information systems that link patient care, finance, nursing services, and ancillary departments are decreasing costs by lessening lost charges, costs of forms, data entry time, and time handling and retrieving information. Also, MISs are increasing productivity in nonclerical duties and fostering improved decision-making capabilities. They can record patient classification input, then calculate staffing requirements, and assign and schedule staff by computer. Attendance, payroll, staff performance, and other personnel matters are recorded and stored. Costs related to nursing hours, supplies used, and overtime are calculated. Present and future staffing needs can be determined; budget planning, information for contract negotiations, utilization summaries, licensing information, continuing education, and research are a few of the many uses for computerized MISs.

Resourceful and effective MISs can, however, be developed without computerization. The key is to develop effective communication systems, identify sources of data, and formulate mechanisms for processing timely, relevant, and appropriate information in a useful form. Supervisory reports, patient acuity summaries, and payroll reports are all a part of MISs. Whatever method is used, the nurse-administrator must utilize current information for effective human resource management, and must keep up with change and involve nursing management and staff to maximize all information for decision making.

In addition to expertise in financial and business management, the nurse-administrator must develop *political savvy* to effectively manage the staff. As facilities expand and become part of multihospital systems, hierarchical structures can become more complex than that of the independent facility. Often the nurse-administrator must answer to the chief executive officer, as well as to a corporate board or a group of executives. Policy making and long-range decision making is most often administered from this corporate level. The nurse-administrator must have expertise in politics and persuasion, as well as an understanding of the acquisition and use of power. Cooperating, sharing, negotiating, and influencing are necessary tools for success in today's world. Nurse-administrators must prove their worth in dollars and cents, supplementing their clinical knowledge with financial expertise and substantiating all planning with facts.

The Changing Roles of Women and the Nursing Workforce

The nature of the workforce in nursing, as well as the direction of the profession as a whole, is affected by the *changing roles of women*. In the past, women's top priority was the home, and nursing was just a means of earning a living. Active participation in the profession has been lacking by the majority of nurses, and because of this, many decisions concerning health care have been made by other professions and interest groups. Rather than taking control of their professions, nurses allowed others to do so.

Another problem is that many nurses have transferred their female, submissive self-images to their work. Physicians and hospital administrators have been mostly male and dominant, while nurses have been passive and unquestioning. Many nurses have felt that taking a stand or fighting for what they believed in was unfeminine, unattractive, and would cause disapproval. This, along with a lack of career commitment, caused nurses to ignore issues and problems. The unhappy nurses simply quit and moved to another institution.

Women now have unlimited career opportunities, and nursing as a profession will have to compete to attract recruits. Issues concerning pay, working conditions, image, and autonomy must be addressed and resolved, so that nursing will be an attractive profession for both men and women. Young women in all professions are more assertive and informed of their rights. Although many women do not share the feminist philosophy, media exposure to the fight for the Equal Rights Amendment, the National Organization of Women, and collective bargaining have provoked an awareness of women's rights, as well as higher expectations from the employer–employee relationship. Nurse-administrators can expect a labor force that seeks more satisfaction, career mobility, professional respect, and independence in decision making than in the past. This need for independence, satisfaction, and respect can be used to achieve both the organization's and the individual's goals.

Autonomy

In general, the nursing work force is seeking more *autonomy in practice.* Increasingly, nurses have more academic training, seek a more professional image, and expect opportunities for advancement and career mobility. Nurse-administrators must adapt to and change with this trend in order to ensure the viability of the organization. As the worker changes, so must human resource management.

One response to this change is the emergence of new organizations for nursing services, which promote a creative environment and provide more satisfaction for the professional nurse. Self-governing, self-disciplining nursing organizations with management teams, nursing councils, and joint practice are some of the developments in hospital nursing. The National Commission on Nursing's *Models for Successful Organizational Change*[10] is one of many publications describing recent trends in this area. Two examples of progressive organizations are the Mount Sinai Medical Center in Miami, Florida, and the Rose Medical Center in Denver, Colorado. The Mount Sinai Medical Center divides nursing into two organizations: administrative and clinical. A nursing administrative committee reviews all administrative activities, while a nurse executive committee, composed of physicians and other health care providers, collaborates for clinical review.

The Rose Medical Center has a nursing congress with bylaws, standards, peer review, credentialing, and a multidisciplinary collaborative practice. A professional review committee, human resources council, and patient care council review monitor, represent, and recommend actions for various aspects of the organization. The nursing congress is managed by seven officers who serve two-year terms and represent the total nursing division.

Joint practice is an example of the trend toward increased autonomy; it is a collaborative relationship between a nurse and a physician that serves to coordinate the approach to patient care. Roles are complemented, based on mutual respect, and involve the nurse and the physician jointly evaluating patient care.

The relationships and roles in a joint practice are defined by both the physician and the nurse, in accord with state law and hospital policy. Effective practices usually occur when there is primary care and a staff comprised mostly of R.N.s. A committee for joint practice monitors relationships and recommends actions. The nurse is encouraged to use independent clinical decision making, and the patient record is integrated.[11]

Another recent development is the concept of *shared governance.* This concept is best defined by an example—in this case, St. Joseph's Hospital in Baltimore, Maryland.[12] At St. Joseph's, all nursing staff members are involved in administrative decisions. Various councils are formed where the staff discusses issues, problems, and alternatives, and comes to agreement. Councils include all aspects of nursing, from policies and procedures to standards of practice and peer review. The planning, evaluation, and management of nursing service occurs at the level closest to the functioning of that service. Budgeting and management are decentralized to this level. Each area and staff nurse can participate in top-level management decisions. The nurse-administrator, in turn, attends board meetings and is part of the medical staff and chief executive officer's management team.

Although the developments in joint practice and shared governance reflect growth in nursing autonomy and participation, many hospital administrators are opposed to nursing's drive for professional autonomy. Nurses are beginning to gather the influence and knowledge necessary to face these challenges. They are looking to one another for strength and support, through networking and mentorships.

Networking

The concept of *networking* has been around for years, especially in business circles. The "old-boy network" was an administrative tool whereby men collaborated, exchanged ideas, and made decisions on an informal basis, away from the work area. On the golf course, at elite men's clubs, or at special gatherings, top-level decisions were made among expert and powerful men. Women were excluded from these circles. and consequently were left out of this network of information. Women in business have now begun to form their own networks for support, information, and the exchange of ideas.

Networking involves developing and maintaining contacts for advice and help in career development. Many nursing leaders recognize the need to share information. They realize how isolation, distrust, and lack of support have contributed to nursing's lack of professional growth. Nurses are just beginning to use existing and new networks to support one another and to accomplish their goals.

One such network is the Arizona Nursing Network, which meets monthly to discuss legislative issues.[13] This group receives up-to-date legislative information, and comes to agreements on legislative issues and courses of action. These nurses collaborate and plan strategies for political effectiveness. Another network is the National Identification Program for Advancement of Women in Higher Education Administration.[14] This network searches out and recommends women for administrative positions, and strengthens information sharing and mentor systems.

Mentorship

Mentorship is another old concept that has gained new recognition and popularity. Nursing is realizing that in order to develop creative practitioners, administrators, educators, and researchers, it must provide role models and mentors. A mentor offers nurturing, guidance, and teaching to a less experienced person, in return for satisfaction and personal growth. The relationship is aimed toward personal and career development, and can involve a teacher and a student, a preceptor and a new graduate, an employer and an employee, or a variety of other relationships.

Mentoring is not only job-focused, but is also used in education for the development of scholarliness and professionalism. It is concerned with the emergence of personal as well as professional development. As with networking, mentoring is an important trend in nursing today. When nurses cease to compete and work against one another, and begin to share and support personal and career development, the results can only produce more satisfied and fulfilled persons.

Other Opportunities

With the expansion and extension of hospital services, and development of new trends in health care delivery, other *opportunities are opening up for nurses.* Although the need for highly specialized, acute-care nurses remains high, the areas of hospice, home health, and ambulatory clinics are growing rapidly. Nurse-administrators will have more options to offer staff nurses who wish to extend their practices from acute-care settings and develop other skills. Specialties in gerontological and family-centered nursing will emerge and be in demand. Opportunities for transfer within multihospital systems and among clinics and expanded facilities, while still maintaining benefits and seniority, will be a plus for nurses.

CHALLENGES FOR NURSING ADMINISTRATORS

Trends and developments in health care point to several challenges that may lie ahead for the nurse-administrator and the profession as a whole. These challenges include alternative providers, institutional licensure, restrictions in independent nursing roles, and nursing education.

Institutional Licensure

Another attempt to exert control over health care providers is seen in the issue of institutional licensure. This involves an institution being given one license and being legally accountable for its services. Many institutions realized that accountability was already on their shoulders, because the professional's individual licensure had not served as an institution's defense against malpractice suits. Supporters of institutional licensure believe that personnel could be better used, costs contained, and quality control monitored to each facility's standards. Definition and qualifications, as well as training for each role, would be defined by the institution.

Accountability for patient care is placed entirely upon the institution and not upon the individual provider. Advocates for institutional licensure point out that under such a system, unskilled workers could enter, learn skills, and demonstrate knowledge for advancement. Thus, career advancement and mobility would be promoted within one institution.

Opponents of institutional licensure argue that costs for education and training would be high, that each institution would have varying standards, and that too much power would be given to hospital administrators. Mobility between institutions would be more difficult. The chief concern is that accountability *must* be placed upon the individual providing the care, in order to ensure patient protection. Opponents of this system claim that it is not concerned with service, but with administrational needs.

Alternative Providers

Alternative providers could pose a threat to nursing and patient care in the wake of cost containment. Nursing has often been manipulated so that facilities can adjust to environmental changes in the health care field. During the nursing shortage, technicians and aides were used in place of R.N.s; in some areas technicians were trained to perform nursing duties, such as administering medications. Emergency medical technicians (EMTs) have been placed in emergency rooms and operating theaters under the R.N.s supervision. Critical-care technicians and respiratory care technicians have replaced R.N.s in monitoring patient care. During times of economic struggle and rapid change, nursing positions are often cut, and R.N.s are substituted for by less expensive or unlicensed personnel. Efforts must be made for nurses to control nursing practice.

Restriction in Independent Nursing Roles

Nurses have functioned in expanded roles for years, but recent developments in health care such as HMOs, and an increased aging population have made this an important issue. New opportunities in prevention and health promotion will cause an increase in the number of nurses functioning in independent practice. But with the physician surplus and intense competition, the functions of nurse-practitioners are being questioned: are they "within the scope of nursing?" At the same time, nurses are being recognized by both the government and consumers as performing a valuable service at a reasonable cost. More states are legislating reimbursement for expanded nursing services, independent of a physician. This recognition is due partly to nursing marketing and growth in political effectiveness and power, as well as due to a public need for alternative health care delivery.

In response to environmental need, masters-prepared clinical nurse specialists, especially in mental health clinics, along with nurse-anesthetists, nurse-midwives, and nurse-practitioners, have begun to move more into independent practice or to form group practices. These nurses have proved competent, as well as satisfying to the consumer. But many physicians see nurse-practitioners as a threat to their economic survival, and are fighting to control and limit their practice. Nurse practice acts and state laws allowing expanded nursing practice have become the target of attack from physicians and, in some cases, hospital associations.

In order to function as independent practitioners, nurses will have to receive compensation for their services through third-party payers. In addition to the Rural Health Clinic Act of 1977, the 1980 Omnibus Reconciliation Act legislated the reimbursement of nurse-midwives' services to the needy, either directly or through an institution. Some states are mandating that private and commercial insurance companies offer the services of nurse-practitioners and midwives. Many insurance companies are reimbursing nurses in expanded roles without requiring physician supervision. Approximately 26 states recognize these nurses as reimbursable by Medicaid.[15]

The key to these reimbursement issues lies with state laws and regulations. Nurse practice acts must adequately define the independent nursing role and the scope of their practice.

Nursing Education

Nursing schools are also having to adapt and adjust in order to survive; they must also respond to the changing workforce and the cost-containment efforts of the government. Nursing education is facing serious cutbacks in federal, state, and local support, as well as in financial aid to students. In addition, rising tuition rates and women entering other careers have caused nursing programs to expect a decline in enrollment. It is even speculated that the least expensive programs, such as the associate degree, will attract the most students.[16]

Several options are available to nurses who wish to continue their education and obtain a baccalaureate degree. Nursing schools now have to compete for their recruits by marketing their services and offering classes and programs that fit the schedules of many working students. Many hospitals and colleges will work together for work-study, career ladder, and extern programs, owing to a shortage of funds for education. Educational programs need to have easy access, offering correspondence courses, part-time courses, videotaping, independent study, and work-study programs. Nurses returning to school need day-care facilities, on-the-job evaluation for clinical credit, credit for work experience, and ladder programs for articulation.

Many developments are occurring to help decrease costs and increase the income of nursing schools. Sharing faculty among neighboring nursing programs, establishing regional nursing education centers, accelerating nursing programs of study, and marketing faculty expertise and program offerings to nonnursing students are a few of these developments.

Allison has discussed an approach to improve university-based nursing education by the unification model.[17] An *affiliation model* of unification consists of joint appointments where university faculty both teach and perform patient care at the affiliated hospital. The *medical model* of unification involves the teaching hospital's dean of nursing education also serving as the director of nursing service. Nursing service personnel hold appointments at the school, and the nurses contract their services and responsibilities. The hospital and nursing school must have one owner for the medical model to work. In both models, the nurses within the institutions must practice primary nursing, and be academically and professionally oriented.

Whatever the approach, nursing education is responding to the challenge of change, and this response has a definite effect on nursing practice. As organizational complexities, economic restraints, intense competition, and other environmental factors alter the nature of health care, nursing education and service must join forces to ensure the future stability and progress of the nursing profession.

CONCLUSION

The effects of change on the health care system must be continually assessed. Then, as information is interpreted and synthesized, it can be put to use through purposeful and deliberate planning. Planning is critical to all functions, and is dependent upon a perception of environmental change. The understanding of trends and prediction of potential developments will dictate the focus of all plans. And this leads to the subject of the next chapter.

REFERENCES

1. Riffer, J. Elderly 21 percent of population by 2040. *Hospitals,* 1985, *59*(5), 41–44.
2. Heckler, M. Medicare turns 20 as america grays. *Hospitals,* 1985, *59*(3), 59–60.
3. Bauknecht, V. L. Capital commentary. *The American Nurse,* Nov./Dec. 1986, p. 2.
4. Jacobson, S. F. Psychosocial stressors of working women. *Nursing Clinics of North America,* 1982, *17*(1), 138–141.
5. American Hospital Association. *Hospital Week,* 1985, *21*(25), 1.
6. Dentzer, S., Hager, M., Zuckerman, S., et al. The big business of medicine. *Newsweek,* October 31, 1983, pp. 62–74.
7. Van Slyck, A. Models of practice: Variable charges for nursing care. In *Professionalism and the Empowerment of Nursing.* Missouri: ANA, 1982, pp. 47–57.
8. Brewer, C. Variable billing: Is it worth it? *Nursing Outlook,* 1984, *32*(1), 38–41.
9. Caterinicchio, R. P. A debate: RIMs and the cost of nursing care. *Nursing Management,* 1983, *14*(5), 36–39.
10. National Commission on Nursing. *Nursing in transition: Models for successful organizational change.* Chicago: The Hospital Research and Education Trust, August 1982, p. 10.
11. National Joint Practice Commission. *Guidelines for establishing joint or collaborative practice in hospitals.* Chicago: National Joint Practice Commission, 1981, pp. 4–12.

12. Carroll, M. Hospital framework for shared governance in nursing. On the scene: St. Joseph's Hospital. *Nursing Administration Quarterly*, 1982, *7*(1), 27.
13. Bagwell, M. The nursing network—A united front. *Nursing Leadership*, 1980, *3*(2), 5–8.
14. Felton, G. On women, networks, patronage and sponsorship. *Image*, 1978, *10*(3), 58, 59.
15. Powell, P. J. Fee-for-service. *Nursing Management*, March *14*(3) 1983, pp. 13–15.
16. Morton, P. G. The financial distress of higher education: Impact on nursing. *Image*, 1983, *15*(4), 102–106.
17. Allison, R. J. Nursing unification in principal teaching hospitals. *Health Care Management Review*, Summer 1981, pp. 55–57.

SUGGESTED READING

Adams, R., & Johnson, B. Acuity and staffing under prospective payment. *JONA*, 1986, *16*(10), 21.

Aikens, L. Nursing priorities for the 1980s: Hospitals and nursing homes. *AJN*, Feb. 1981.

Aiken, L. Nursing's future: Public policies, private actions. Shortage or surplus? *AJN*, 1983, *83*(10), 1440–1444.

AJN news. How DRGs work in a hospital: Issues & answers for providers. *AJN*, 1983, *83*(11), 1608–1611.

AJN news. Evidence mounts that quality of care is slipping under DRGS. *AJN*, 1986, *85*(5), 600.

AJN news. Recruiters abound as shortage escalates. *AJN*, 1986, *86*(9), 1054.

AJN news. Nursing enrollments, applications fall again; closures seen but some schools hold their own. *AJN*, 1986, *86*(10), 1178.

Alley, L. Nursing shortage? Turnover? Maldistribution? *Imprint*, 1982, *29*(4), 20–23.

Alward, R. R. A marketing approach to nursing administration—Part I. *JONA*, March 1983, pp. 9–12.

Archer, S. E. National health service: Rationale and implementation. *Nursing Outlook*, June 1981, pp. 364–368.

Bandura, F. K. Nurse acceptance of a computerized arrhythmia monitoring system. *Heart & Lung*, 1982, *9*(6), 1044–1045.

Barney, D. R. Regulation of health service advertising. *Hospital and Health Service Administration*, 1983, *28*(3), 85–102.

Barrell, L. M., & Hamric, A. B. Collaboration can work. *Nursing and Health Care*, 1986, *7*(9), 496.

Beck, M., & Buckley, J. Nurses with bad habits. *Newsweek*, Aug. 22, 1982, p. 54.

Bell, N. K. Whose autonomy is at stake? *AJN*, June 1981, pp. 1170–1173.

Bennett, N. E., & Fisher, B. W. Looking back, looking forward: Last year's changes are future financing. *Hospitals*, April 1, 1983, pp. 87–90.

Bowman, M. Which cap today? *Nursing Mirror*, Feb. 3, 1982, pp. viii–x.

Bryan, N. E. Administrative manpower utilization in community nursing: A key to better health care. *Australian Nurses Journal*, 1983, *12*(9), 41–43.

Bryant, B. E. Issues on the distribution of health care: Some lessons from Canada. *Public Health Reports*, 1981, *96*(5), 442–447.

Bullough, B. (Ed.) *The law and the expanding nursing role* (2nd ed.). New York: Appleton-Century-Crofts, 1980.

Buys, D. Nursing management must be strengthened. *Modern Health Care,* Aug. 1981, pp. 100–102.

Campbell-Heider, N. Do nurses need mentors? *Image,* 1986, *18*(3), 110.

Chickadoz, G. H., & Keenan, M. J. Share governance. *Nursing & Health Care,* 86, *7*(8), 432.

Chow, R. K. The problem of financing the Social Security system. *Journal of Gerontological Nursing,* Sep. 1982, pp. 524–525.

Coelen, C., & Sullivan, D. An analysis of the effects of prospective reimbursement programs on hospital expenditures. *H. C. Finance Review,* 1981, *2*(3), 1, 2.

Collier, P. Health behaviors of women. *Nursing Clinics of North America,* 1982, *17*(1), 121–126.

Corona, D. The nursing shortage. *Nursing Leadership,* 1983, *6*(1), 344.

Cushing, M. Legal side: How courts look at nursing practice. *AJN, 86*(2), 131.

Diehl, D. H. Private practice—Out on a limb and loving it. *AJN, 86*(8), 907.

Diers, D. Nursing reclaims its role. *Nursing Outlook,* Sept./Oct. 1982, pp. 459–463.

Edmunds, L. Computer-assisted nursing care. *AJN,* 82(7), 1076–1079.

Edmunds, L. Teaching nurses to use computers. *Nurse Educator,* Autumn 1982, pp. 32–38.

Ellis, P. J. Matching students with clinical experience by computer. *Nursing Outlook,* Jan. 1982, pp. 29–30.

Ellis, R. Conceptual issues in nursing. *Nursing Outlook,* July/Aug. 1982, pp. 406–410.

Endo, A. S. Using computers in newborn intensive care settings. *AJN,* 1981, *81*(7), 1336–1337.

Falk, D. The challenge of change. *Hospitals,* April 1, 1983, p. 98.

Feldstein, P. J. Economic success for hospitals depends on their adaptability. *Hospitals,* Jan. 16, 1981, pp. 77–80.

Finch, L. E., & Christianson, J. B. Rural hospital costs: An analysis with policy implications. *Public Health Report,* 1981, *96*(5), 423–433.

Flaherty, M. J. Professional ideas and idealism. *Nursing Management,* Jan. 1982, pp. 49–50.

Ginzberg, E. The economics of health care and the future of nursing. *JONA,* March 1981, pp. 28–32.

Griffin, H. Competition in health care. *Nursing Outlook,* Sept./Oct. 1983, pp. 262–265.

Grimaldi, P. L. DRGs and nursing administration. *Nursing Management,* 1982, *13*(1), 30–34.

Hamilton, M. S. Mentorship: A key to nursing leadership. *Nursing Leadership,* 1981, *4*(1), 5–13.

Hayes, L. V. Hospital nursing is in danger: Will it survive? *Nursing Life,* 1982, *2*(4), 48, 49.

Hendricks, D. E. The power problem. *Nursing Management,* Oct. 1982, pp. 23, 24.

Housley, C. E. Material management: A fertile environment for hospital cost containment. *Hospital Topics,* Sept./Oct. 1982, pp. 42–49.

Hughes, S. J. Installing a computer-based patient information system. *JONA,* 1980, *10*(5), 7–10.

Jenkins, S. The right to fight. *Nursing and Health Care,* 1986, *7*(9). 476.

Johnson, K. A. Hospital economic forecast. *Hospitals,* April 1, 1983. pp. 65–72.

Kranstaker, S. M. Establishing a nursing journal club for professional education & certification. *Journal of Continuing Education in Nursing,* 1982, *13*(1), 167–168.

Krebs, P. ICN's programme on nursing in primary health care: Present and future. *International Nursing Review,* 1982, *29*(6), 246, pp. 167–168.

Kuntz, E. F. States out of whack with federal deregulation, considers rate setting. *Modern Health Care,* March 1982, p. 83.

Lackner, B. J., & Rosenberg, D. O. Environmental change faces hospital CEO's. *Hospitals,* Jan. 1, 1980, pp. 75–78.

LaViolette, S. Nurses have best case for equal pay. *Modern Health Care,* Aug. 1982, pp. 50–52.

Lawrence, M. M. Baccalaureate degree: The issue of entry into nursing practice. *Australian Nurses Journal,* 1983, *12*(8), 50, 51.

McCauley, M. Health care trends and issues in the 1980's. *Cross-Reference on Human Resource Management,* Sept./Oct. 1981, pp. 5–8.

McGillick, K., & Fernandez, R. L. Reaching for the stars. *Nursing Management,* 1983, *14*(1), 24–26.

Maher, A. B., & Dolan, B. Determining cost of nursing services. *Nursing Management,* Sept. 1982, pp. 17, 18.

Morganthan, Han T. & Cooper, N. The case of Baby Jane Doe, continued. *Newsweek,* Dec. 12, 1983, p. 47.

Neuhauser, D. The future of technology & manpower in medical care. In J. B. Silbers, W. N. Zelman, & C. N. Kahn (Eds.), *Health Care Financial Management in the 1980s.* Ann Arbor, Michigan: AUPHA Press, 1983.

Nixon, J. E. The right to health care: Reflections and implications for nursing administrators. *NAQ,* Summer 1982, pp. 1–6.

Penberth-Valentine, M. It could happen in your state—Senate bill 666. *Nursing Management,* 1982, *13*(11), 34–39.

Peterson, M. E. Shared governance: A strategy for transforming organizations. *JONA,* 1986, *16*(1), 9.

Pfeiffer, E., & Cohen, E. S. Assessment: The long term care issue of the '80s. *The Coordinator,* July 1983, pp. 16–18.

Priest, S. L., & O'Sullivan, V. J. The computer is coming—What should I do? *Health Care Supervisor,* 1983, *1*(4), 75–90.

Pritchard, K. Computers—Possible applications in nursing. *Nursing Times,* March 17, 1982, pp. 465–466.

Ralph, C. Angels by any other name. *Nursing Mirror,* Feb. 3, 1982, pp. 24–27.

Robbins, H. L. Teaching technologies for the 1980s. In J. B. Silvers, W. N. Zelman, & C. N. Kahn (Eds.), *Health Care Financial Management in the 1980s.* Ann Arbor, Michigan: AUPHA Press, 1983, pp. 156–157.

Rose, M. A. Factors affecting nurse supply and demand: An exploration. *JONA,* Feb. 1982, pp. 31–34.

Rzasa, C. B. Prospective rate system for Medicare reimbursement. *QRB,* June 1983, pp. 158–160.

Saba, V. The computer in public health: Today and tomorrow. *Nursing Outlook,* Nov./Dec. 1982, pp. 510–514.

Sandrick, K. M. Cost containment. *QRB,* Feb. 1983, pp. 36–38.

Schmied, E. Living with cost containment. *JONA,* May 1980, pp. 11–17.

Shaheen, P. P. Nationalizing health care: A humanitarian approach. *Nursing Outlook,* June 1981, pp. 358–363.

Shenkin, B. N. Change in Swedish health care: What lessons for us? *NEJOM,* 1980, *302*(9), 526–527.

Slack, P. Survival of the fittest? *Nursing Times,* Sept. 1, 1982, pp. 1459, 1460.

Smits, H. L. The PSRO in perspective. *The NEJOM,* 1981, *305*(5), pp. 253–259.

Sorenson, L. Hospitals and doctors compete for patients with rising bitterness. *Wall Street Journal,* July 19, 1983.

Steinwald, B. Hospital-based physicians: Current issues & descriptive evidence. *H. C. Finance Review,* Summer 1980, 2(1), 63–75.

Taylor, M. The effect of DRG's on home health care. *Nursing Outlook* 1985, *33*(6), 288.

Trandel-Korenchuk, D. M., & Trandel-Korenchuk, K. M. Current legal issues facing nursing practice. *NAQ,* Fall 1980, *5,* pp. 37–55.

Turban, E. Decision support systems in hospitals. *HCM Review,* Summer 1982, *7*(3), 35–42.

Turnball, E. N. Interdisciplinarism—Problems and promises. *J. of N.E., 21*(2), Feb. 1982, pp. 24–31.

Waterstradt, C. Computers: Bringing nursing service "on-line." *Nursing Management,* 1981, *12*(12), 18, 19.

Whitman, M. Towards a new psychology for nurses. *Nursing Outlook,* 1982, pp. 48–52.

Winslow, W. W. Changing trends in CMHCs: Keys to survival in the eighties. *Hospital & Community Psychiatry,* 1982, *33*(4), 273–276.

4 Planning

Planning is necessary in order to implement purposeful change effectively, as well as to respond to the increasing complexities and changes in the internal and external environment. In today's competitive climate, with its shrinking resources, planning has become essential to establishing a posture for the future, appropriately allocating resources, and increasing the chances of success.

Although planning is a major component of the administrative function, it can be a relatively simple procedure, despite all of the confusing jargon and complicated tools and models. It can be seen as deciding what is wanted, and then determining what must be done to get it. The key point to remember in planning, as in all management processes, is to *keep it simple.* Adapt systems and methodology that work. The following chapter offers an overview of some of the current planning concepts and methodologies.

THE PLANNING PROCESS

Planning is a process involving the development of new services, optimizing human resources, and enhancing patient outcomes. As a process, it must be flexible in response to environmental change, be acceptable or include those who will be implementing the plans, and be realistic.

Assessment is the first step in the planning process. It is ongoing, and can be directed by an identified need or problem. Information is gathered from the internal and external environments in regard to present and potential resources, present and changing conditions, forecasting, and other input pertinent to the identified need or problem. Following information analysis and synthesis, a diagnosis is made concerning (1) the future desired state, (2) the present status or state, and (3) the gap of deficiency between the present and the desired states. The gap represents obstacles, deficiencies, or needed strategies that are then listed and explicitly defined.

The *planning phase* involves prescribing solutions to reach the desired future state. This entails developing measurable objectives that are aimed at effecting the necessary changes to fill the gap. Specific tactics are then developed to direct actions necessary to achieve the objectives. Each tactic explains what work is to be done, how, by whom, and whom it will affect, as well as timetables and control systems.

The *implementation phase* involves actualizing the tactics. The outcome of these activities is *evaluated* according to the criteria outlined in the objectives and tactics. *Revisions* are made as conditions change, and as actions are effective or ineffective in achieving the desired results. The planning process operates with each component being interrelated to and interacting with the other components. Change in one area produces change in some other area, or in the total process. Therefore, assessment must be a continuous process.

TYPES OF PLANNING

Basically, planning can be grouped into three categories that interrelate to achieve the organization's future desired state: strategic, intermediate, and short-term planning. *Strategic* planning concerns projecting conditions and needs for a 5 to 10-year future. It is ongoing and includes technological planning, determining missions and aims, expansion plans, divestment plans, total resource allocation, and long-range positioning of the organization. Intermediate, short-term, and contingency planning also make up the corporate strategic plans.

Due to the rapid rate of change, many believe that a future of over 5 years is exceedingly difficult, if not impossible, to predict. A mission may aim toward a 5- to 10-year future, but this plan is annually reviewed and revised according to environmental trends. Environmental assessment is integral to effective planning.

Intermediate planning covers a 1- to 5-year period and is designed to achieve strategic plans. It includes program or project planning, which focuses on one event such as developing a specific service or building a new facility. It also includes plans for marketing and annual budgeting.

Short-term planning consists of specific tactics and operations designed to achieve an objective and meet intermediate plans. It is narrow in scope, a means to an end. The time span is 3 months to a year and must include budget plans, timetables and mechanisms of control, and contingency plans for alternative actions for possible changes and altered events. Contingency plans are built in to deal with rapid change.

ORGANIZING FOR PLANNING

Directives for all planning are set by the governing board, which defines hospital policy for planning, delegates strategy formulation to administration, then approves or disapproves and revises hospital missions and strategies. Planning may be implemented in many ways; the following is an example for integrating strategic, intermediate, and short-term planning within the organization.

Strategic planning may be implemented through a *steering committee*, consisting of top-level administration, the chief of medical staff, and a governing board representative. This committee may meet monthly, review information from hospital and operational planning committees, and synthesize assessment data from these reports, as well as from the organized information system.

The steering committee determines and revises the mission and overall strategies for the hospital, and reports these to the board for final decision. The mission and overall strategies, with recommendations and assessment analysis, then go to the *hospital planning committee* for intermediate planning.

The hospital planning committee may consist of the chief executive officer (CEO) as chairperson, selected department heads, and should include the vice-president for nursing and the director of medical records. This committee may also meet monthly, review information from the steering committee, and determine objectives for the hospital. The hospital planning committee should recognize the need for communication and input from those who are implementing the plans, and should allow individuals with ideas and recommendations to attend meetings and to explain their suggestions. Personnel and committees can also submit ideas and suggestions to individual members of the committee.

The hospital planning committee can analyze assessment data, develop objectives, and supply this information and recommendations to the delegated department heads. These department heads may choose to chair the projects themselves, or to appoint staff members as chairpersons on specific projects. The department head should, however, remain ultimately responsible for the implementation, evaluation, and communication of the objective or project.

Short-term or operational planning may occur within each department, through a *departmental planning system.* Ad hoc committees may be organized to plan, direct, and control operations for a delegated objective; these committees should consist of both management and staff representatives, and be self-terminating once objectives are reached. Or the department may choose to have a standing planning committee, with both permanent and rotating members; the permanent members may represent management and staff personnel, while the rotating members could vary among clinical specialties, shifts, and/or areas of expertise. Rotating members would, of course, be appointed for specific projects only.

Another workable system in the nursing department is to combine the nursing planning committee with the nursing quality assurance committee; the combined committee would then review pertinent activities, outcomes, reports, and problems occurring within the nursing department for quality assurance as well as planning purposes.

It is important to note that the nursing planning committee can do more than just achieve predetermined objectives. Through representation from the nursing staff, it can involve all personnel in the planning process; it can also strive to develop talent, skills, and potential within the nursing service, and to foster new ideas and solutions.

THE HOSPITAL-WIDE INFORMATION SYSTEM

All data, consultants, and support personnel from the hospital's information system should be available for each department's planning functions. This hospital-wide information storehouse can be centralized in order to avoid duplication and inefficiency. Any additional needed information may be supplied through this system, or retrieved by the individual planning participants.

Just as the planning process is dependent upon information, so must it in turn feed information and results back into the information system. A nursing department can also maintain its own information system by compiling and reviewing all minutes, reports, studies, and outcomes from committees, projects, functions, shift supervisors, as well as patient classification, census, and feedback information. This information may be organized in a set of notebooks, a filing cabinet, or may be computerized; it is important, however, that it be current and easy to retrieve.

CONSIDERATIONS IN PLANNING

Values, attitudes, and environmental change all affect successful planning. Research has shown that different segments of the worker population are motivated by different incentives. For example, older, dedicated workers want job security whereas ambitious, young workers want a challenge, as well as increased responsibility and financial reward. As the "baby boomers" mature and the age of retirement rises, there will be fewer management positions. One positive response to this dilemma is restructuring of organizations, using autonomous work groups and increased flexibility in functions. A need to create opportunities for participation and responsibility by this large group of experienced workers is emerging. Union representatives are joining governing boards, workers in some areas are electing board members, and work groups are making organizational decisions.[1] Where planning was once strictly from the top down, future planning systems must focus on the individual's role in achieving excellence and receive input from the bottom up. As organizations restructure to adapt to change, so must planning systems.

The *time period, impact, and priority* of certain plans is another consideration, and will dictate the approach. Another problem may take top priority, employee negative response may have been underestimated, and the benefits may no longer outweigh the effort and risks. These types of variables will change the focus of planning to one of satisfying, or making the fastest, easiest decision to achieve results to "get by." High-impact needs may call for optimizing, where the best possible solution must be reached, utilizing a thorough environmental assessment.[2] The nurse-administrator must know when "getting by" is sufficient, when a combination approach may be used, or when only an optimal decision is acceptable.

The *existing system of planning* is an important consideration for the nurse-administrator. The existing hospital planning system usually reflects the style and philosophy of the *chief executive officer*. Does the CEO practice an autocratic type of management, where planning and decisions are secretive and made by the chief and perhaps an assistant or a small executive team? Or does the CEO practice a more participative style of management, where all department heads are involved in administrative decision making, and planning is an ongoing communicative and sharing experience? Chances are the answer lies somewhere in between. Is the nurse-administrator included in strategic planning and executive-level decision making? Is there any formal planning system, or is any planning done at all? The nurse-administrator must be aware of the CEO's style of management and philosophy of planning and nurse involvement. Relations and interactions with the governing board should be examined: are interactions secretive, excluding nursing, or is nursing input sought and recognized as valuable in determining future planning?

If nursing is a key part of executive decision making, nursing planning systems must be organized consistently with executive-level planning systems, and must serve to facilitate and continue the plans of top management. The whole idea of planning is, after all, to carry out the aims and mission of the organization. Ideally, all planning should be coordinated, communicated, and interrelated.

If there is no formal or recognized type of planning at all on the top executive level, the nurse-administrator must establish realistic and workable planning systems within the nursing department, based upon whatever information can be obtained. With access to information about organizational activities, status, and unwritten plans or strategies, the nurse-administrator can integrate nursing planning into these overall plans.

If there is a top executive planning system or team, but nursing is not included, then the nurse-administrator must strive to obtain information about organizational plans, and make nursing planning consistent with these plans. At the same time, the nurse-administrator must continue efforts for nursing involvement in decision making, but expectations must remain realistic. Constant frustration can only serve as an emotional drain and obstacle to effective management. If excluded from top-level involvement and information, the nurse-administrator must work toward optimal results within the nursing department—planning and working toward *what can be controlled,* within the constraints of the executive administration.

In planning, those involved in formulating, communicating, and implementing the plans must also be considered. This includes the *nursing management team* and the nursing staff. The nurse-administrator must know everything about the management team, which serves as an extension of himself or herself. If they misunderstand and miscommunicate messages, if they disagree philosophically or work to undermine the nurse-administrator, if they are unable to grasp new concepts and learn new skills—then there is a problem that must be alleviated. The management team must be able to change, learn, perceive, and communicate, and they should share a similar or common philosophy with the nurse-administrator concerning the importance of human resources to the organization and a fundamental understanding of the workings of change.

The nurse-administrator must communicate these expectations to the management team, and demand first-rate performance of management practices at all times. It is up to this team to involve the nursing staff and provide the creative, growth-producing environment that fosters job satisfaction and quality service.

The nursing staff as a whole must be considered when formulating plans: their talents, educational backgrounds, attitudes toward change, ability to accept change, and skill and performance capabilities are all important factors in planning. The nurse-administrator cannot plan in isolation, but must consider both the entire organization and who will be implementing the plans. There should be a system for receiving feedback from all levels of the nursing staff involved in any change.

DECISION MAKING

Decision making occurs within every phase of planning, from the selection of assessment factors to the choosing of an implementation approach. Decision making is inherent within the planning process, and therefore expertise in making decisions goes hand in hand with the success of such planning.

Lancaster and Lancaster[3] define the decision-making process by the following steps:

1. Problem identification
2. Assessment
3. Development of alternatives
4. Implementation and evaluation.

Bailey and Claus[4] describe a useful model for decision making: the following outlines this model:

1. Define overall ends and objectives.
2. Determine the problem: delineate between what is desired and the present status.
3. Assess the internal and external environments and generate hypotheses about the cause of the problem and its nature. Then narrow down these hypotheses and define the problem.
4. Analyze available resources and constraints pertaining to the problem. Get input from any potentially affected group.
5. Write objectives or expected outcomes in performance terms. Prioritize, separating the critical from the noncritical.
6. Generate alternative plans and solutions.
7. Analyze alternatives.
8. Choose an alternative.
9. Implement the solution; correct deficiencies.

Ehrat[5] has described some important factors for consideration in hospital decision making:

1. Most organizations are run by their history of past experiences, tradition, and the market forces. The decision maker should know the history of past experiences and outcomes.
2. Hospitals use simple indicators to predict complex events, such as nurse turnover and absenteeism. The decision maker should know what indicators are used and monitor them.
3. All departments believe in equity and fairness, and the decision maker should remember that they expect equal treatment.
4. Change is best received during times of crisis and uncertainty. Only small change is accepted during stable times.
5. The decision maker should always test ideas informally first, and then on a small scale.

Planning is ultimately decision making. What distinguishes it from simple problem solving or decision making is its orientation to the future, its coordination of multiple decisions, and its focus on organizational functions and goals. But the steps in the planning process correlate to the steps in decision making, and as plans become more tactical or specific, they more closely resemble the decision-making process.

Tools for Decision Making

Many analytical tools are available to assist with key decision points in the planning process. Computer simulators forecast probable outcomes, decision trees plot out contingency plans, and graphs and charts are used to identify progress, flow of operations, and activities that are critical to results.

A *contingency planning model* is based on the understanding that decisions are dependent upon the situation, and that situations change. Alternative plans are therefore developed in the event that certain changes may occur. Short-term contingency plans often help to restore equilibrium during times of crisis, but contingency plans should not be used as the sole planning approach.

Forecasting is predicting the future using scientific methods. It is only a part of the entire planning process, rather than a process in and of itself. Because the future cannot be predicted with great accuracy, care should be used concerning the role of forecasting in individual planning. One forecasting method is the *alternate scenario method,* where various types of probable futures are generated, and contingency plans are created for each possible future. These scenarios can be pared down to the best, worst, and most possible futures, and contingency plans made for these three.

Riggs[6] describes two approaches to decision making. One approach is the *comparison of alternatives.* Each alternative is rated numerically, according to its effects, as if it has already occurred. Then it is compared to the other alternatives. The highest-ranking alternative is chosen. This approach is effective when decisions are self-contained and when there is little uncertainty of variables.

The second approach, *conditional decisions,* involves various alternatives at each stage of planning. depending upon conditions. The same as contingency planning, this creates a decision tree where various alternate courses of action are mapped out.

Many analytical tools are available for planning and decision making. *Linear programming* assigns math symbols to problems and solves them mathematically or by plotting them on a graph. *Gantt or bar charts* are models for scheduling projects with times and dates to reflect degree of completion. *Networking* maps out activities on a flow chart, indicating each activity with estimated time periods for completion of a project, and what must be done to finish on time and within budget.[6] Though they are useful in reducing the chance of error and in coordinating decision making, the nurse-administrator must not become overdependent on these tools, or overconfident of their accuracy. As humans we are subjective, and tend to slant even analytical information to suit our needs. Circumstances must not be overanalyzed, nor must plans be made only in a detached, methodical manner. Planning must involve intuition along with analysis, and *focus on the end result* of quality and excellence.

HUMAN RESOURCE MANAGEMENT PLANNING

Human resource management stems from strategic, intermediate, and short-term planning, and is integrated into the total organizational planning system. Specific personnel plans concerning activities such as recruitment, selection, salary scales, and so on involve human resource management planning (HRMP), which is centralized within the nursing planning system and receives input from all hospital sources.

The following questions are addressed by HRMP: What human resources are needed to achieve the organization's goals? How can the organization recruit and retain these human resources? How might future competition for human resources change?

In HRMP, the planner tries to match employee competency with organizational needs, and to develop a fit between the employee and the organization. The status of human resources within the organization must be inventoried, and plans made to develop, promote, transfer, or hire human resources congruent with organizational plans.

Steps in HRMP include[7]:

1. Developing a purpose or philosophy for the human resource management program.
2. Formulating assumptions about the organizational growth rate, external factors affecting organizational plans, future human resource needs, financial considerations, and the advantage of human resources versus capital resources.
3. Defining organizational responsibility: how do all employees fit into the organization in terms of roles, authority, and structure?
4. Developing an inventory of resources.
5. Evaluating the processes of compensation, administration of benefits, training, recruitment, and performance evaluation.
6. Evaluating and compiling information concerning ways to assess, analyze, and manage human resource issues that affect the organization; ways to identify human resource needs from organizational plans; career development; and feedback and communication to administration by attitude surveys, exit interviews, etc.
7. Analyzing major trends, such as increased expectations by the work force, high technology, and aging baby boomers.
8. Analyzing internal trends such as a decrease in promotable workers, poor union relationships, or the availability of needed skills.
9. Deciding upon human resource needs.
10. Developing action plans to meet goals.

Human resource planning involves the continuous staffing of positions with qualified personnel. While short-term plans may include filling existing positions, long-term HRMP involves determining the gap between the present and desired status: this gap is the human resource requirement. According to Castetter,[8] HRMP involves the following:

1. Developing assumptions based on goals, knowledge of the organization, division of labor, number of positions, job requirements and responsibilities, position design, roles, administrative roles, staffing, and scheduling.
2. Projecting organizational structure and corresponding human resource needs; knowledge of future plans of the organization is essential.
3. Making a personnel or current inventory of human resources, including ages, special skills, size, characteristics and composition of staff, present and future positions, morale, and any other available information. How can existing personnel satisfy projected needs?
4. Forecasting likely changes in personnel, such as retirement, resignation, leaves of absence, layoffs, transfer, and promotions. Compare these forecasts to projected needs.
5. Developing programs to meet future needs, such as recruitment, matching current employees with future positions, long-term development, and a time frame for various plans.
6. Creating control plans. Review, compare to objectives, correct deviations, update information, find causes of problems. Ongoing assessment and evaluation is required here.

In conclusion, planning is a creative process. Creative planning leads to the practical application of innovative ideas, and helps to make ideas work. Creativity is essential for controlling the forces of change, and all aspects of human resource management should be blended with creative and innovative thinking.

REFERENCES

1. Fulma, R. M., & Franklin, S. G. Planning paradoxes for managers in the 80s. *Managerial Planning*, 1983, *31*(3), 19–24.
2. Jeager, B. J. The concept of corporate planning. *Health Care Management Review*, 1982, *7*(3), 21–22.
3. Lancaster, J., & Lancaster, W. Rational decision making: Managing uncertainty. *JONA*, Sept. 1982, pp. 22–28.
4. Baily, J. T., & Claus, K. E. *Decision making in nursing—Tools for change*. St. Louis: Mosby, 1975, pp. 18–112.
5. Ehrat, K. S. A model for politically astute planning and decision making. *JONA*, 1983, *13*(9), 29–35.
6. Riggs, J. L. *Economic decision models*. New York: McGraw-Hill, 1968.

7. Smith, E. C. How to tie human resource planning to strategic business planning. *Managerial Planning*, 1983, *32*(2), 29–34.
8. Castetter, W. B. *The personnel function in educational administration* (3rd ed.). New York: Macmillan, 1981, pp. 75–124.

SUGGESTED READING

Barnard, C. The environment of decision. *JONA*, March 1982, pp. 25–29.

Bodzek, J. W. Corporate approach lends control over complex environment. In J. M. Kraegel (Ed.), *Planning Strategies for Nurse Managers*. Germantown, Maryland: Aspen, 1983, pp. 85–93.

Bolles, R. N. Life/work planning, change and constancy in the world of work. *The Futurist*, 1983, *13*(16), 7–11.

Brown, J. L., & Agnew, N. M. Corporate agility. *Business Horizons*, 1982, *25*(2), 29–33.

Curtin, L. Editorial opinion. *Nursing Management*, 1984, *15*(3), 7, 8.

Dale, R. L., & Mable, R. J. Nursing classification system: Foundation for personnel planning and control. *JONA*, 1983, *13*(2), 10–13.

Drucker, P. *Management: Tasks, responsibilities, policies.* New York: Harper & Row, 1974.

Dyck, M. H., & Woodruff, A. Goal setting in hospital departments. *HCM Review*, Summer 1981, pp. 37–47.

Edwards, L. H. Health planning: Opportunities for nurses. *Nursing Outlook*, 1983, *31*(6), 322–325.

Emery, J. C. *Organizational planning and control systems.* London: Macmillan, 1969.

Erickson, E. H., & Bormeyer. V. Simulated decision-making experience via case analysis. *JONA*, 1979, *9*(5), 10–15.

Fingerhut, E. C., & Hatano, D. G. Principles of strategic planning applied to international corporations. *Managerial Planning*, 1983, *32*(5), 4.

Friedman, E. Voluntary communitywide health planning. *Hospitals*, 1981, *55*(2), 61, 62.

Goodwin, I. H. A guide to planning critical care units. *JONA*, 1979, *9*(6), 20–25.

Griffith, J. *Quantitative techniques for hospital planning and control.* Lexington, Mass.: Lexington Books, 1972.

Harris, R. *Precedence and arrow networking techniques for construction.* Ann Arbor: University of Michigan Press, 1973.

Hayes, R. L., & Radosevich, R. Designing information systems for strategic decisions. *Long-Range Planning*, 1974, *7*(4), 45–48.

Hein, L. W. *The quantitative approach to managerial decisions.* Engelwood Cliffs, New Jersey: Prentice-Hall, 1967.

Hopkins, M., & Vander Hoeven, R. Basic-needs planning and forecasting: Policy & scenario analysis in four countries. *International Labor Review*, 1982, *14*(6), 689–712.

Hubbard, B. M. The future of futurism—Creating a new synthesis. *The Futurist*, 1983, *17*(2), 52–58.

Katz, G., Zavodnick, L., & Markezin, E. Strategic planning in a restrictive and competitive environment. *HCM Review*, 1983, *8*(4), 7–12.

Kraegel, J. M. *Planning strategies for nurse managers.* Germantown, Maryland: Aspen, 1983.

Lorsch, J. W., & Lawrence, P. R. (Eds.) *Organizational planning: Cases and concepts.* Homewood, Illinois: Irwin, 1972, pp. 38–48.

Makridakis, S., & Wheelright, S. C. *Forecasting: Methods and applications.* New York: Wiley, 1978.

Mascarenhas, B. Coping with uncertainty in international business. *Journal of International Business Studies,* 1982, *13*(2), 87–98.

Melum, M. M. 10 "lessons" point the way toward successful hospital planning. *Hospitals,* 1981, *55*(23), 58–61.

Michnich, M. E., Shortell, S. M., & Richardson, W. C. Program evaluation: Resource for decision making. *HCM Review,* Summer 1981, pp. 25–35.

Mitroff, I., & Emshoff, J. R. On strategic assumption making: A dialectical approach to policy and planning. *Academy of Management Review,* 1979, *4,* 1–12.

Monson, T. Mastering the art of planning by committee. *JONA,* Nov./Dec. 1981, pp. 71–72.

Naylor, T. H. The effective use of strategic planning, forecasting and modeling in the executive suite. *Management Planning,* 1982, *30*(4), 4–11.

Naylor, T. H. The strategy matrix. *Managerial Planning,* 1983, *31*(4), 4–9.

O'Donnell, J. A planning process for hospitals and service organizations. *Managerial Planning,* 1983, *32*(5), 28–31.

O'Donnell, M., & O'Donnell, R. J. MBO—Is it passe? *H&HSA,* 1983, *28*(5), 46–58.

Peters, J. P., & Wacker, R. C. Strategic planning. *Hospitals,* 1982, *56*(12), 90–98.

Pollok, C. S. Adopting management by objectives to nursing. *Nursing Clinics of North America,* 1983, *18*(3), 481–490.

Porter-O'Grady, T. Planning: A framework for action. *Health Care Supervisor,* 1983, *1*(4), 29–41.

Quinn, J. B. Formulating strategy one step at a time. *Journal of Business Strategy, 1,* Winter 1981, pp. 42–63.

Riggs, J. L. *Economic decision models.* New York: McGraw-Hill, 1968.

Schechter, D. S. A chance to start over for hospital planning. *Hospitals,* 1981, *55*(21), 61, 62.

Simon, H. *Administrative behavior.* New York: The Free Press, 1979.

Stevens, B. J. First-line nursing management. *Nurse as executive* (2nd ed.). Wakefield, Mass.: Nursing Resource, 1980, pp. 213–224.

Stokes, J. F. Quality patient care and cost control too. *Health Care Supervisor,* 1983, *1*(4), 60–63.

Toohey, E. M., Shillinger, F. L., & Baronowski, S. L. Planning alternative delivery systems. *JONA,* 1985, *15*(12), 9–15.

Watson, H. J. *Computer simulation in business.* New York: Wiley, 1981.

Wilson, P. A. Health planning: Structure, processes and social work involvement. *Social Work in Health Care,* 1981, *1*(1), 87–97.

Zilm, F., Arch, D., & Hollis, R. B. An application of simulation modeling to surgical intensive care bed need analysis in a university hospital. *H&HSA,* 1983, *28*(5), 82–101.

5 Creativity

Creativity and innovation are our tools for controlling change, and they are essential to the success of any organization. Although programmed problem-solving and past habits may be adequate for survival, progress and success can be attained only by developing inner potentials for creativity. In this world of constant change, human resources that are flexible, can improvise, and can develop creative responses to change are needed.

FOSTERING CREATIVE POTENTIAL

What do you do when you get a flash of an idea that, at the moment, seems brilliant? Nine times out of ten you will not follow the idea through to reality. You think of a hundred reasons why it will not work and then dismiss it from your mind. How many times have you squelched someone else's ideas? What about all those new nurses who "just about drove you crazy" with their ideas for change? Do you remember feeling irritated by their "unrealistic" enthusiasm?

Many businesses and corporations are starting to take these flashes of ideas seriously. Creativity is no longer viewed as something to be pursued outside of the work environment; it is now seen as an important ingredient to success. Businesses are setting the stage for freer and more flexible thought, fostering interorganizational competition for ideas, and developing communication channels for creative suggestions. The days of the autocratic manager are gone. The most effective leaders are not those who have simply learned and practiced management theory and techniques, but those who are in tune with their own intuition, have a deep understanding of human nature, and possess the ability to draw upon the potentials and talents of others. We must all be smarter, more daring, unique, and creative to compete in today's world.

You may now be asking, "How can I be creative? I don't have a creative bone in my body!" Well, you *are* creative. Everyone is born with some creative abilities and still possesses vast amounts of creative talents. Somewhere along the way you learned to suppress your subconscious thoughts with rational and logical thinking; you were programmed to conform and to follow the rules of conventional thought. Researchers have discovered that overanalyzing and logical reasoning are no more effective than pure intuitive decision making.[1] Corporate executives are going back to the intuitive areas of thought that were once dismissed as useless; it is now realized that the best results come from a blend of creative, intuitive thought and rational, analytical thought. The mind must be open to imaginative thought and the generation of ideas first, and then these ideas can be evaluated, analyzed, and refined for application.

What exactly is creativity? It is both originality and new ideas, and the results of these ideas put to work. An illuminating hunch is captured and then applied, resulting in the creative act. Creativity involves newness and improvement, from product development to personal satisfaction. Newness, however, does not imply *total* originality; it can be using the old in new ways by varying characteristics, order, or combination of elements to generate different results.

OBSTACLES TO CREATIVITY

Your habits and attitudes that are blocking creativity must be broken in order to overcome obstacles to creativity. Table 5-1 lists barriers to creativity. By identifying the positive characteristics and practicing them, you can reprogram yourself and incorporate new habits and behaviors into your everyday life.

FREEING CREATIVITY

The following techniques will help you to free your creative potential. In using them, it is important to be positive; stop criticizing. It is also important not to be distracted or interrupted. Take a few moments to empty your mind of work problems. And remember, you are only as creative as you allow yourself to be.

One of the best ways to unlearn mental blocks and enhance creativity is through *autosuggestion*. By first reaching a state of deep relaxation, and then through concentration, you can unlock barriers and obtain increased

TABLE 5–1. BARRIERS TO CREATIVITY

Barriers	Creativity
Rigid thinking; staying with preconceived thoughts and prior education	Fluid and flexible thinking; open-minded and committed to lifelong learning
Always thinking others' ideas are better	Believing in own instincts and ideas
Only seeing the here and now	Exploring possiblities and testing alternatives; being future-oriented
Afraid to question—don't want to appear stupid	Always asking why; being curious about causes and reasons
Fearing failure or mistakes	Taking risks; learning from mistakes
Conforming—afraid to be different	Purposely veering from the norm
The routine is security; disliking change	Seeking and enjoying change; striving for improvements
Always being realistic and logical	Speculating, fantasizing, and imagining
Cannot let loose; must be mature and reserved at all times	Letting the child out; having fun and being uninhibited
Cannot see the real problem or its relationship to other things	Getting to the heart of the matter; having a holistic view of problems and events

awareness of your inner self. The process is based on two beliefs: (1) that the mind is programmed to accept or reject information and can be reprogrammed by feeding it consistent, continual information; and (2) that there is a vast amount of knowledge in the mind. The process of autosuggestion, however, requires discipline and practice. You must first learn to get in touch with your entire body through progressive relaxation; this involves concentrating on sensing and relaxing each body part, until the entire body is in a state of deep relaxation. When this state is achieved, it is possible to concentrate on activating inner energies. The mind actually wills a certain state, and, through continual feeding of suggestions, can obtain control of its own processes.

Autosuggestion can be learned through independent reading and study, but it is advisable to seek training from an experienced professional. Many universities and medical centers have facilities for biofeedback training. Group classes and audiotapes that teach the basic techniques are also available. Whichever route you choose, it is imperative to practice daily, or you will lose the art of intense concentration. Appendix 5–1 provides an example of an autosuggestion technique.

Self-reliance can also be important in overcoming creative obstacles and freeing creativity. Poet and essayist Ralph Waldo Emerson wrote that you must trust your own thoughts and instincts, and believe in yourself.[2] Do not be afraid to veer from the majority opinion and think for yourself. Listen to your inner voice; trust your impressions. Having confidence and believing in yourself is an important step to unleashing creativity. As with everything else in life, your mental attitude determines the results you get. By believing that you have creative abilities, you will become more creative.

Creativity requires freeing the mind to roam, explore, and ponder. While children are often taught that this is unacceptable, *daydreaming* is important in generating new ideas. It allows the subconscious mind to rise into the conscious mind, and the imagination to wander. While daydreaming, things are seen from a different perspective, and are often visualized in images, rather than in words. Irrational thinking and daydreaming often generate ideas that can later be refined for practical application.

After concentrating on the solution to a problem, get away from the problem for awhile. Go for a walk or engage in a relaxing activity that allows the mind to rest. Your mind will be *incubating,* working unconsciously to solve the problem. Often, when the mind is relaxed, the answer will come forward. The trick is to work diligently on a solution, and then forget it. You have programmed your brain to perform unconscious problem solving.

Another way to free your creativity is by *studying creative people.* Identify their positive qualities and practice them. By continually practicing these behaviors, you incorporate them into your way of life. Read, study, and collect information about creative people—writers, artists, composers, doctors, and businessmen. What made them successful?

Some people feel more creative when they are *learning.* The more reading and studying you do, the more knowledge you have to draw from. Creativity often involves building on someone else's ideas—adapting or changing them to fit a different situation. Draw on ideas from other fields, and relate these to nursing. Be alert for good ideas, regardless of where they crop up. Look for that which is not obvious; observe everything.

Find some means of *self-expression.* Take ballet lessons, play a musical instrument, arrange flowers, embroider, keep a journal, learn to paint, or prepare gourmet meals. Exposure to creative activities is helpful in generating ideas. Along the same line, think in pictures. When you hear an idea or are confronted with a problem, picture it in your mind as a visual image; this sparks the imagination and helps to generate ideas as well.

It is important to *spend time alone,* allowing your mind to wander. Walk on the beach, ride a bike, jog through the park, or simply relax in an isolated part of your house. It is important to have time to reflect inwardly. Meditation is a good way to get in touch with yourself and block out the external world.

While you are spending time on your mind, *do not forget your body as well.* A fit body helps to keep the mind alert. With a busy schedule and family obligations, nurse-administrators often neglect their physical selves. Make health a top priority; forget about junk food and eat vegetables instead. Do not forego your daily exercise; release all that stress and tension, even if you feel tired. At the same time you can be daydreaming.

Know yourself; we all function better under different conditions and at different times of the day. If you are more alert in the morning, then use that time for problem solving. If you work best with music or around other people, then create an environment for this. Learn what conditions have helped your creativity in the past, and recreate them.

DEVELOPING A CREATIVE ORGANIZATION

It is true that some people are more creatively gifted than others, but it is also true that everyone has creative potential that can be developed. When people are assisted in freeing inhibited talents and expressing themselves, they become more productive and satisfied. If you can provide an environment that fosters self-expression and creative thought, you will have a more resourceful, progressive organization, and a more productive and satisfied staff.

Written Policies

Written policies, job descriptions, merit raise systems, and recognition systems can all reflect a commitment to creativity. Although a separate policy for creativity is not necessary, a certain mode of thought should be integrated throughout all policies. For example, your present nursing philosophy statement could contain the following paragraph:

> We believe that creativity and innovation are tools for controlling change. Progress and success can be achieved only by developing inner potentials for creativity, imagination, and innovation. We believe that everyone has creative abilities, talents, and insights that can be fostered to achieve personal satisfaction and organizational progress. We believe that human resources are the most valuable part of the organization and an essential link to organizational success; therefore, we are committed to assisting each individual in creative abilities and contributing ideas for improvement.

Job descriptions and performance evaluations should include the employee's role in creative problem solving. Statements such as "suggests ideas for improvement," "participates in research activities," and "implements planned innovations," reflect the employee's responsibility toward creativity. Of course, evaluation and reward systems must follow accordingly; promotions, merit raises, recognition of achievement, and clinical ladder programs should be based on creative contributions, as well as skills and duties (see Chapter 9).

Written policies alone are not enough; set an example by generating and being open to new ideas, and make sure your management team does the same. The staff will recognize your commitment by its results.

You may want to begin implementing your commitment to creativity by allowing those employees who are currently interested in innovations and change a chance to try out their ideas. Take a look at the creative people who may be frustrated or inhibited by a structured environment, or those who are constantly making suggestions and communicating ideas. These people are telling you that they want change—so let them have it. Ask for volunteers to staff a *special unit,* totally unique and autonomous, where they can experiment with innovations and changes. Take one of your nursing units and place these volunteers there, allowing others to be transferred. Set ground rules and retain final authority, and then leave your special unit to its own devices. The other units will be watching, and will also want to participate, once they see the results.

Those employees who cannot readily accept change should be permitted to work in a traditional, structured unit. There will be many of these employees at first, but they may later want to join a creative unit. Allow for these individual differences. Creativity cannot be forced, but must be allowed to happen.

Recruiting Talent

When you recruit and interview potential employees, make past creative achievements and present creative abilities a criterion for selection. Look for intelligent, unique, and perhaps maverick people who are not afraid to think for themselves, ask questions, or be different. People who are often labeled "mavericks" or "radicals" may have frustrated creative talents. When allowed to function with some control, express and put their ideas to work, these "radicals" will work for you rather than against you.

Creative Task Forces

Form task forces for the sole purpose of generating new ideas on a particular subject; once the goal is achieved, disband the task forces. Rotating the members of task forces is a good idea; always include those who are willing to participate and be flexible. Use brainstorming and synectics to enhance the generation of ideas. You will need some ground rules:

1. No criticism or analysis at this point.
2. Acceptance and encouragement of all ideas and thoughts.
3. Aim for imaginative, wild ideas and illogical thinking.
4. Generate as many ideas as possible.

Free thinking and fun are keys to these task forces. Others will refine and implement ideas; creative task forces generate them.

Brainstorming

Brainstorming is used to elicit a large number of ideas. A question, topic, or problem is posed before a group, and then the group members either call out or write down any and every idea that comes to mind. No criticisms are allowed, and the free flow of imaginative and even ridiculous ideas is encouraged. Brainstorming can be practiced alone, as well as in a group. Set a time frame and decide on a topic, and then list all your thoughts and ideas. The purpose of brainstorming, again, is to generate a vast number of ideas, regardless of the quality of those ideas. Brainstorming can lead to opened creativity and can help overcome creative barriers.

Synectics

Another technique for enhancing creativity is the game of playing with metaphors. This involves taking a particular subject and comparing its similarities and differences to something else. Alexander[3] provides the following procedure for synectics:

1. State and define the problem.
2. Allow the group to restate, redefine, and reinterpret the problem from various perspectives.
3. Ask evocative questions: no analysis or criticism is permitted. Questions include:
   a. Direct analogies—How is this problem like something else?
   b. Personal analogies—How can you put yourself in the problem and actually become it? How does it feel? How will you act?
   c. Symbolic analogies—How can you describe the problem with symbols?
   d. Fantasy analogies—Describe a solution by a fantasy, dream, or wish.

Prince[4] describes the use of purging in synectics. The group has time to call out all thoughts related to the subject, "purging" their brains. The leader of the session then calls a "force-fit" for the group to attempt to fit the analogy back into the original problem. A "viewpoint" is reached when someone sees a way to approach the problem.

The ideas generated at a synectic session may seem impractical, but at this point they are unrefined. They are taken to a planning committee for scrutiny. One synectic session alone may not generate ideas; sessions can be continued at a later time. Appendix 5–2 provides a simplified example of a synectic session.

Stimulating Creative Thought

Both patients and employees are affected by the environment; small changes in environment can go a long way for enhancing creativity. Consider the following ideas, and see if they can apply to your environment.

Decorate the Walls with Artwork. Let your staff contribute personal works, frame art by patients, or bring in children's watercolors. Ask volunteer services to bring in art as well.

Pipe in Classical Music Over the Intercom. Try different types of classical music, such as piano, string, symphony, or woodwinds. The variety itself will be stimulating. You could even post information on the composer and the work on the bulletin board.

Make Work More Fun and Interesting. Have contests and games to stimulate staff participation and teamwork. An interunit competition can be held to stimulate ideas. Recognize outstanding units by throwing a party or giving them a trophy. Whatever you do, make it fun.

Hold Study Sessions. Encourage learning. Have role playing and mini-plays to act out information for the audience. Unit personnel can meet regularly and take turns presenting information on medications, procedures, or special subjects.

Promote Physical and Mental Well-being. Nurses often eat junk food with coffee and neglect their need for proper rest and exercise. Have health food days in the cafeteria where everyone brings a nutritious dish. Have fruit available next to the candy machine. Set up exercise classes so that each shift can exercise before going home; ask staff members to volunteer to lead these classes.

Hold Relaxation Classes. This will promote mental awareness and creative thinking. A good schedule is once a week for four to six weeks, repeating classes three or four times a year.

Open Interdepartmental Communications. Have departments talk to one another about what they do. Try to help your department see problems from another department's perspective. Invite guest speakers from other departments.

Implementing Ideas

Communicating your commitment to creativity is not enough; you must implement ideas that are presented to you. Let staff know you will listen and set aside an appointed time of day or schedule regular meetings to hear new ideas. The suggestion box is also an effective way to receive ideas—if you let the staff know that you both see and use the suggestions. Suggestions may be anonymous or may be signed for personal recognition.

Establish a creative planning committee to go over ideas and refine them. This could be either a standing committee or one that rotates. This committee could rank ideas for implementation in terms of priority, and make recommendations to management. Or you could screen ideas and then present them to the committee for further refinement.

Form a task force for change. If an idea has merit and can solve a problem, then it should be refined and applied. This task is assigned to the task force for implementing change. Objectives are set here, schedules determined, resources evaluated and allocated, procedures delineated and controlled, and results evaluated.

Remember, you do not want to change just for the sake of changing. If what you have is working, then leave it alone. At the same time, creativity has an important place in your organization. Promote self-awareness and self-expression. Open your mind to new possibilities. Strive to satisfy your staff and bring out their best.

REFERENCES

1. Loye, D. The brain and the future. *The Futurist, 16*(5), October 1982, pp. 15–19.
2. Emerson, R. W. Self-reliance. In *Essays of Ralph Waldo Emerson*. New York: A. S. Barnes, p. 15.
3. Alexander, T. Synectics: Inventing by the madness method. In Davis, G. A., and Scott, J. A. (Eds.), *Training creative thinking*. New York: Holt, Rinehart & Winston, 1971, pp. 1–13.
4. Prince, G. M. The operational mechanism of synectics. In Davis, G. A., and Scott, J. A. (Eds.), *Training creative thought*. New York: Holt, Rinehart & Winston, 1971, pp. 33–37.

SUGGESTED READING

Agor, W. H. Tomorrow's intuitive leaders. *The Futurist*, 1984, *17*(4), 49–52.

Arieti, S. *Creativity: The magic synthesis*. New York: Basic Books, Inc., 1976.

Bates, T. How to manage creativity. *Management Today*, June 1983, pp. 82–85.

Brown, B. J. (Ed.) From the editor. *In Nursing Administration Quarterly*, 1982, *6*(3), Spring viii–x.

Cornella, T. Understanding creativity for use in managerial planning. In G. A. Davis, & J. A. Scott (Eds.), *Training creative thinking*. New York: Holt, Rinehart, & Winston, 1971.

Crawford, R. P. The techniques of creative thinking. Charlotte, Vt.: Fraser, 1964.

Gregory, C. E. Planning. In J. M. Kraegel (Ed.), *Planning strategies for nurse managers*. Germantown, Md: Aspen Corp., 1983, pp. 71–81.

Huckabay, L. Nursing administration's role in establishing a creative climate. In B. J. Brown (Ed.), *Nursing Administration Quarterly*. 1982, *6*(3), Spring 64–67.

Johne, G. A. How to lead by innovation. *Management Today*, September 1983, pp. 91–95.

Leininger, M. M. Creativity and challenge for nurse researchers in this economic recession. *JONA*, March 1983, pp. 21–22.

Le Breton, P. P. Determining creative strategies for a nursing service. In B. J. Brown (Ed.), *Nursing Administration Quarterly*, 1982, *6*(3), 1–11.

Maier, N. R., & Hayes, J. J. *Creative management*. New York: Wiley, 1962.

Maslow, A. H. *The farther reaches of human nature*. New York: Penguin Books, 1971.

Mendel, J. S. Must we think harder, smarter, or differently? Metaphysical provocations for planners. *Managerial Planning*, 1983, *31*(6), 10–12.

McIvor, M. Shaping the profession's future. *Nursing Mirror*, July 28, 1982, pp. 47–48.

Mintzberg, H. Planning on the left and managing on the right. *Harvard Business Review*, 1976, *54*(4), 49–58.

Rowland, H. S. & Rowland, B. C. *Nursing administration handbook*. Germantown, Md: Aspen Systems Corp., 1980, pp. 23–26.

Simberg, A. L. Obstacles to creative thinking. In G. A. Davis & J. A. Scott (Eds.), *Training Creative Thinking*. New York: Holt, Rinehart, & Winston, 1971, p. 119.

Steiner, G. A. Intuitive-anticipatory versus formal strategic planning. In J. M. Kraegel (Ed.), *Planning Strategies for Nurse Managers*. Germantown, Md.: Aspen Corp., 1983, pp. 77–81.

Steiner, G. *The creative organization*. Chicago: University of Chicago Press, 1969.

Steinmetz, C. S. Creativity training: A testing program that became a sales training program. In G. A. Davis & J. A. Scott (Eds.), *Training Creative Thinking*. New York: Holt, Rinehart, & Winston, 1971, p. 165.

Winer, L. How to add goal-directed creativity to planning. *Managerial Planning*, 1983, *32*(3), 30–36.

APPENDIX 5–1

An Example of the Procedure for Autosuggestion

Find a quiet, comfortable spot to lie down. At first provide one hour of uninterrupted time (it is important psychologically to know you will not be interrupted).

Lie on your back with arms and legs extended comfortably. A small pillow may be used to elevate the head slightly; do not choose a time when you are sleepy.

Begin by talking mentally to yourself in a calm, slow, reassuring, *inner* voice. Your voice will be your guide, and you will follow its directions. At first this may seem strange, but after a time you will find that it works.

The voice will say your name, and tell you to relax your mind and body. Your mental conversation will go something like this: "Jane, you will hear my voice, and concentrate upon it. You will only hear my voice, and do exactly what I say. Completely empty your mind of all thoughts. You will think of nothing but my voice." (Allow time between each statement and speak slowly.)

"Your mind is floating through your body, down to your toes. Your toes feel the air, the pulsations, and even an occasional twitching. You are within every toe and can relax every muscle of every toe." (Pause-time is allowed to concentrate on feeling each toe, experiencing the sensations, and relaxing every muscle. Then the voice proceeds.) "Your mind is moving into your feet. The skin and muscles feel good, relaxed, and warm. You are totally aware of all sensations within your feet and they are totally relaxed." (Again, time is allowed for concentration.) Each part of the body is approached in this manner until the entire body is completely relaxed. Your mental voice guides the process while you become totally emerged in the sensations of your body. In the first session, just the feet and legs should be relaxed. The mind must practice concentrating, so go very slowly. Only after one body part can be mentally "felt" and relaxed should the process be continued. A good test of total concentration is to will the feet to *tingle*. When a tingling sensation can be elicited in both feet, a good state of concentration has been obtained.

When the abdomen is reached, the voice guides the mind into the internal organs, to relax the inner nerves and muscles. When the chest is reached, the heart can actually be felt. The mind concentrates on every pulsation, which projects blood throughout the body. This process is envisioned and mentally enacted. When the voice reaches the lungs, slow, deep breaths are begun, and the mind envisions the clean air coming into the body, and stress, tension, and waste products leaving with every exhalation. Each muscle group, up to the neck and face, are sensed and then relaxed. The head is relaxed by starting with the lips, nose, and eyes. Envision a band being released around the head, until every muscle is totally relaxed.

Throughout the process, the voice continues to remind you that you are becoming more deeply relaxed. It continues to say, "You will not lose my voice. Though you are becoming deeply relaxed, you will continue to hear my voice." This will prevent falling asleep.

This process takes about an hour at first, but in time you will be able to reach a state of complete relaxation much sooner. This comes with practice and discipline. Once a completely relaxed state is reached, the voice begins making the predetermined suggestions: "You are now completely and deeply relaxed. You will take three slow, deep breaths, and on each exhalation, you will become even more deeply relaxed . . . on the count of three you will be completely asleep, but you will still hear my voice. You will be completely asleep on the count of three. One, two, three. . . ." Your body will then experience an actual feeling of deep sleep. The eyes will flutter and your mind will continue to hear the voice:

"You have many creative talents and abilities within your brain. You have the capacity for invention, innovations, and a vast number of creative ideas within you. All of these talents and potential lie within your brain."

"You are completely and deeply relaxed." (This is repeated at intervals throughout the entire process.) "You have total control over your mind. You have the power to unleash your creative abilities. Concentrate on this voice, and remember—you have total control over your mind."

"Now, concentrate totally on the creative processes within your brain. You can feel the excitement, the energy, the talents and ideas beginning to emerge. You can feel the deep sensitivity to life, the artistic imagination, and the dreams being released. You feel the urge to explore, to search for meaning, and you feel a connection with all of your previous subconscious knowledge."

"You have complete control over your mind. At will you can delve into your brain and bring out your imaginative ideas and creative thoughts. You are in touch with your intuition and have access to your subconscious creative thoughts, and can activate them at will."

"You are an imaginative, creative person and you are confident of your creative abilities." These words are repeated.

At the completion of the autosuggestive message, the voice says, "When you awaken, you will feel refreshed and enthusiastic about life. You will have the ability for total mind control. Your imagination and creativity will be open and available to you. You will enjoy your creative and intuitive abilities. All of the messages you have heard will stay with you. On the count of 10, you will wake up. Slowly begin to awaken with each count. One . . . two . . . three . . ." (Slowly count to 10.)

APPENDIX 5–2

Example of a Synectic Session

To use the technique of synectics, a group must be carefully chosen, with a leader who preferably has knowledge, training, or experience in creativity training. It does not really matter what procedure is followed, as long as responses are elicited. The idea is to go for quantity of ideas and solutions, and later work on analysis, specifics, and refinement. The purpose of this group is to generate creative thoughts and ideas on a particular problem or situation.

The most productive group will be predominantly intuitive-minded or creative thinkers. People who are spontaneous, nonconformists, uninhibited, and "feel deeply" are the type needed for this creative purpose. If the goal is development of creative thinking, or overcoming obstacles to creativity, then the group would consist of anyone interested. For solidifying plans and choosing alternatives, it is good to have an even mix of creative and analytical thinkers.

The purpose of the group leader is to guide the entire process and elicit responses from the group. The leader ensures a relaxed, nonthreatening environment, and that the right stimulus is provided to evoke a large number of ideas. When the discussion becomes nonproductive and is not progressing, he or she refocuses by asking different questions and prevents the group from getting discouraged, ending the session when it does not seem to be working. He or she decides when the group needs a rest. The group may have to meet several times, with different perspectives each time, before any solutions are generated.

The following demonstrates a simplistic example of synectics at work.

Problem Identification and Explanation

Group leader: As you know, with DRGs, our hospital may be in financial difficulty. Administration is asking each department to reduce costs. We, as a group, need to come up with ideas for how nursing service can reduce operating costs and still provide quality care. *Problem:* How can we decrease costs while providing quality care?

Restatement of Problem and Reinterpretation

Group member A: I see the problem as being how to have less people do more work, or be more productive.

Group member B: I see it as being how to put less money into the nursing service, but continue providing the same services. Simply how to spend less.

Group member D: I see the problem as how to change the work being done so that it is less costly, but still of good quality.

Group leader: Okay, purge.

Purge

Group member A: Robots can do some of the monotonous stuff, and run errands, to save time for more productive work. Have people who are smarter, better trained, so there will be less wasted time and mistakes.

Group member C: Spend less—tighter budget, tighter wallets, buy cheaper products, look for better bargains.

Group member D: Condense things—when you make something smaller, there is less of it and therefore takes less effort (money) to do things.

Evocative Questions

Group leader: Give me a *direct analogy* to condensing the work.

Group member B: When I think of condensing, I think of Campbell's soup. It comes condensed, but when you add water to it, it turns into the real thing.

Group leader: Give me a *fantasy.*

Group member B: When patients come into the hospital, robots do their histories and physical exams, then triage them to a unit. Those not as sick or more independent patients take care of themselves, and the family may stay with them. No nursing staff is needed on these units other than a secretary to do the paperwork. Severely ill patients are confined to ICU-type situations. This way patients are condensed. But each patient's vital signs, body metabolism, ECG, brain waves, and dreams are monitored by a computer. Any deviations automatically cause the *A Team* to appear. This team can only be seen by the patients with "problems." The A Team takes care of the patient, implements the nursing process, communicates with the physician, and does whatever is necessary, both physically and psychologically to correct the problem. Anything not corrected dictates transferring the patient to a different unit. Once the patient is okay, the A Team disappears.

Group leader: Symbolic analogy.

Group member C: Superman and Wonder Woman are watching over the people. When anyone gets into trouble, they swoop down and straighten everything out. The title would read: "Superman and Wonder Woman Save the Day!"

Group leader: Direct analogy.

Group member A: These superpeople are like butterflies. The butterfly flutters over the patient, watching for any problems. It does not appear to be there, but is there all along. The butterfly flutters all over, from room to room, gently caressing the patient with its wings. When the patient needs someone, he reaches out for the butterfly and grasps him in his hands. At that moment, the butterfly turns into a caterpillar and comes down to earth. All of his many legs are used to soothe the patient and correct his problems.

Group leader: Okay, getting back to condensing—give me a *personal analogy.*

Group member C: I feel like I'm shrinking. I'm getting smaller. I'm becoming more concentrated. This concentration makes me stronger and more powerful, and I work faster.

Group leader: Force-fit!

Group member C: Patients can be organized so that work is more concentrated, and the staff's time will be more productive and efficient. This will be less costly.

Group member D: Viewpoint.

Group leader: Go ahead.

Group member D: One way to condense the work would be to match up roommates in such a way that one can watch over the other. This could be figured into their bills some way for a discount. One could even be responsible for helping the roommate to get up, go to the bathroom, and so on. The roommate could be like the butterfly, watching over the other patient.

Group member E: We could also set up wards, like years ago, where patients could be grouped and watched by a sort of roving camera—similar to monitoring patients in ICU.

Group member B: We could even have patients "graduate" to different wards, like they go from the ICU to a stepdown unit. As they progress, they are moved to a more independent unit, until they are eventually seen on an outpatient basis, then totally discharged.

Group member A: Each unit would have staff specially train for that particular level of illness. A nursing team could even be used to float through the independent units—or just be called in if needed.

Group leader: Any other comments? Well, that's enough for one day. Good work; you came up with a lot of ideas that just might work. See you next week.

The ideas from this session went to the planning committee for further discussion and development. Plans were made for a "buddy" system for elderly and dependent patients. Several patient wards were formed with camera monitors and a special team of nurses for each ward. Future plans include a system for stepdown units from critical care to independent care, each with various levels of nursing staffing for each level of care.

Though synectic sessions normally are less "logical" than the one presented in this example, it still provides an idea of the synectic process. It is best to limit the topic to one specific thing or needed product, and not use any logical thoughts until a "viewpoint" is reached or a "force-fit" is called.

PART

II The Personnel Process

The second half of this book is devoted exclusively to the nuts and bolts of human resource management. Chapters 6 through 13 focus on each of the eight personnel processes that together form the major aspects of utilizing, managing, and maximizing the human talent, potential, and resources within the organization. Each personnel process uses and builds upon the concepts presented in the first section of this book. The remainder of these pages will explore recruitment, selection, orientation, performance evaluation, counseling and coaching, retention and productivity, staff development, and labor relations. Each progressively builds upon the preceding process, and together comprise the fundamental personnel processes for human resource management.

6 The Recruitment Process

The success of any organization depends upon the quality of personnel that it can attract and retain. The recruitment process is integral to organizational success; its goal is to ensure a steady supply of qualified employees to meet organizational needs and to promote the proper placement, retention, and growth of these employees within the organization. Effective recruitment yields candidates available for selection and placement, and results in satisfied employees who have adapted to the organizational milieu.

Recruitment is both a short-term and long-term process. Short-term recruitment plans concern current needs for immediate openings. Long-term plans concern developing a potential pool of personnel who will be qualified to work in the system. The need for recruitment is ongoing and must respond to environmental change. Even in times of full employment, or reductions in force, plans must be developed and implemented to ensure a continual supply of qualified employees.

Recruitment methods will change according to the environment. For instance, in times of economic limitations, recruitment efforts may be tied to rehiring laid-off employees, or granting permanent status to temporary help. In times of short labor supply, recruitment efforts have included special bonuses, supplying automobiles, attraction of foreign students, and other extreme methods. In times of increased labor supply and decreased demand, efforts may be geared to recruiting specialized, highly educated, or creative individuals who will contribute to the evolution of the organization. During these times, organizations can afford to be more selective and set higher standards. Even during hiring freezes, a source of expert candidates must be maintained for the future, because the time will always come when they will be needed.

Recruitment not only involves seeking outside sources of applicants; it also involves a system for attracting, developing, and selecting employees from within the organization for present and future vacancies. This process must be continuous with other personnel processes, such as staff development and selection, and must be ongoing. Proper selection, placement, orientation, and management practices to retain employees will affect the success or failure of recruitment efforts. The right nurse must be recruited and selected for the right job, and become satisfied and challenged with that job. Recruitment is integrated with and interdependent upon the other personnel processes for success.

The following demonstrates guidelines and procedures for developing and implementing the recruitment process in the organization. It discusses organizing for recruitment and the basic functions of the recruiters, and presents ways to meet short-term and long-term recruitment needs.

ORGANIZING FOR RECRUITMENT

The responsibilities for recruitment processes can be organized in various ways. They may be implemented by the nurse-administrator and top assistants, by an individual nurse-recruiter, or through a recruitment committee. The following briefly describes some ways to organize the recruitment process.

The Nurse Executive Committee

The nurse-administrator is ultimately responsible for the results of recruitment processes and human resources management. Often, then, the nurse-administrator forms a small committee of top aides and implements these processes personally. Because recruitment is such a crucial activity, the nurse-executive may want to be personally involved. A small committee consisting of the nurse executive, the assistant, the nursing education coordinator, and one or two key nursing department heads or supervisors can plan recruitment processes in coordination with the other human resource functions.

The Nurse-Recruiter

In some institutions a specific nurse is responsible for recruitment. In these difficult economic times, not all facilities maintain a position solely for this purpose. The nurse-recruiter usually is involved in screening and placement, orientation, staff development, and a variety of other roles, and answers to a nurse-administrator.

The Nursing Recruitment Committee

This committee, consisting of five to eight nursing management personnel, plans and implements the recruitment process and reports to a nurse-administrator. Other key staff members may participate on this committee.

The Special Committee

While the nurse-administrator and team may perform recruitment planning and implementation, the formation of special ad hoc committees is useful for problem solving and generating ideas in specific areas. For example, if there is a problem of rapid turnover or a staff shortage in a particular unit, nurses on that unit would form a committee to address the problems and make recommendations. A task force is also helpful to search for candidates for a management position, or to set up policies and procedures for internal recruitment and development. The general recruitment processes are centralized in one area, such as those listed, but various aspects of recruitment, such as job analysis, require input from the staff level. The more involvement of nurses at all levels, the better the chances for acceptance of the new employee. In addition, indirect rewards of improved morale can also result from this participation.

Personnel Departments

Facilities with personnel departments (now called human resource divisions in some areas) will have built-in recruitment, but will still require coordination, consultation, and information from the nursing division. Although part of the responsibility of the personnel department is recruitment of employees, they cannot recruit nursing personnel without information and participation from the nursing department. A recruitment process should be organized within nursing and be closely coordinated with the personnel department. The nursing department can provide the needs, plans, recommendations, and information, while the personnel department does the legwork and initial screening of applicants. Then the nursing department can select and place the new employee. The personnel department can greatly reduce the time and necessary paperwork for the nurse-recruiters, and can also provide extensive assistance and support for the recruitment process. Without mutual cooperation, coordination, planning, and communication between the two departments, the processes cannot be effectively implemented.

FUNCTIONS OF THE RECRUITMENT PROCESS

Ten basic functions can be identified in the recruitment process:

1. Environmental scanning and analysis of trends affecting supply and demand

2. Analysis of future internal changes and trends relating to human resource planning
3. Development of a philosophy
4. Ongoing assessment and inventory of human resources
5. Assessment of current internal factors pertinent to recruitment and retention
6. Recruitment planning
7. Job analysis
8. Ensuring a continual supply of qualified candidates
9. Attracting and reaching the candidate market
10. Evaluating the recruitment process

These functions are interdependent and closely coordinated with other personnel processes. They are organized and directed from a centralized mechanism, such as through a recruitment committee or the nurse executive committee (in the remainder of this chapter, these mechanisms will be referred to simply as "the nurse-recruiters"). Although aspects of each function may involve taskforce participation, input from other departments, or staff collaboration, these functions are the responsibilities of nurse-recruiters and, ultimately, of the nurse-administrator. These ten functions, when effectively organized, planned and implemented, facilitate a successful recruitment process.

The remainder of this chapter will focus upon and explore each of these ten functions within the recruitment process. Involvement and responsibilities of recruiters in strategic human resource management planning can be readily identified in the first five functions.

Environmental Scanning and Analysis of Trends Affecting Supply and Demand

Nurse-recruiters want to assess current and future conditions that affect supply and demand; they want to anticipate future trends affecting the nature of work and the characteristics of the workers. Environmental factors affecting retention are also pertinent to recruitment because they affect the worker's attraction to and satisfaction with an organization. External environmental assessment is ongoing and focused on trends and changes affecting the balance of labor supply and demand.

The Demand Side. Nurse-recruiters must study future developments in supply and demand, as recruitment involves maintaining a steady balancing of the two. *Demand* refers to the need for (number of position vacancies) and value of a specific product, and the willingness to pay for it. Demand is also related to the available work force, or supply, as well as to the changing nature of the work.

The number of staff nurse position vacancies, or the "need," should be based upon a patient classification system that calculates the nursing manpower needs according to patient requirements. The number of staff nurse "positions" should be related to the needs of the patient population. Other vacancies, such as nurse management positions, will depend upon the job requirements, organizational structure, and optimum span of control. Then, when the services of nurses are *valued* as contributing to the efficiency of patient outcomes, and as improving productivity and quality of health care services, the demand for nurses increases. Increased value determines and enhances need and also the demand. If the supply or number of nurses in the work force is low or unavailable, then the demand becomes even higher. Conversely, if the supply is low and the value is also low, then alternatives to increasing the supply by changing the work and substituting the worker can take place. That is why nursing has become committed to proving its worth to outcomes of health care, efficiency within the hospital, and productivity to patient care by decreasing complications and length of stay. Efforts to prove nursing's contribution will serve to increase the value of and demand for nursing as a profession.

The other aspect of demand, in addition to need, value, and supply, is "willingness to pay." High value often coincides with a willingness to pay. But, despite a high value for a commodity, the facility must be able to pay. With the advent of prospective payment, high competition among health care providers, and other cost-containment efforts, hospitals are under a great financial burden. This, coupled with low occupancy rates, can cause a decreased need for *and* ability to pay nursing personnel, and therefore a decreased demand. Facilities may have the need for nursing personnel, but, due to poor financial status, they may have cut positions and frozen hiring, or have laid off nurses in order to meet financial objectives.

Another perspective to demand for nursing services is the willingness and ability to pay for *quality* personnel. As the labor supply increases and the demand decreases, the facility can be more selective about the quality of its personnel. It may even be able to obtain highly educated and expert personnel at a lower cost. As demand increases and supply decreases, recruitment becomes more difficult and competitive. In addition to its number of vacancies, a facility's value regarding its nursing service, *and* its willingness to pay, will determine the type of personnel it attracts and hires into the organization. Though the need may be high, the institution may not choose to or be able to pay the price, and therefore elect to recruit less experienced, skilled, or educated personnel.

It must be noted that a commitment to obtain high-quality personnel is not only dependent upon financial resources. The facility must make efforts to maintain competitive salaries, improve working conditions, allow independent and autonomous decision-making, participative management, and organizational structures conducive to job satisfaction, and promote employee growth and development. All of these things signify a facility's interest in quality nurses. These factors often can compensate for just "fair" salaries and benefits. Good working conditions play a large part in attracting and retaining quality personnel.

Recruitment must be aimed at retaining employees in the system at all times. Unfortunately, in times of increased supply, areas of retention and satisfaction are often overlooked. The facility often assumes an attitude of "there are plenty more where these came from," and so puts little effort into retention and job satisfaction. This only serves to lower the productivity of the employees. Poor morale, low productivity, and high turnover eventually lead to a decreased future supply of personnel for the facility. This can create future shortages and increased demand. If recruitment is geared at attracting qualified workers to meet organizational needs, it must also be actively engaged in *retaining* these employees. This will decrease the cost of continually refilling positions and retraining, as well as enhance the future attraction of expert people who are willing to work in the facility.

Another factor that affects demand is the nature of the work itself. As environmental changes cause changing needs within the health care facility, the nature of the work also changes. An ongoing assessment and synthesis of environmental change is necessary to predict future work force supply and demand. With the growth of and increase in technology, a greater demand is created for personnel trained in computers and management of specialized equipment. The increased aging population changes the focus of patient care and demands a knowledge of gerontological nursing. With increased diagnostic complexities, patient turnover, and acuity of illness, more specialized and experienced nurses are in demand. These are just a few environmental changes that affect the demand for personnel. Expanded hospital services that include home health care, increased preventative and health maintenance services, health maintenance organizations, and outpatient clinics all affect the demand.

The physician surplus can also affect the role and work of the nurse within the health care facility. Physicians are beginning to reclaim much of the work previously delegated to the nurse.

Supply and demand are more complex than the number of available nurses or position vacancies. The patient population may determine the number of vacancies, but supply, value, financial ability to pay, as well as the nature of the work, all contribute to the demand for a product or service.

The Supply Side. Environmental assessment must also focus on the current and future supply of labor. The supply of labor includes the number, type, characteristics, and location of workers and potential workers.

Number. In determining the supply of nurses, a facility should first look at the number of available and potential nurses and their location. To do this, it must determine geographic boundaries. If under consideration are R.N.s who can be employed without relocation, the boundaries might include a circumference of up to 25 miles from the facility, depending upon the availability of transportation. Or the facility may examine the number of R.N.s in the boundaries of its city. If a facility is considering a master's-prepared management position, it may consider a nationwide search and examine the total number of master's-prepared nurses in a given specialty.

In examining the number of nurses available, the full-time, part-time, unemployed, and number of new graduates per year should be identified. The facility should also consider those employed in fields other than nursing. In some cases facilities focus on the number of retired nurses and ways to promote their re-entry into the workplace.

Trends and changes related to the number of workers must be considered in future planning. With the trend toward a smaller percent of high school graduates and increased career options for women, the future possibility of a decline in new nursing graduates is real. Cuts in federal and state educational assistance will also contribute to this decline. Ways to counterbalance this future shortage may include recruitment of an older work force into nursing as a second but new career choice. Health care facilities may begin more extensive career recruitment in schools and become actively involved in students' career development.

The retention and longevity of the worker in the workplace is also to be considered in examining the number of nurses. Recruitment efforts must zero in on keeping the worker longer and satisfying his or her needs, to compensate for predictions of a decreased supply. Not to be overlooked in the "supply number" is the internal source of labor; staff education and training can develop future sources and supplies of labor needed to meet future needs.

Type. In assessing nursing supply, the type of available workers should be considered. This refers to:

1. Clinical specialty or area of practice
2. Educational preparation
3. Male, female, and minority groups (for affirmative action)
4. Age group, i.e., older workers re-entering the work force
5. New graduates versus experienced nurses

The type of worker that comprises the nursing work force gives important information concerning meeting the needs of the organization. For example, if there is an internal shortage of coronary care nurses and the external supply indicates a large number of nurses trained and practicing in coronary care, then recruitment efforts would be focused on tapping this supply, rather than training and developing inexperienced R.N.s. Identifying the ages, years of experience, and educational backgrounds of the supply of nurses will direct organizational planning. While the bachelor's degree in nursing (B.S.N.) may be a requirement for a management position in one facility, this may not be an appropriate requirement in a rural setting that lacks educational advancement opportunities and consists of predominately associate degree (A.D.) nurses. The nursing service must consider the type of nurses available when planning recruitment and retention strategies. Nurses with various educational backgrounds, experiences, and ages will respond differently because of their diverse needs. An internship program as a recruitment mechanism may be ineffective in an area with a large supply of older and seasoned nurses, but a teaching facility where new graduates comprise the largest recruitment source would find this very helpful. In facilities seeking to recruit retired nurses, a series of refresher courses might be included in their strategies.

Studying changing trends in the types of workers can provide good information for future sources of labor and recruitment tactics. The fact that nurses are specializing more would affect a general rural hospital that has no separate specialty units. These hospitals may consider organizing patient care in a manner to better match the supply of nurses as well as to enhance patient needs. More older women are entering or reentering the nursing job market after raising their families. In an area with a large supply of this type of nurse, benefits such as child-care may be substituted with other benefits, such as exercise facilities or good retirement benefits. The recruitment efforts of the facility must respond to the present and future type of work force.

Characteristics. Assessment of the nursing supply also includes determining the characteristics of the work force. This involves anything that affects the wants, needs, perceptions, and expectations of the work force, and is closely related to the "type" of worker. Attitudes, values, family and socioeconomical background, types of work experience, special skills, personality traits, level of motivation, intellectual ability, and personal priorities all make up the characteristics of workers.

The characteristics or nature of the work force has changed greatly in recent years, mainly due to consumerism and women's liberation. As the public has become more aware of its rights, people have become more assertive in demanding that their needs be met. Women are now working longer, are more committed to their careers, and are rejecting past stereotypes. They expect to be treated with respect and equality. This changing work force creates new demands on the organization. The need for increased autonomy and independence, self-development, career advancement opportunities, and participation in administrative decision-making has become evident in health care facilities. Nurse-administrators must respond to these needs in order to recruit and retain nursing staff. The changing nature of the work force is changing the organizational structures and decision making to a more decentralized and "shared-governance" approach in many areas. In order to maintain maximum use and development of human resources, organizations must meet their changing needs.

Another factor that should be considered in the characteristics of the workforce is the nurses who have returned to the workforce out of financial necessity. Their spouses may be unemployed or underemployed, and with a higher cost of living it often takes two salaries to make ends meet. These nurses have been forced to return and were not previously willing, nor did they have the desire, to practice nursing. They can create a special need within the organization for maintaining productivity, participation, and morale. Many of these nurses experience depression and do not wish to be working anywhere. Their financial burdens and problematic family situations often make them difficult to manage. Although they may contribute to the "supply," their contribution to the organization becomes a challenge for the nurse-administrator; this will be addressed in the chapter on counseling and coaching.

Data Collection. Information regarding the nursing work force can be obtained through recent research and studies performed by national and state agencies, as well as through individual marketing research by the facility. Before initiating expensive and extensive research, the following sources should be explored: American Nurses' Association, American Hospital Association, United States Department of Health and Human Services, National League for Nursing, Department of Health and Human Services—Bureau of Health Professions—Division of Nursing, state boards of nursing, and state and local nursing schools and universities. These sources compile statistics concerning nursing and should be contacted to determine information, studies, and reports they have available on this subject. Efforts to further explore local or statewide work force characteristics and information can be initiated by individual research. Marketing consultants are available to assist the nurse-administrator in this endeavor. Simple surveys, questionnaires, or interviews can also elicit much helpful information in this area without great expense. The extent of marketing research is dependent upon budgetary allowances, as well as upon supply and demand factors. If there is a ready supply of current and future qualified applicants, rather than collect detailed statistics on work force supply, this time and money may be spent on other areas of the recruitment and retention processes.

Analysis of Future Internal Changes and Trends

To plan the recruitment of human resources effectively, changing internal organizational plans must be recognized and anticipated. This assessment is ongoing, as is scanning of the external environment, and together they are synthesized to formulate a philosophy and general direction for the recruitment process.

Organizational Plans. Assessment of organizational strategic plans, mission, and philosophy is essential to ensure consistency when formulating recruitment planning. Recruitment plans must exchange information with the hospital planning and information systems. Especially important is assessment of different services, changing organizational structures, automation, expansion, and changing relationships or roles. Organizational plans that affect current or future position roles or responsibilities must be included in recruitment plans, as must future financial resources and capabilities.

Nursing Department Plans. Recruiters must also be fully aware of any future changes in nursing services or patient care. Future plans for instigating primary nursing or requiring a B.S.N. for certain positions would affect recruitment plans. Nursing budgeting plans and allocations must also be assessed.

Developing Trends. Developing attitudes and expectations from patients, nurses, and other members of the health care team should be considered in recruitment plans. Consideration of a changing internal work force will help in choosing new employees who will fit in and adjust to the organization, as well as in planning strategies to maintain morale and productivity. Through attitude surveys, observation, and interviews, the evolving "culture" of the staff can be identified. As nurses assert themselves in administrative decision making and become more outspoken patient advocates, the organization must respond to meet their needs.

Development of a Philosophy

In planning recruitment processes, a purpose or direction for action is needed, as it is needed in any planning process. From assessment and synthesis of external and internal changes, a diagnosis concerning future directions and missions can be determined. This mission or philosophy should be consistent with the aims and philosophy of the organization, and reflect evolving environmental and internal changes and needs. Table 6–1 provides an example of such a philosophy.

Ongoing Assessment and Inventory of Human Resources

Once the philosophy and direction for the recruitment process is established, a thorough inventory of human resources must be compiled. This provides information concerning the present human resource status, and is continually revised and updated as the status changes. From this inventory, future planning for internal and external recruitment can take place. The human resource inventory consists of the following elements, and should be compiled in such a way as to be easily accessible, current, centralized, and accurate.

- Total number of full-time equivalents for each job classification (R.N., L.P.N., etc.). Number of part-time and full-time employees in each classification. Total number and type of vacancies and location.

TABLE 6–1. RECRUITMENT PHILOSOPHY: A COMPONENT OF THE PHILOSOPHY FOR HUMAN RESOURCE MANAGEMENT

- This organization values its human resources as being the most important element to organizational success. Recruiting, fostering, and developing human talents, creativity, and skill is the primary goal of management.
- The role of recruitment within the organization is to meet current and future human resource needs by planning ways to use and develop existing personnel, or to attract and hire new personnel into the organization in a cost-effective manner.
- The recruitment process is ongoing and responds to internal and external forces of change.
- This organization is committed to the recruitment and development of creative, talented, and innovative people who will contribute to the growth of the organization.
- This organization is committed to recruiting a variety and mix of individuals with diverse backgrounds, ideas, and experience. It is our belief that a good mix of employees contributes to creative growth within the organization.
- It is our belief that the best recruitment is through the satisfaction, retention, and development of current employees. Good morale and job satisfaction set the climate to recruit creative and expert talent into the organization, as well as to develop and retain current talent and potential.
- Personnel are recruited into our organization based upon job requirements and expectations, work experiences and skills, and potential for future growth and development. Recruitment processes offer equal opportunity to all qualified persons, and are not based upon age, sex, race, creed, color, or national origin.
- Our organization recruits and assists individuals in minority groups to develop the necessary skills for selection and advancement in the organization.
- The recruitment process is tuned to the needs of the work force, and supply and demand, and makes efforts and recommendations for change within the organization to respond and meet these needs. Staff participation in innovative and progressive recruitment and retention practices is encouraged and fostered.
- This organization believes that career opportunities and promotions should first be offered to current employees. Every measure should be taken to develop necessary skills and select from within the organization. Only following internal recruitment attempts should external recruitment be undertaken.

- Temporary employees; sex of employees; number of minorities.
- Educational background of R.N.s (B.S.N., A.D.N., M.S.N., etc.).
- Years to retirement.
- Number and type of employees in each work area—ICU, OB, ER, medical-surgical unit, etc.—also break down into full-time equivalents.
- Employees with special training, skills, and talents.
- Employees working toward advanced degrees or additional training.
- Anticipated employee changes, such as leaves of absence, separation due to retirement or moving, dismissals, promotions, transfers.
- Personnel preferences for transfer, shift change, position changes; special employee needs, such as special scheduling due to school-age children.
- Scheduling policies and procedures: weekends only, 12-hour shifts, 7 on and 7 off, 10-hour shifts, job sharing (split shifts), and special scheduling in certain areas

	R.N.s	L.P.N.s	Aides	Orderlies	Unit Secretaries	Administration	Total
Full-time equivalents							
Full-time employees (List minorities, sex)							
Part-time employees							
Temporary employees							
FTE vacancies (List location)							

R.N.s' Educational Background	ICCU	OB	ER	OR	RR	2East	2West	2South	2North	Admin	Total
A.D.											
Diploma											
B.S.N.											
Other											
Progress toward a degree											
Special advanced training, skills or talents											

Figure 6–1. Sample human resource inventory sheet.

	R.N.s	L.P.N.s	Aides	Orderlies	Unit Secretaries	Administration
Employees planning retirement— position, unit, shift, and years to retirement						

	ICCU	OB	ER	OR	RR	Other
Special Scheduling	(i.e., 12-hour shifts)					

Anticipated personnel changes—Shift and position:	**ICCU**	**OB**	**ER**	**OR**	**RR**	**2East**	**2West**	**2South**	**2North**	**Admin**	**Total**
LOA											
Separation											
Promotions											
Transfers											
Potential dismissals/probationary employees											

Special requests for shift changes, transfers, promotions or other:

Management recommendations for employee transfer/promotion:

Figure 6–1. *(Continued)*

Data: __________ Revised: __________

Name: __________ Title: __________ Position and location: __________

Years with the organization: __________ Salary: __________

Preference for shift, unit, or position: __________

Special experiences desired: __________

Special growth and development needs: __________

Long-term goals: __________

Special talents, experiences, background, skills, and continuing education: __________

Figure 6–2. Sample personnel data form.

The nursing recruiters must have ready access to the above information, and ensure that it is current. Standardized forms, tables, or graphs should be used to document data, as shown in Figure 6–1.

In addition to the forms shown in Figure 6–1, an individual filing system should be established to maintain a current inventory of internal and external talent. Each employee, applicant, or new employee should fill out a form similar to the one shown in Figure 6–2. These forms can be cross-referenced by name, job classification, unit, talent, or skill, (such as enterostomal therapist or diabetic specialist), and be utilized for recruitment, selection, placement, and retention. Previous applicants' preferences and skills can be recalled at a later date when various positions become open.

The form shown in Figure 6–2 may be attached on the employee application form. Employees are encouraged to bring resumes and CVs with them for completing this summary, and to update it as necessary. Management may review this with staff during the performance evaluation interview. This personal data form facilitates the matching of talent and special training with current and potential job openings, or to plan special training and development needs of individual staff members.

Assessment of Current Internal Factors Pertinent to Recruitment and Retention

Another necessary function within the recruitment process is to assess and monitor factors within the organization that affect recruitment and retention. Through existing information systems and by direct means, information can be gathered and analyzed for recruitment planning. The following are a few of the internal factors to be examined.

1. Organizational roles, relationships, hierarchy, communication, and structure. These can be obtained through job descriptions, policy and procedure manuals, and organizational charts.
2. Employee attitudes and morale, needs, and expectations. Surveys

and questionnaires, exit interviews, grievances, observations, and word of mouth are several ways of obtaining information about employee morale. Attitudes, job satisfaction, and the work environment are important factors to recruitment and retention, so must be closely monitored.

3. Quality of services as evidenced by quality assurance reports, patient outcomes, monitoring of standards of care, patient satisfaction, and performance appraisal systems. This is important information for determining competency and productivity of current staff, and need for further recruitment and planning.
4. Turnover rates, absenteeism, vacancies, overtime due to vacancies, and recruitment, training, and orientation costs to fill new positions, all are important sources of information related to morale, job satisfaction, and effectiveness of recruitment and selection. If the appropriate employee is recruited and placed into the right position, and the working environment is conducive to job satisfaction, then the turnover, absenteeism, and orientation costs should be low. Individuals starting a recruitment and retention program should measure these rates before and after the program has been implemented to evaluate results. Other reasons for turnover, such as transportation problems, need for child care, interference of rotating shifts with family obligations, and noncompetitive salaries/benefits, must be identified and addressed.
5. Salary scale and benefits. These must be compared to those of other hospitals and facilities within the area to determine whether or not they are competitive.
6. Philosophy and practices of administration, as well as the support of and communication with the staff, should be examined. Problems in this area can be pinpointed in studies of morale and by implementing the assessments listed under 4.
7. The work environment and working conditions must be assessed. Nurse-to-patient ratio; staff mix; use of P.R.N. and float pools; division of labor, i.e., primary or team nursing; method of assignments; nature of services per unit; method of scheduling (by whom and staff input); quality of support services and amount of non-nursing duties; available resources; physician attitudes and practices with nursing; patient acuity; automation; attractiveness and conveniences of the work environment—all are important to planning recruitment and retention strategies and must be evaluated.

Recruitment Planning

The nursing recruiters must maintain a current recruitment plan that is consistent with the organizational and nursing plans. From assessment and scanning of the environment, and assessment of future internal trends and changes, a prediction can be made regarding the future need for recruitment directions. This determination was shown as the philosophy for the recruitment process.

Then synthesis from the assessment of the current organization, including a human resource inventory and assessment of internal factors related to recruitment and retention, results in diagnosis of the present state of the organization. The gap between the first three recruitment functions (the future anticipated direction of change) and the fourth and fifth recruitment functions—the present status—would determine areas in need of change. For example, the planning of an open-heart unit (future organizational change) would put definite requirements on the recruitment process. Examination of human resource inventory and personal data forms (present internal states) may reveal a lack of expertise in open-heart surgery. Specific plans must be made either to develop existing personnel or recruit external candidates for the job. From studies of supply and demand (environmental assessment), the availability of nurses with specific expertise in open-heart surgery can be determined. This availability would affect the type and scope of recruitment advertising planned for these positions. From studies of demand and competitive salaries and benefits (environmental assessment), recruiters can recognize competitive obstacles or capabilities that would affect their method of promoting the institution and aspects upon which they will capitalize to attract applicants.

In line with the philosophy formulated for the recruitment process, planning would include developing objectives to obtain these desired results. Recruitment plans would include objectives such as:

1. Provide financial and material resources for recruitment, and measure and evaluate the cost effectiveness of recruitment processes.
2. Identify and recommend organizational changes necessary to improving the retention and supply of qualified personnel for the future. These recommendations may relate to salary and benefits, flexible scheduling, morale and job satisfaction, or other areas of concern to recruitment.
3. Set an application ratio, i.e., to provide a minimum of five qualified applicants (internal or external) per vacancy, to promote optimum selection and placement.
4. Coordinate recruitment plans with all personnel processes for maximum continuity and effectiveness.
5. Demonstrate to employees a management commitment to fostering, developing, and satisfying human resources.
6. Establish specific policies and procedures regarding the priority for internal recruitment and development.
7. Develop cost-effective procedures and methodology for external recruitment processes.
8. Develop and recruit creative, talented, and unique individuals for the growth and development of the organization.
9. Ensure equal employment opportunity to all applicants and em-

ployees in regard to salary or benefits, advancement opportunities, and other employment conditions.*

10. Foster job satisfaction and staff participation in recruitment processes.
11. Ensure ongoing and current external and internal scanning, assessment, and synthesis of information pertinent to recruitment and retention.
12. Match the supply of human resources with current future needs to "fill the gap" over a designated time frame.

Operational Recruitment Planning. Following the assessment and identification of strategies and objectives, specific operational planning must take place in order to implement the recruitment process effectively. Operational recruitment planning involves job analysis, strategies to ensure a continual supply of qualified candidates, and attracting and reaching the candidate market.

Job Analysis

Prior to determining the recruitment strategy for a potential position vacancy, nurse-recruiters must know more about the job. An in-depth analysis of the nature of the work and factors affecting the work must be undertaken. Then a job description, specifying roles, responsibilities, relationships, personal specifications, and job requirements, must be available and consistent with the job analysis.

Job analysis can be an in-depth process involving job classification and evaluation for determining salary ranges and comparable worth. For the purpose of this discussion, job analysis is limited to eliciting and utilizing job-related information to help attract, select, and retain the right person for the right job. This analysis of the job in a given position is accomplished by a combination of several methods: observation of the work being done, interviewing those doing the work, interviewing those managing the workers, and exit interviews with those who have done the work. The results from these methods should elicit the following information:

- General description of the job and how it fits into the organizational chart; how it helps achieve organizational objectives
- Authority, roles, chain of command, and communication hierarchy for the job
- Specific responsibilities, tasks, and work to be done in the position

*Equal employment opportunities and discrimination in employment will be discussed in the following chapter on selection. Recruitment affirmative action plans may be voluntarily instituted by the facility to ensure the hiring and advancement of minority employees. These recruitment plans must also monitor employment practices for all applicants and employees to avoid *reverse* discrimination.[1]

- Staffing information such as mix, patient ratio, patient acuity, and expected productivity for the position
- Management policies and practices surrounding the position
- Social environment and culture surrounding the position
- Personal requirements for the position
- Expected standards of practice for the position
- Current and long-term expectations for the job, and needed changes from performance by previous employees
- Personal rewards of the job—hidden benefits, opportunities, and positive aspects
- Negative aspects of the job—limited manpower or funds, rigid thinkers, or physician frustrations
- Work routine and assignments
- Salary and raise schedule
- Ideas and suggestions from management and staff regarding recruitment, retention, and need for special training
- Identification of need to alter salary scale, restructure position, or change work environment

The nurse-recruiters synthesize this information and compare their results to the existing job description. Prior to recruitment planning, they must have an accurate job description reflecting this information, and a list of the desired characteristics for the candidate most likely to successfully fill the position and adjust to the work environment.

The Job Description. The job description for a particular position must contain certain elements, as it may serve as the contract for the new employee. The job description should be derived directly from the standards of practice, be the basis for the performance evaluation, and reflect the expectations for the job. A signed job description prior to hiring can be the new employee's agreement to carry out these expectations. Jernigan and Young's *Standards, Job Descriptions, and Performance Evaluations for Nursing Practice* provides detailed examples of job descriptions and relates them to the nursing standards and performance evaluation. An example of an R.N. job description from this book is provided in Appendix 6–1.[2]

Components of the Job Description

- Job title. Job classification such as R.N., L.P.N., and so on, with specific location, such as Obstetrics or Coronary Care.
- Position requirement: Minimum and preferred educational level, skills, and experience requirements for the job. (A B.S.N. may be "preferred" but not required; ability to perform thorough physical assessment may be a required skill; experience in management and supervision may be preferred. These requirements will be based on job analysis information and assessment of supply and demand.)

- Professional requirements (for the professional nurse): Professional requirements pertaining to personal growth and development or continuing education, affiliation with professional organizations, certification, publishing, or community activities.
- Accountability: To whom the nurse reports and for what the nurse is accountable.
- Job summary: A synopsis of the nature of the work, areas of responsibility, and role within the organization.
- Job responsibilities: A list of responsibilities that provide explicit information regarding what is to be done in the job. This is a series of statements that should include nursing standards and personal requirements.

As seen in Appendix 6–1, the job responsibilities can be divided into components that correspond to nursing standards and nursing process. This emphasizes the importance of assessment, planning, implementation, and evaluation, and sets forth the requirements for each.

Following analysis of the job description, the nurse-recruiters must ensure that its information and requirements are consistent with the analysis of the job. Revisions may be made as approved by nursing administration. In addition, the recruiters should complete a special list of personal requirements, job strengths and weaknesses, opportunity for advancement, special scheduling requirements, and salary scale and schedule with the job description. This information will pertain specifically to that unit and work environment in which the job will take place, and provide needed information to recruiters *and* applicants for decision making. See Appendix 6–2 and below.

Specific Information Concerning the Job

Personal Requirements. Given an assessment of the social and physical environment, and strengths, weaknesses, and special needs on the unit, the desired characteristics of the potential candidate can be determined. This list of characteristics can be used for comparison in selecting the appropriate individual for the job. It will provide insight into personal requirements needed by the applicant to adjust and succeed in the unit's environment.

Job Strengths and Weaknesses. The recruiter and applicant must recognize positive and negative aspects of the job. This information will ensure that the applicant's "eyes are open" and promote a better complement with the organization. Recruiters can also utilize job strengths in promotional advertising.

Opportunities for Advancement. Given present trends in needs and expectations of the work force, opportunities for promotions, or advancement through career ladder programs have become an important issue with today's nurses. Applicants will desire this information, and recruiters can utilize it in promotional advertising.

Salary Scale and Schedule. The pay scale or salary range for the job should be attached, or the information should be readily available. Administration must ensure that salary scales are based upon specific criteria, and not individual preference, or they could be charged with discrimination. This salary scale must be standard for all personnel. A copy of the personnel handbook or list of employee benefits should also be attached to this information.

Special Scheduling Requirements. Split shifts, rotating, 12-hour shifts, and other flexible staffing utilized on a unit should be identified and listed with the job description. A specific shift vacancy, such as on the 3 P.M. to 11 P.M. shift, should also be documented. Recruiters must know this information to find the appropriate candidate; applicants must know this information to determine their decision regarding the job.

Plan of Action. The information pertaining to job analysis, job descriptions, and special job requirements must be examined for each vacancy. Once this information is compiled, it can simply be updated. Management personnel are responsible for helping the recruiters keep accurate and current information.

After this information is assessed for a vacant position, recruiters must recommend a plan of action to the nurse-administrator. This plan would concern filling the existing position, changing or restructuring the position, changing aspects of the unit or organization, or changing job expectations and requirements.

Filling the Existing Position. If approval is given by the nurse-administrator to fill the existing position as it is, then the recruiters begin planning their methodology for recruitment.

Restructuring the Position. If the nurse-administrator determines from the information that the job should be changed, it may be abolished or integrated into another position.

Changing Aspects of the Unit/Organization. Salary scale, benefits, management practices, or special programs such as internships may be altered or upgraded to respond to identified needs and problems that result from the job analysis.

Changing Job Expectations or Requirements. Additional requirements pertaining to education, skills, or experience may be added to or deleted from the job description. Roles and responsibilities of the job may also be altered. These alterations must be made prior to implementing recruitment efforts.

Ensuring a Continual Supply of Qualified Candidates

Plans to match needs with candidates involve ensuring a current and continual supply or pool of qualified people who are willing to work within the organization. This supply pertains to internal recruitment of existing personnel, and external recruitment of existing and potential candidates. These plans are continuous and closely related to the strategy to attract candidates to the organization.

Internal Recruitment. Internal recruitment refers to two processes: (1) matching or preparing existing personnel to meet human resource requirements, and (2) retaining personnel who will grow and develop with the organization. As described earlier, retention of personnel results in decreased turnover, lower staffing expenditures, and improved productivity. This in turn facilitates the attraction and hiring of outside talent and resources into the organization. Retention will be further explored in Chapter 11.

Matching or Preparing Existing Personnel to Meet Human Resource Requirements. There must be a fair and effective system for recruiting from within the organization. It must be nondiscriminatory, objective, based upon specific standards, policies, and procedures, and be accepted by the personnel.[3] Some specific methods for internal recruitment include job posting, skills inventory matching, internal search efforts, management recommendations as part of the performance evaluation and/or career ladder program, and specific staff development or training projects.

JOB POSTING. Clark describes the following job posting procedure as being an effective means for internal recruitment.[3]

1. *Criteria for eligibility and selection:*
   a. Minimum of one year with the organization and six months in the present job is required for promotion or transfer
   b. A maximum of two bids is allowed for promotion or transfer per year
   c. Only one bid is allowable at a time
   d. Must have a minimum of "satisfactory" on performance evaluation
   e. Cannot be on probation
2. *Additional criteria for selection*
   a. Supervisor's recommendations
   b. Seniority (preferred but not required)
   c. Satisfactory attendance record
   d. Possesses qualifications for specific job requirements and ability to meet job and personal expectations
3. *Procedure*
   a. Job vacancies are posted in centralized locations at 11 A.M. each day, for a two-week period. Application deadline and instructions

are posted along with the following: job title, department, shift, job description, and requirements with specific information concerning the job.

b. Type and location of interview should be described, and the time period during which candidates will be notified of the decision (usually three weeks).

c. Job posting may also be included on various bulletin boards, in meetings, and in employee publications.

4. *Decision making*

a. Applicants who are rejected are notified in writing, with specific reasons. Further counseling and career planning is made available, with suggestions and ways to improve performance. Appeals procedures are also provided upon request and according to policy.

b. The selected employee must notify the supervisor of the job change 30 days to 6 weeks prior to assuming the new position.

c. Some facilities may choose to notify supervisors of the bid for promotion, and others may wish to include the supervisor in the interview. Employees are encouraged to communicate their bids for promotion to their immediate supervisors. Some facilities do not inform the supervisor until an employee is selected or being seriously considered. Consideration and measures must be taken not to penalize an employee for bidding for a change.

SKILLS INVENTORY MATCHING. According to Kaumeyer, when organizational size causes management not to know all of the individuals' capabilities and preferences, the skills inventory matching system is effective for internal recruitment. By utilizing the human resource inventory assessment described earlier, management can search for people with varying backgrounds, experiences, and talents to fill a position. Computerized systems can match people's skills, work histories, *and* preferences with specific positions, creating a pool of qualified candidates. Noncomputerized systems are also effective if organization and cross referencing are thorough, especially in smaller institutions.[4]

INTERNAL SEARCH EFFORTS. In addition to skills matching or job posting, the recruiters may formulate a special committee to search out the right individual for a position. This committee may be on a particular unit that has had a staff shortage, or may be a cross-section of nursing personnel to provide input and objectivity to the recruitment process. The staff participation will facilitate acceptance of the new person in the position, as well as improve morale. The committee would determine policies and procedures, eligibility, and selection criteria for the position, and methods of notifying personnel of the vacancy and application procedures.

The internal search committee can be a highly effective mechanism for selecting a unit management person. Nursing staff on the unit who do not wish to bid for the promotion can be involved in setting criteria, interviewing, and selection of their own head nurses or supervisors. It is interesting to see that these nurses want an assertive, expert leader who will enforce policies and maintain standards. When they are involved in recruiting this individual, the transition and acceptance process is greatly facilitated.

MANAGEMENT RECOMMENDATIONS

1. *Performance evaluation.* As part of the performance evaluation system, management submits recommendations to administration concerning the performance and future development of the employee. The nurse-administrator then keeps a centralized record of recommendations for promotion or transfer. From this list, eligible candidates are considered for position vacancies. Recruiters and search committees can obtain a pool of candidates from this list.
2. *Career ladder.* As part of a career development and advancement program, nurses who have achieved certain skills or advanced degrees or have reached certain goals are rewarded by a salary increase or recognition. A mechanism for entering these nurses into the pool of employees recommended for new positions could be managed in a manner similar to the one described above. Also, level of achievement on the career ladder should become a component for eligibility and selection.

STAFF DEVELOPMENT AND TRAINING PROGRAMS. It may be determined from assessment of the organization that needed skills or talents are not available among the existing staff. A decision regarding the cost and benefit of developing these personnel or recruiting from outside the organization must be made. If the external supply of people with this particular specialty is low, or if adequate time and resources are available within the organization, the decision may be made to recruit by staff development from within. Recruiters may also recognize a long-range need for a particular skill, and for morale and retention purposes choose to provide the existing staff the opportunity to obtain these needed skills. Training programs may be set up on a group or individual basis. If a particular individual has shown potential and demonstrates the qualifications and preference for a job, an individual development program may be developed. This program may involve classes in a nearby school, home study, completion of a self-learning module, or clinical training within the organization. Following completion of this individualized development program, the nurse must demonstrate the required skills for the job prior to being selected.

If a new service is to be developed within the organization, or several vacancies exist in one specialty area, a training course may be initiated to develop a group of nurses to fill these positions. Acceptance into the training course would be based upon meeting eligibility criteria.

External Recruitment. When attempts to fill a position through internal recruitment have been exhausted, recruiters turn to the external candidate market. The needs and characteristics of the market specific to this vacancy must be identified and measures taken to meet those needs. Efforts must be made to capitalize on job strengths and benefits, and beat the competition in order to "sell" the job. These attempts and methods also work to enhance job satisfaction, retention, and morale.

From environmental assessment of supply and demand, much information should already be available to recruiters regarding the candidate population. However, when a particular position becomes available, the exact candidate market for this position must be pinpointed and further examined. Any special needs, expectations, attitudes, and characteristics should be identified. Furthermore, the location of this population should be determined and become the target. Recruiters may plan first to look for local candidates, then extend the efforts to larger boundaries. Plans may first include new graduates, those actively seeking employment, or those employed but "possibly interested in a change." They may later focus on the "nonjob seekers," and unemployed population. The extent of the efforts will depend on the supply, the demand, and the recruitment budgetary allowance.

Meeting the Needs of the Candidate Market. Following the assessment of the specific market, recruiters will plan ways to meet their needs. Some of these measures have been mentioned earlier in the text and will be further explored in later chapters. The following are examples of some of the benefit programs and methods instituted in organizations for recruitment and retention purposes. These methods are incorporated into the recruitment advertising plans:

- Child care services: The facility may provide these services or find suitable child care for the employee.
- Flexible scheduling: A variety of scheduling mechanisms may be made available to the nurse. Each one must be evaluated for its effects on continuity and quality of patient care. Job sharing for split shifts, work weeks, or weekends may be available. Repetitive scheduling cycles to provide predictability, along with a variety of other plans, may serve to meet employees' needs. Some organizations institute a method of self-scheduling by staff members on a unit, to improve participation and acceptance of scheduling.
- Self–governance and joint practice: These are measures to involve staff nurses in administrative decisions, and to promote collaboration in patient care decisions. Some example of self-governance and joint practice were given in Chapter 3.
- Career ladder: To facilitate career advancement, continued growth and development, and avenues for clinical as well as administrative promotions.

- Staff development and continuing education programs: Extensive and comprehensive opportunities to expand skills and knowledge are important to nurses. An educational department that provides expert consultants, instructional assistance, and ongoing continuing education programs to the staff will assist in recruitment efforts.
- Orientation: A thorough orientation program that provides a smooth transition to the new job is important to new employees. This program may include *refresher courses* for nurses returning to work; *preceptorships,* where new personnel are assigned to experienced employees for a period of time; *internships,* where new employees are provided varied clinical experiences and classroom instruction over a period of months to a year to assist in gaining needed skills and confidence, and *externship programs,* where nursing students are allowed to work within the facility as part of their school experience. These students are paid to provide care under supervision, and in some instances receive school credit for their work. The externship program allows the student to learn and decide about the facility, and the facility to evaluate the student. Often extern programs are a major means for recruitment and cut down on orientation and internship needs.
- Tuition reimbursement: Facilities may pay a student's tuition through school in return for a commitment to work within the facility (usually 1 year for every 1 year of tuition paid); they may provide financial assistance to employees seeking advanced degrees. This is an important recruitment incentive to nurses who wish to work toward their bachelor of science degree in nursing.
- Competitive salaries/benefits: Though this is not a major motivator, nurses need to know their salaries and benefits are at least competitive with other facilities. A slight difference may be compensated by other pluses, but major differences will most likely deter recruitment and retention.
- Transportation: In instances of heavy traffic or long distances to travel, the facility may provide a car pool or bus to assist employees in getting to work. This benefit would aid recruitment efforts in outlying areas.

Other than specific methods or benefits, recruiters will capitalize on other strengths within the organization; some examples follow.

1. A small hospital may promote its warm, relaxed atmosphere, flexibility, and close teamwork. A large firm would promote its security, stability, higher salaries, advancement opportunities, and variety of work experiences within its expanded services. The aim is to blend the two. Small facilities may combine positions or titles and add duties to increase pay. Large firms can work toward decentralization and creating a more flexible, warm environment.[5]
2. A progressive and caring image in the community is promoted by recruiters to attract candidates.

3. Organizing services into specialty units, such as pediatrics, orthopedics, urology, and so on, may facilitate the recruitment of today's nurses. More nurses are specializing, and many do not want to work on general units.
4. Establishment of float pools on call-in is helpful in recruitment. Nurses fear being "pulled" to units where they feel insecure, and this has been the cause for much dissatisfaction and dissent.

Use of Temporary or Supplemental Nursing Agencies. Though these agencies would only provide a temporary means to filling a vacancy, they do provide a pool of qualified employees. There are some disadvantages to utilizing these agencies, among which are:

- Temporary staff often lack commitment and teamwork within the organization, due to their temporary status. They do not participate in in-service education and nursing committees and activities.
- Temporary staff can reduce continuity of patient care, as several agency nurses may be utilized to fill one particular position on an unpopular shift (i.e., 11 P.M. to 7 A.M.).
- Temporary staff nurses must be supervised by an experienced nurse within the facility because they are not familiar with many aspects of the unit and organization. They cannot be placed in supervisory positions. This is often a problem when there is an R.N. shortage.
- Agency nurses make more per hour than the hospital nurses, creating resentment in employees who must supervise them (though without paying benefits to temporary staff the organizational costs are less then they appear to be).
- Often agency nurses cannot fill an 11 P.M. to 7 A.M. position, resulting in the employee nurses working these shifts while agency nurses work the day and evening shifts.
- It is difficult to evaluate the performance of temporary staff and ensure compliance with standards.
- Though policies and procedures are followed, it is still difficult to ensure that the agency nurse is prepared and qualified to work in a particular area.

Many times nurses turn to temporary agencies for higher salaries, more flexibility, and input into their work schedule and areas. Nurse-administrators are finding that they can offer nurses many of these same incentives and keep them in the organization. It is less expensive for the organization to recruit and retain satisfied nurses than it is to staff with agency nurses who perpetuate the shortages by frustrating the existing staff.

If, due to unforeseen events, the nurse-administrator must utilize a supplemental agency, the following should be kept in mind: use an accredited agency that is organized to achieve the Joint Commission Accreditation Standards. This agency will request specific information from your organization for development of an orientation packet for its nurses, and will ensure that these nurses receive the orientation packet. It will show evidence of licensure checks, qualification of its nurses, and require an evaluation of their performance for their files (and yours). It will also provide specific policies concerning conditions under which their nurses can work, and responsibilities of the hospital and facility.

Alternatives. One alternative to the use of temporary nurses is to develop an "in-house" P.R.N. or float team. These nurses could be hired under the same conditions as that of the agency nurses, but be part of the organization. Another approach is the use of part-time workers to cover busy times of the day or parts of an 8-hour shift. (Salaries may be higher for nurses working a minimum number of hours, "on-call," or on unpopular shifts, and they may receive a percentage of the fringe benefits.) These types of P.R.N. and part-time people still receive orientation and in-service, and over time can become part of the organization's culture.

Attracting and Reaching the Candidate Market

The next function of the recruitment process is aimed at communicating with the specific external market in a manner that will attract candidates to the organization. Attracting and reaching the specified market involves identifying sources for recruiting candidates, utilizing appropriate advertising media and content to attract the intended audience, and searching out specific talent.

Sources for Recruiting Candidates. Though assessment information is available from previous studies regarding location of nurses in the work force, recruiters must determine specific sources that can bring in qualified candidates to the organization. These sources will either be directly associated with potential candidates, or can be utilized to communicate with the specified market. Examples of sources for potential candidates include employee referral systems, professional contacts and networks, college and school campuses, and employment agencies. Recruiters may use one or a combination of these approaches, along with advertising and talent searches. The extent of efforts may depend on the value of the position, the costs, and the results.

Employee Referral Systems. According to Rick Stoops, applicants referred by current employees are the most effective and least costly recruitment approach.[6] Stidger[5] states that employees should be utilized in recruiting and selling jobs. If they are included in management decisions and involved with committees, their enthusiasm and concern for the organization will be a selling point to potential employees.

An employee referral system is an organized means to involve employees in recruitment. It involves employees contacting friends and colleagues about a job opportunity within the organization, and promoting the organization through word of mouth. Through their contacts with their specialty associations, ties from nursing school, and their involvement in the community, employees can locate qualified applicants for position vacancies. An employee referral system should be organized to include the following:

- Meetings and staff development to emphasize the employee's importance and role in the success of the organization.
- Stressing the importance of projecting the organization's image in a positive manner to the public. This can be the most important promotional tool.
- Ensuring that employees are knowledgeable about all employee benefits.
- Teaching that continual promotion of and recruitment for the organization is a job shared by all people within the organization.
- Teaching employees how to identify and communicate with potential candidates for a position.
- Providing incentives for employees who recruit qualified personnel. Incentives may be in the form of recognition, additional benefits such as paid time off, or monetary bonuses.

In an employee bonus system described by Levine,[7] an employee is given a cash bonus for recruiting new employees who remain in the organization for a certain length of time (usually three months to one year). Some facilities pay $25 to the recruiter when the new employee finishes orientation, then $100 following the first six months.[7] Bonuses range from $100 to $500. Other organizations pay the recruiter a percent of the new employee's first year's salary, or of the employment agency fees; this sum may be divided over a period of months. Other benefits such as tuition reimbursement for one year, a week of paid vacation, and other rewards are also effective.

Professional Contacts and Networks. Nurse-administrators make it a point to become involved in professional associations and groups. In some areas, special networking groups are formed by administrators strictly for sharing, continuing education, problem solving, and pooling ideas. Through these associations, nurse-administrators can let the word out about specific job opportunities, especially for management personnel. Though some members in these associations may be the "competition," they may have received an exceptional application for which they had no vacancy. Meetings at regional and national levels are also very helpful, because the nurse-administrator may learn of nurses relocating, and can also publicize special job opportunities.

College Campuses. College students are an important source of potential employees. Recruiters in organizations that are affiliated with nursing schools have automatic recruitment mechanisms if they provide the proper environment. Recruiters who are not affiliated with nursing schools should make plans to become involved with schools and colleges of nursing. Recruiters can promote the organization in school publications, become active in career planning and guidance counseling, and maintain close communication with student faculty and placement counselors.

College recruitment is becoming a very important recruitment tactic. It focuses on the future available labor supply and attracting this supply to the organization. The process involves scheduling and promoting a college visit, providing brochures and information about the organization, and setting up interviews with students on campus. In these interviews, information about salary and benefits, growth potential, job security, and career advancement is provided. This initial interview provides a chance for both the student and recruiter to evaluate and screen each other. Then, following a one- to three-week period, specific students are requested to interview with the organization. Travel expenses are reimbursed. This second interview involves specific job content, tours of the facility, and exchange of further information. Offers can be made for tuition reimbursement, joining externship programs, or, if close enough to graduation, for specific position openings.[8]

Employment Agencies. For certain types of personnel, especially clerical and ancillary workers, employment agencies may provide a pool of potential candidates. Stidger recommends the following when using an employment agency[5]:

1. Send detailed job descriptions and require that they only send qualified applicants.
2. Test each applicant's skill or knowledge, using the same test for each job.
3. Always check references.
4. Investigate agency fees—they may be 5 to 15 percent of the employee's first-year salary; they may charge applicants a fee.
5. Do not use an agency that does not send qualified people.

Walk-ins. Walk-in applicants should never be overlooked as a source of potential employees. Though immediate vacancies may not be available, a mechanism for interviewing and future recruiting of these applicants should be developed. Record systems with applicants' skills and experience should be available, accessible, and cross referenced by name, specialty areas, and special talent. These applicants can be a vital source of future candidates and should be recruited actively, regardless of position vacancies. Efforts must be made to *maintain communication with all high-quality candidates* for future openings.

Recruitment Advertising. There are many methods for advertising job opportunities. The most common include newspaper ads, ads in professional journals, radio, and exhibits at career days or conventions.

According to Frank Coss, journal and newspaper ads are the most effective means for recruiting.[9] "Reply by mail" or "send resume" ads in newspapers are widely read, convenient, fast, and reach job seekers. (Large newspaper display ads are the most effective in attracting attention.) Journal display ads get national coverage and are specific to a field. They also get fewer responses than newspaper ads and require increased cost and time to publish. Coss also recommends radio advertising as a means to supplement newspaper ads. The message should be simple and repeated at least ten times per day in order to reach the audience.

Career days and conventions are also opportune times for recruiters to promote their organization. Potential job seekers will come by the booth to receive literature and information about nursing services and the facility. Recruiters may use various mechanisms to provide this information, including audiovisual aids. Baptist Medical Center in Birmingham, Alabama, developed a sound system with a 6½-minute message about the facility to go along with a brochure. This proved to be a simple and cost-effective means of advertising.[10]

Ad Content. It is important to plan the content for recruitment advertising carefully to ensure that it communicates the appropriate message to the appropriate audience. The audience's values and needs, the purpose of the ad, appropriate media, time period for responses, number of applicants needed, and method of screening and interviewing applicants should be determined prior to placing the ad.[9]

Ads must be written at the educational level of the intended audience and be placed in media that communicate with this audience. They should appear attractive and unique, if display ads, and serve to catch attention. Contents of ads should state necessary information about the job, such as title, name of organization, location, summary of responsibilities, essential requirements, and some incentive statement regarding salary, advancement opportunities, work environment, or special benefits. Instructions for applying or sending resumes should also be included.

Ads should be seen as part of the entire marketing plan, geared to address and meet the needs of an intended market, and to promote the image of the organization and its employees. They should be accurate, personal, and written from the reader's point of view. Some organizations maintain continual display ads in newspapers and professional journals, to project a certain image as well as to remind readers of what the organizations can offer. The extent and type of recruitment advertising will depend on urgency of filling the need (need quick response), size and competition for the intended market, quality and quantity of past responses, and budgetary allowances. The number of quality responses to specific strategies must be evaluated for future use.

The Talent Search. Talent search involves seeking out specific individuals with known talents and skills and enticing them to interview with the organization. Special committees can be formed within the organization to develop lists of potential candidates and contact these individuals. Thorough and accurate record keeping by personnel or the nursing service will facilitate contacting individuals and past applicants with the needed skills and talents. Personal telephone calling proves to be very effective for attracting the interest of individuals, though it is a time-consuming procedure. Other approaches to the individual talent search are through consulting firms and direct mail.

Consulting Firms. Consulting firms, recruiting agencies, and management search firms all provide "headhunting" services. For a fee, usually based upon the new employee's first year's salary, they will search out, screen, and provide the organization with needed candidates who possess the desired skills and talents.

Recruitment firms are geared toward middle- and upper-level management positions. Whereas employment and placement agencies represent the individual, recruitment and search firms represent the employer. They will provide confidentiality, objectivity, maximum exposure, and thorough search of numerous sources and contacts. In turn, the organization must provide detailed information about the job, the facility, and the requirements. Fees may be established per day, per hour (around $50 to $100), percentage of salary (25 to 30 percent), or by monthly fee for providing continual (retainer) consulting and search services.[11]

Direct Mail. Qualified candidates may not respond to newspaper and magazine ads because they are not actively job hunting. They may be successful and happy, but also enticed and motivated by new and challenging opportunities. These individuals are best reached by direct mail. The list of potential candidates and addresses must be sufficient in quantity to elicit the desired number of responses, and contain accurate mailing information. Only home addresses should be used.[12] A supply of names and addresses should be continuously recorded and updated, to be used at the appropriate time.

One company using the direct mail approach mailed out 2000 cover letters with job descriptions. Forty people applied for the position, and five were very promising. Of these five, one was hired. This company was impressed with the quality of the applicants and the contacts this procedure developed. They had developed detailed target mailing lists, and were prepared to handle all inquiries.[13]

Stoops[12] describes a procedure for the direct mail approach: plan to mail in phases, sending a batch to the closest locations first. If responses are inadequate, then mail a second batch to further geographic locations. Design the outer envelope to attract attention, and include an attractive brochure describing the company's successes. Enclose location, important policies, employee benefits, and the job description with the job requirements. Also enclose a small reply card for name, present job, credentials, correct home address, phone number, and a place for candidates to indicate their interest in being contacted.

When reply cards are received, a system must be ready to process the information quickly and contact the individual. Phone contacts to interested parties concern discussing job opportunities, the individual's interests and goals, and the possibility of matching the two. Interviews are then scheduled for promising and interested candidates.

Professional Recruitment Services. In addition to the above talent search methods, some professional associations and organizations provide recruitment information. The American Nurses' Association and some individual states have professional networking and placement services. State and national professional organizations should be contacted regarding provision of recruitment services.

Evaluating the Recruitment Process

Following assessment, planning, and implementation of the recruitment plans comes the last function of the recruitment process—evaluation. As with all planning systems and activities, evaluation is an *ongoing process* that *occurs at every stage* of the recruitment process and within every function. Recruiters must evaluate the outcome of an entire recruitment effort, according to costs and effectiveness, and then reassess and revise specific functions.

The effectiveness of the recruitment process is ultimately evaluated by the quality candidates who are hired *and retained* in the facility. If the recruitment process is achieving its purpose in a cost-effective manner, then the results will be less cost per employee hired. Of course, this cost figure will be the result of many personnel processes, such as selection and placement, orientation, retention, staff development, and performance evaluation. Each function plays a part in employee adjustment and retention in the system.

Cost Per R.N. Hired. The following procedure outlines the steps necessary to calculating the cost per R.N. hired; it is reprinted with permission from Frances M. Hoffman's *Financial Management for Nurse Managers.*[14] The cost per R.N. hired is computed as follows (figures and percentages are only examples):

$$\frac{\text{Total costs}}{\text{Total R.N.s hired}} = \text{Cost per R.N. hired}$$

Figures for 1983–1984 yield a cost per R.N. hired of:

$$\frac{\$380{,}725}{250 \text{ R.N.s hired}} = \$1{,}522.90 \text{ per R.N. hired}$$

Detailed cost factors are presented below.

Recruitment Costs

Nursing Recruiter Salaries	**% Time**	**Salary ($)**
Recruitment specialist	100	25,000
Nurse recruiter	50	10,500
Secretary	100	12,000
Fringe benefits at 18%		8,550
Total		56,050
Supplies		
Printing brochures		8,000
Office supplies		1,000
Total		9,000
School and Job Fair Visits		
School visits		1,800
Project Tomorrow		400
State Nurses Association		100
Chicago Job Fair		100
State Student Nurses Convention		200
National Student Nurses Convention		500
Association of Nursing Students		50
Oncology Nursing Society		300
Total		3,450
Advertising		
Professional journals		2,500
Convention booklets		200
Newspapers		1,800
Nursing newspapers		1,500
Flyers		10
Audiovisual display		700
Nursing directory		3,500
Total		10,210
Student Visitation Days (2)		
Invitations		250
Decorations, etc.		200
Food		2,000
Total		2,450

Recruitment Costs *(cont.)*

Student Nurse Summer Program	**% Time**	**Salary ($)**
Hourly wages for ten weeks for 20 students		40,000
Seminars		
Recruitment seminar		500

Indirect Costs of Offices

	Number of sq. ft.	Cost ($) per sq. ft.	Total cost ($)
Recruitment specialist (100%)	120	5.00	600
Nurse recruiter (50%)	100	5.00	250
Secretary (100%)	120	5.00	600
Total	340		1,450

Orientation and Training Costs

Staff Development Salaries—Centralized	**% Time**	**Salary ($)**
Assistant in staff development	100	21,000
Assistant in staff development	50	9,200
Fringe benefits at 18%		5,436
Total		35,636

Staff Development Salaries—Decentralized	**% Time**	**Salary ($)**
Nursing specialist—Pediatrics	50	9,500
Nursing specialist—Obstetrics—Gynecology	50	11,300
Nursing specialist—Surgery	50	10,300
Nursing specialist—Medicine	50	10,600
Nursing specialist—Specialties	50	10,400
Fringe benefits at 18%		9,378
Total		61,478

Audiovisual Materials

Prorated audiovisual costs $200

Indirect Costs of Classrooms

	Number of sq. ft.	Cost ($) per sq. ft.	Total cost ($)
Classroom 1	190	9.25	1,757.50
Classroom 2	400	9.25	4,700.00
Classroom 3	250	9.25	2,312.50
Total	840		7,770.00

Turnover Costs

Unused Vacation/Sick Time Paid to R.N.s

Avg. hours of unused vacation/sick time per R.N.:	74 hours
Avg. hourly rate of pay upon termination:	$9.50
Terminations during 1983–84:	200
74 hours × $9.50 = $703 per R.N.	
$703 × 200 R.N.s =	$140,600

Exit Interviews

(Face to face with an administrator)		
Administrator's salary (5% of total)		$1,000
Fringe benefits at 18%		$180
Total		$1,180
R.N. hours (200 R.N.s × 20 minutes each):	67 hours	
Average hourly rate of pay upon termination:	$9.50	
R.N. cost of time		$636.50
Fringe benefits at 18%		$114.57
Total		$751.07
Exit interviews: Total		$1,931.07

Costs Attributable to Unfilled Positions	
Overtime Expenses	$10,000
GRAND TOTAL OF ALL COSTS	$380,725.07

As can be observed here, reducing turnover is the key. The more nurses that must be recruited and oriented, the greater the cost per R.N. So recruitment is definitely geared to *finding the right person for the right job and retaining that person.*

From the comparison of these figures with those of previous years, recruiters can focus their evaluation on each specific recruitment function. For example, how cost-effective is the advertising plan? Does it elicit enough quality respondents from which to choose? If qualified applicants are not being hired to fill vacancies, was the appropriate candidate market reached? Were candidates' needs addressed in promotional materials? Was the proper medium utilized to reach them? Were assessment data accurate? Are the organization's salaries competitive, and is the organization responsive to trends in market needs and expectations?

A written evaluation of the recruitment process should be completed each year. Included in this evaluation should be:

1. A comparison of the past two years' cost-per-hire figures with the present year's.
2. Statistics showing the average number of *qualified* (according to job description) applicants recruited per position vacancy.
3. The exact number of qualified responses to specific recruitment plans (i.e., college recruitment, advertising, referral by recruitment firm).
4. The ratio of application to hire (i.e., five applied, one was hired).
5. The reasons for applicants rejecting a job offer.
6. The exact recruitment expenditures.
7. Recruitment costs should be divided by the number of nurses hired to determine the recruitment cost per new nurse.
8. Analysis of the above information, rationale, and recommendations should be made for revising recruitment processes and revising

other areas of the organization. Projected budgets can also be developed from this analysis and information.

CONCLUSION

The recruitment process is an ongoing, systematic interaction of ten basic functions: environmental scanning, analysis of future internal changes, development of a philosophy, development of a human resource inventory, assessment of the current internal environment, recruitment planning, job analysis, ensuring a continual supply of qualified candidates, attracting and reaching the candidate market, and evaluating the recruitment process. Each function is interdependent within the recruitment system and with the other personnel processes. The nurse-administrator is ultimately responsible for the implementation of each function and for ensuring coordination and integration into selection processes.

Selection is closely linked to and builds upon the recruitment process. Selecting the right person for the right job is dependent on effective recruitment, and in turn affects the success of recruitment efforts. Recruitment produces the pool of qualified candidates from which to choose. Selection processes then determine the optimum job match—a match that will result in a satisfying and productive relationship between the employee and the organization. Selection is the process that carries recruitment plans to completion, and is the subject of the next chapter.

REFERENCES

1. Shepard, I. M., & Doudera, A. E. *Health care labor law.* Ann Arbor, Michigan: AUPHA Press, 1981, pp. 179, 185.
2. Jernigan, D. K., & Young, A. P. *Standards, job descriptions, and performance evaluations for nursing practice.* E. Norwalk, Conn.: Appleton-Century-Crofts, 1983.
3. Clark, K. J. Recruitment—An effective job posting system. *Personnel Journal.* 1984, *63*(2), 20–25.
4. Kaumeyer, R. *Planning and using skills inventory systems.* New York: Van Nostrand Reinhold, 1979, pp. 6–27.
5. Stidger, R. W. *The competence game—How to find, use, and keep competent employees.* New York: Thomond Press, 1980, pp. 65, 71–73.
6. Stoops, R. Recruitment ads that get results. *Personnel Journal,* 1984, *63*(4), p. 24.
7. Levine, H. Z. Consensus—Recruitment and selection programs. *Personnel,* 1984, *61*(1), 4–6.
8. Bergman, T., & Taylor, S. College recruitment: What attracts students to organizations? *Personnel,* 1984, *61*(3), 34–46.
9. Coss, F. *Recruitment advertising.* New York: American Management Association, 1968, pp. 47–70, 72–78.
10. Buzachero, V., & Parker, M. Sound recruiting with BMC soundsheets. *Personnel Administration,* 1984, *29*(5), 116–117.

11. Williams, R. *How to evaluate, select and work with executive recruiters.* Fitzwilliam, New Hampshire: Consultants News, 1981, pp. 1–27.
12. Stoops, R. Recruitment-direct mail: Luring the isolated professionals. *Personnel Journal,* 1984, *63*(6), pp. 34–36.
13. Zemke, R. Want to hire a trainee? Try the U.S. mail. *Training,* 1984, *21*(3), 8, 10.
14. Hoffman, F. *Financial management for nurse managers* E. Norwalk, Conn.: Appleton-Century-Crofts, 1984, pp. 107–110.

SUGGESTED READING

Achatz, H. E. How to gain control over your nominator recruiter. *Managers Magazine,* 1984, *59*(3), 22–23.

Aiken, L. The nurse labor market. *JONA,* 1984, *14*(1), 18–23.

Beauchamp, S. P. Use supervisory personnel to recruit nurses. *Supervisor Nurse,* Dec. 1980, p. 36.

Brinckerhoff, J. H. The job interview as a marketing tool. *Marketing Communications,* 1983, *8*(12), 74–75.

Cohen, S. The basis of sex bias in the job recruitment situation. *Human Resource Management,* 1976, *15*(3), 8–10.

Cowton, C. J. To advertise or to use a recruitment bureau. *Management Decision,* 1983, *21*(6), 31–38.

Crawford, J. C., & Lumpkin, J. R. The choice of selling a career. *Industrial Marketing Management,* 1983, *12*(4), 257–261.

Deets, C., & Froebe, D. J. Incentives for nurse employment. *Nursing Research,* 1984, *33*(4), 242–246.

DeSatnick, R. L. *The expanding role of the human resource manager.* New York: American Management Association, 1979.

Drake, L. Organizational performance: A function of recruitment criteria and effectiveness. *Personnel Journal,* 1973, *52*(10), 885–891.

Dunkelberger, J. E., & Aadland, S. C. Expectation and attainment of nursing career. *Nursing Research,* 1984, *33*(4), 235–240.

Edwards, J., Leek, C., Loveridge, R., et al. (Eds.), *Manpower planning.* New York: Wiley, 1982, pp. 4, 5.

Fox, H. W. Better hiring decisions. *Personnel Journal,* 1983, *62*(12), 966–970.

Gerson, H. E. Hiring—The dangers of promising too much. *Personnel Administrator,* 1983, *29*(3), 5–8.

Greenleaf, N. P. Labor force participation among registered nurses and women in comparable occupations. *Nursing Research,* 1984, *32*(5), 306–311.

Hunt, J. W. The shifting focus of the personnel function. *Personnel Management,* 1984, *16*(2), 14–18.

Jones, M. A. Job descriptions made easy. *Personnel Journal,* 1984, *63*(5), 31–34.

Kropf, L. Registered nurses fifteen years after graduation: Findings from the nurse career-pattern study. *Nursing & Health Care,* 1983, *4*(2), 72–76.

Levine, H. Consensus: Recruitment and selection programs. *Personnel,* 1984, *61*(1), 4–10.

Lewis, B. Recruitment of trainee nurses—The role of school of nursing. Part 1. *Nursing Times,* Sept. 25, 1980, pp. 1694–1696.

Mangan, J. & Silver, M. The demand for and supply of labour. In J. Edwards (Ed.),

Manpower Planning: Strategy and Techniques in an Organizational Context. New York: Wiley, 1983, pp. 13–34.

Miller, C. Dual careers: Impact on individuals, families, organizations. *National Association of Bank Women*, 1984, *60*(3), 4–9.

Mottram, R. A. Executive search firms as an alternative to search committee. *Educational Record*, 1983, *64*(1), 38–40.

Pascale, R. Fitting new employees into the company culture. *Fortune*, 1984, *109*(11), 28–43.

Peterson, G. G. Structuring company personnel policies and procedures. *Aging and Work*, 1982, *5*(4), 275–281.

Pincus, J. Recruitment and selection. . . . Guidelines to help nurses choose new employees. *Nursing Mirror*, 1982, *155*(19), 42–43.

Rayfield, R. E. Setting goals: The public relations outreach program. *Public Relations Review*, 1984, *10*(1), 59–67.

Scharffe, W. G. Layoff is a dirty word. *Phi Beta Kappan*, 1983, *65*(1), 60–61.

Scott-Brown, C. Management mobility. *Management Services*, 1984, *28*(1), 18, 20.

Shearer, K. M. Contingency nursing. *Nursing Management, 1982, 13*(3), 56, 58.

Stoops, R. Reader survey supports market approach to recruitment. *Personnel Journal*, 1984, *63*(3), 5–8.

Storholm, G. College graduates: An untapped source of talent. *Direct Marketing*, 1984, *46*(9), 64–66.

Taylor, M. S., & Schmidt, D. W. A process-oriented investigation of recruitment source effectiveness. *Personnel Psychology*, 1983, *36*(2), 343–354.

Teel, K. S. Estimating employee replacement costs. *Personnel Journal*, 1983, *62*(12), 956–960.

Trembly, A. C. How to land top talent. *Computer Decisions*, 1984, *16*(2), 173–178.

Van Meter, E. J. Eight ways to recruit the teachers you want for the jobs you've got. *American School Board Journal*, 1984, *171*(2), 27–28.

Warner, E. Novel recruiting methods targeting DP professionals. *Computerworld*, 1984, *18*(20), 22.

Wernimont, P. Recruitment policies and practice. In D. Yoder & H. Heneman (Eds.), *Staffing Policies and Strategies. Vol. 1. ASPA Handbook of Personnel and Industrial Relations*. Washington, D.C.: Bureau of National Affairs, 1974.

Wojahn, E. In search of the retention incentive. *INC*, 1984, *6*(5), 211–216.

APPENDIX 6–1

Medical-Surgical Registered Nurse: Job Description*

Position requirements	Graduate from an accredited school of nursing with current licensure as a registered nurse in the state of Alabama.
Professional requirements	Pursues programs of continuing education consistent with requirements of the Alabama Nurses' Association; participates in educational conferences, and updates and maintains professional knowledge and skills related to areas of responsibilities.
Position accountable for	All nursing care behaviors described in the Medical-Surgical R.N. job description.
Position accountable to	Head Nurse, Supervisor, Director of Nursing, the patient, and family.
Position summary	Performs the primary functions of an R.N. in assessing, planning, implementing, and evaluating the care of all assigned patients on the unit during the shift. Is responsible for meeting the established Medical-Surgical Standards of Nursing Practice, for managing all assigned personnel, supplies and equipment on the unit, and for promoting team work with physicians and personnel of other departments.

I. Assessment
   A. Assesses the number and level of personnel needed to provide quality patient care on the unit and collaborates with the Head Nurse or Supervisor in adjusting staffing and assignments.
   B. Assesses the delivery of nursing care on the unit and identifies problems and any need for improvements and changes.
   C. Assesses the health status of assigned patients on the unit as outlined in the nursing standards.
      1. Completes a comprehensive patient history and physical including patient interview, psychological and physical assessment, as well as patient's perception of illness.
      2. Collects data from the patient, family and significant others, health care providers, individuals, and/or agencies in the community.

*Reprinted with permission from Jernigan, D.K., and Young, A.P. *Standards, Job Descriptions, and Performance Evaluations for Nursing Practice.* East Norwalk, Conn.: Appleton-Century-Crofts, 1983, pp. 88–91.

3. Collects data by: interview, observation, inspection, auscultation, palpatation, and reports and records.
4. Organizes assessment data so that they are accurate, complete, accessible, and so that they remain confidential.
5. Communicates assessment data in an orderly fashion by recording, updating, and communicating among the health team daily and revising as appropriate.

II. Planning
- A. Serves on hospital committees and helps to review and revise policies and procedures, as directed by Head Nurse or Supervisor.
- B. Plans and develops self-objectives.
- C. Plans ways to creatively solve problems and make innovative changes and improvements on the unit in collaboration with supervisory personnel.
- D. Completes a written care plan for assigned patients on the unit. Plans the care for individual patients as well as directs and supervises others in the planning of patient's care.
  1. Identifies the patient's present/potential problems from the patient assessment.
     Patient's health status is determined,
     Health status is compared to the norms,
     Problems are given priority according to impact upon the patient's health status.
  2. Formulates desired outcomes specific to the patient problems and established norms.
  3. Ensures that desired outcomes are mutually agreed upon by the patient and nurse and are: (a) specific, (b) measurable within a certain time frame, and (c) consistent with other health providers' expectations.
  4. Incorporates home health care into the patient's desired outcomes. This includes but is not limited to teaching about the disease process and complications, medications, diet, exercise/activity, self-care techniques and materials, and available support systems and resources.

III. Implementation
- A. Implements activities necessary to meeting self-objectives.
- B. Participates in implementing planned creative changes and activities to improve nursing service.
- C. Holds self accountable for the delivery of quality nursing care.
- D. Promotes harmonious relationships and favorable attitudes among the health care team.
- E. Supports and adheres to administrative and nursing service policies and procedures.
- F. Assists with orientation of new employees.

G. Acts rapidly and effectively; manages self, patients, and other employees during any emergency situation.
H. Attends required inservice education programs.
I. Formulates nursing prescriptions that delineate actions to be taken.
Prescribed actions:
1. Are specific to the patient's problems and the desired outcomes.
2. Are based on scientific knowledge.
3. Are based of principles of patient teaching.
4. Are based on principles of psychosocial interactions.
5. Are based on environmental factors influencing the patient's health.
6. Include human, material, and community resources.
7. Include keeping patient knowledgeable of health status and total health care plan.
J. Implements the actions delineated in the nursing prescriptions.
Actions implemented:
1. Actively involve the patient and family.
2. Are based on current scientific knowledge.
3. Are flexible and individualized for each patient.
4. Include principles of safety.
5. Include principles of infection control.
K. Conforms to hospital dress code.
L. Is rarely sick or absent from work due to health.
M. Is prompt and attends report.

IV. Evaluation
A. Evaluates self-objectives; revises and formulates new objectives.
B. Evaluates the effectiveness of problem-solving techniques and the activities implemented to improve nursing services.
C. Contributes to the performance evaluation of nursing service personnel on the unit.
D. Participates in evaluation of RN orientation policies and procedures and recommends revisions to Supervisor or Head Nurse.
E. Participates in the evaluation of inservice education programs.
F. Evaluates achievement or lack of achievement of desired outcomes.
1. Data are collected concerning the patient's health status.
2. Data are compared to the specific desired outcomes.
3. Includes the patient's evaluation of the achievement of desired outcomes.
G. From evaluation of achievement or lack of achievement of desired outcomes, reassesses and revises the nursing care plan.
From evaluation:
1. Reassesses the patient problems.

2. Reassesses desired outcomes to determine if appropriate, realistic, and in correct priority.
3. Reassesses nursing prescriptions to determine if appropriate, realistic, and stated accurately.

From reassessment:

4. Determines new patient present/potential problems.
5. From new patient problems, formulates and revises desired outcomes.
6. Revises nursing prescriptions.
7. Implements new actions in order to carry out revised prescriptions.
8. Continually evaluates desired outcomes for achievement or lack of achievement.
9. Continually evaluates and revises the nursing care plan according to changes in the patient's health status.

APPENDIX 6–2

Specific Information Concerning the Job

Personal Requirements. The nursing staff on Two North has recently instigated primary nursing and developed an innovative diabetic patient teaching program. The R.N. employed on this unit must be physically able to provide baths, make beds, and perform other physical aspects of primary nursing. In order to fit into the innovative culture on this unit, the R.N. must be challenged by problems, be flexible and willing to change, be a risk-taker, possess effective communication skills, be perceptive to alternatives and opportunities, and be an intuitive, creative individual. Considering the wide variety of personalities and the assertiveness of the nurses on this unit, this individual must be responsive to criticism, work well under pressure, and be assertive; must be willing to assert creative ideas, but also to be a "team player." This new employee must be evaluated as "highly recommended," prior to selection.*

Job Strengths. Co-workers are innovative and enthusiastic; physician support is strong; management of the unit is under a participative system involving its staff nurses.

Job Weaknesses. Layout of the unit requires much walking; due to fast patient turnover plus high acuity level of patients, nurses are put under great pressure to provide all care, document, and participate in management of the unit; low socioeconomic/educational level of this patient population creates special problems and frustrations for patient education and discharge planning.

Opportunity for Advancement. In the past the opportunity for advancement was low without transfer to another unit. The only promotable positions are Head Nurse and Supervisor. At present a career ladder program is being instituted whereby the nurse can advance clinically and receive salary increases, based upon the designated achievement of criteria. Refer to clinical ladder program for details.

Salary Scale and Schedule. The base salary for this R.N. position is $10 per hour for a new A.D.N. graduate. Additional experience or education (B.S.N., M.S.N.) would be compensated according to the standard nursing salary scale. Salary increases are considered yearly, and are according to the merit raise system. (Refer to policy.) Other than cost-of-living increases, salary raises are dependent upon performance evaluation and may be 3 percent or 5 percent raises per year.

*See Chapter 7.

Schedule Requirements. Two North schedules according to fixed shifts. This position calls for a *straight* 11 P.M. to 7 A.M. shift. Schedules provide every other weekend off, and flexibility in off days to meet personal needs. Opportunity for shift change is available, and is based upon seniority. Requests should be made at the earliest possible date, in order to place you on the waiting list.

7 The Selection Process

The selection process involves choosing the most qualified candidate for the job—the candidate who will grow, develop, and contribute his or her best to the organization. This process is one of the most difficult of all personnel processes. Not only must you find the best-qualified person who is willing to work for your salary and on the needed shift, but you must also predict successful performance from an application form, some rather slanted references, and a few moments of conversation. In addition, you are searching for a good "cultural fit," where the candidate's values, personality, style of working, and attitudes fit those values and the general "personality" of the unit where he or she will be assigned.

Sound like a tall order? Well, indeed it is! And yet the selection process is often the most underrated in terms of systematic procedures, training of interviewers, and objective rating scales. Nursing administrators will develop elaborate research methodologies to determine patient outcomes and cost savings as rationale for increasing nursing salaries. And they will utilize creative recruitment strategies and pay high consultant fees for management search procedures to bring in a large pool of qualified candidates. And yet the selection procedures are often conducted hurriedly, with little preplanning or preparation. Decisions concerning selection are made on the spot, sometimes based upon first impressions or personality preferences.

Selection plays a big role in retention processes. If the right person is not hired for the right job, then costs begin to rise for sick time, low productivity, low morale, and eventually, turnover. If the selection process fails to select the appropriate person for the job, then recruitment costs will be wasted. If the selection process is ineffective, and a new employee is not right for the job or the organization, then orientation and staff development will also be ineffective. Proper selection efforts affect every personnel process and the successful operations of the organization.

Speaking realistically, success in selection is limited by human errors in judgment and interpretation of behavior. The final selection decision is based on subjective as well as objective data and must involve some degree of insight and hunch about an individual. But only after systematic elimination of applicants, using consistent and uniform procedures that produce a number of *equally* qualified candidates, can intuition be called upon. Up until that point, objectivity is the name of the game.

The need for systematic and objective selection procedures is necessary for two reasons:

1. A well-planned, systematic selection process will result in a better job match, and therefore in improved productivity, creative contributions, and longevity.
2. Equal employment opportunity laws require equal treatment of applicants and prohibit discrimination. Nurse-administrators need documentation and reasoning for choosing Nurse A over Nurse B, especially when Nurse B is 55 years old.

EFFECTIVE SELECTION

Just as effective selection affects all areas of the organization, selection processes are affected by certain factors:

Human Resource Management Planning (HRMP)

These plans will map out the future human resource needs, expectations, and roles, mold job vacancies and requirements, and determine the type of individuals selected to fill those vacancies.

Recruitment

The outcome of recruitment efforts produces the pool of candidates from which to choose. Selection can only be as good as the quality of the applicants. A large number of highly qualified applicants will enable a more "selective" choice, whereas a minimum number of marginally qualified applicants may cause a change in selection and recruitment plans.

Unsolicited Applicants

The number of qualified applicants who "walk in" and apply for a job contributes to this pool of candidates. These unsolicited, unpredicted applicants can prove to be successful and valuable employees. A mechanism must be worked out with recruiters to tap this supply and ensure follow-up when no vacancies exist. Administrators must prevent qualified applicants from being "filed away," and see that recruiters and selectors maintain ready access to all qualified applicants' files.

Job Descriptions and Expectations

As in the recruitment process, accurate and explicit information must be available concerning the requirements for the job vacancy. Effective selection will depend on an understanding of the responsibilities and needs of the job. The selection process must be finely tuned to the culture on the unit and the staff's expectations. That is why selection procedures are often placed on the management level closest to the vacancy. In many cases the staff on the unit are actively involved in selecting the new employee for that unit.

Job Satisfaction and Morale

As with recruitment efforts, successful selection of new employees is affected by the atmosphere and satisfaction within the organization. Few applicants can be "sold" on a facility that generates the impression of unhappy, discontented, or even unfriendly employees. Unless retention and job satisfaction efforts are successful, time and expense for screening and evaluating applicants can result in failure of the chosen applicant to take your job offer. In addition, the factors affecting successful recruitment, such as orientation procedures, benefits, and staff development, also affect the obtainment of a mutual agreement between your facility and a highly qualified candidate.

Sound Selection Procedures

The effectiveness of the selection process will depend upon the institution of systematic, consistent, and thorough selection procedures and policies. As stated earlier, this is necessary to enhance objectivity, procure a good job match, and conform to equal opportunity regulations. As with any endeavor, a well-planned, controlled procedure will produce better results.

Interview and Selection Personnel

Last, but not least, the people doing the selecting will determine the outcome of the selection process. Interviewers and evaluators must be knowledgeable about policies and procedures, communication skills, legal requirements, interviewing techniques, and the philosophy of the organization. They must be aware of the job expectations and the needs of the unit. Extensive preparation, training, and coaching are critical. The selection process must be executed as planned, in a fair and consistent manner that will generate good feelings about the organization.

THE STEPS IN THE SELECTION PROCESS

The entire selection process consists of several interrelated and progressive steps or procedures. It is guided, as are all processes, by an overall plan, based upon organizational goals and objectives. The selection "plan" is continuous with and springs directly from the recruitment plan. Recruitment plans, comprised of personnel inventories, staffing plans, and other personnel information, spring directly from human resource management plans. These are the blueprint for current and future human resources and guide decision making. The selection process is the step that carries recruitment plans to completion.

Due to this relationship, recruitment personnel work very closely with selection personnel. Nurse-recruiters may counsel and train interviewers, conduct initial screening or preliminary interviews, and assist in evaluating candidates. Recruiters closely follow selection procedures and ensure continuation of the process. Selection personnel provide feedback to recruiters concerning the quality of applicants and report any needed changes in the recruitment process. The two processes must work as one in order to get results. Therefore, continuation of recruitment planning is considered the first step of the selection process. Figure 7–1* outlines the components of the selection process and the text to follow. The discussion and examples of these components are guides for implementing effective selection, and are not intended to be the only way. Utilize these examples by adapting and altering them to fit your unique organizational setting.

ORGANIZING THE SELECTION PROCESS

Organizing for the selection process basically involves arranging a structure for selecting personnel. This structure should delineate the four "Ws" *w*ho, *w*hat, *w*here, and under *w*hat conditions. Who should be responsible for selecting new personnel? What are their specific responsibilities? Where do the selection procedures take place? What are the conditions of the selection process? This involves ground rules for final approval by the nurse-administrator, monitoring for equal employment opportunity, testing rating scales for validity and reliability, and other evaluations to control quality.

The structure for organizing selection must be delineated by the nurse-administrator in a policy statement and communicated to current and prospective employees. This structure is dependent upon the organizational structure of the nursing department and reflects the management styles,

---

*All figures referred to in Chapter 7 can be found at the end of the chapter text.

philosophy, and needs of the nursing service. Although a number of modifications in structure exist, the following examples summarize three different organizational structures. Each structure is based upon specific needs and has strengths and weaknesses. On the one extreme is the autonomous, self-governing organization. On the other extreme is the completely centralized structure. Then a modified, "middle-of-the-road" approach is offered as an example. These are guides for examining your own organization and how the selection process fits into this structure.

The Autonomous Approach to Selection

In this example, the nursing staff on the unit selects the new employee and is autonomous in its decisions. This participative and decentralized approach takes place in self-governing facilities, where the staff nurses maintain authority and control of all decisions regarding their unit. Unit coordinators or administration may be rotated or elected, and serve more as facilitators and resource people than as authority figures. The nurses are highly professional, make decisions by democratic rule, and usually are involved in collaborative practice and primary nursing. The staff determines "who, what, where," and the conditions are only that quality be monitored and controlled and that all practices promote equal employment opportunity.

Pros. This management approach can be very effective and satisfying for the nursing department. It can improve morale and productivity through increased job satisfaction and autonomy. Changes are accepted and implemented effectively due to staff participation. New employees are readily accepted due to the participatory selection process. The staff learns to negotiate and compromise on issues, and cohesiveness and teamwork are enhanced. Energies focus on quality and professionalism, and staff turnover decreases.

Cons. This type of approach calls for a very unique type of individual. The nurse on this unit must value professionalism, quality, and innovations, and have deep insight into human behavior and group dynamics. Unfortunately, some nurses function more effectively under clearly defined authority and a more structured environment. The nurse-administrator must consider the type and characteristics of the staff before implementing an autonomous-type unit. Otherwise he or she may find power struggles versus unity, subjective selection based on favoritism versus objective criteria, and decisions based on personal interest versus quality patient care. If the majority of nurses on the unit are technically oriented, they will be unable truly to grasp the concepts of professionalism, autonomy, and self-governance. The nurse-administrator should then choose an organizational structure that will match the needs and characteristics of the staff.

Centralized Approach to Selection

On the other extreme is the completely centralized approach to selection. This is where decision making occurs within the top administrative structure of the organization, and there is very strict control. The flow of decision making is essentially from the top down. The nursing staff answers to the shift assistant head nurse, who answers to the head nurse of the unit. The head nurse reports to the division director of nursing, who reports to the vice-president of nursing. The structure of this organization is not what necessarily makes it centralized. It is the amount of authority and autonomy delegated to the unit level, along with the degree of staff participation. There are degrees of centralization. A totally centralized organization would be a replica of the military, where orders come from the top and are irreversible. There is little or no upward communication. Few organizations practice this type of management approach today. But most centralized organizations consider the vice-president for nursing and the directors of nursing as the decision makers. The authority and decision-making process flows from the top-level administrator and the management team.

Pros. There are times when a centralized approach to management and selection is not only effective, but necessary. For example, a new nurse administrator is hired and needs to develop a new management team. A complete change in leadership due to poor performance, inefficiencies, or unacceptable management practices should hardly be left to democratic vote. Staff nurses must provide patient care and should not be involved in all administrative decisions. In addition, difficult problems that must be handled in a rapid, quiet, and assertive manner should be solved in a centralized manner. During times of turmoil, the staff will seek strong leadership and look to the administrator for strength, security, and decisive action.

Another example of effective centralized management often occurs in a small hospital. The nurse-administrator may be the only qualified person to recruit and select new personnel. The management team may be composed of "working" supervisors who, in addition to supervisory responsibilities, provide total patient care. In this circumstance, the nurse-administrator works closely with the staff nurses and supervisors, and often helps with patient care. The administrator is aware of unit needs, constantly receives input and information from the staff, and informally discusses ideas and problems, thus maintaining active communication with the personnel. Then the administrator makes decisions, selects personnel for all areas, and communicates decisions and rationale to the staff. Due to the size, expertise, and professional background of the staff, this may be the best approach.

Many large organizations also function well under a centralized approach to management. Centralization can facilitate standardization in policies and procedures, controlled and efficient operations, and a predictable, structured work environment. Again, the success of any structure will depend on the needs and characteristics of the staff, as well as the management style and the needs of the organization.

Cons. The negative aspects of a centralized approach can include the following: firstly, two heads can be better than one for decision-making. Receiving input from the staff level can improve the success of selection processes and decision-making. Secondly, in many cases, the top-level nursing administrators do not truly know the needs of a nursing unit. Due to the centralized authority, nurses may be reluctant to share their thoughts and problems, and the nurse-administrator can lack the information needed to make the best decision. In the selection process this can result in a poor job match, which later leads to increased turnover. Also, nurses may be less likely to accept a new employee who does not fit well into their unit culture and who was selected without their input. Today's nurses resent the "dictator" approach and want some control over decisions on their units. And a head nurse and assistant head nurse must be given the authority to do their jobs. If not, they soon adapt a passive attitude and nonassertive management approach.

Modified Participative Approach to Selection

This is an example of an intermediate approach, which blends the self-governing, autonomous method with the centralized approach. It provides decentralized decision making and top administrative control. The management style is fairly flexible, allowing variation in structure and procedures among the units. The focus is freedom to try new methods, individuality, and flexibility, and the unit management is determined solely by the head nurse* or the unit coordinator.* If the head nurse develops a self-governing type of unit, with complete participative management, this is acceptable. The only difference is that the head nurse is held accountable to the vice-president for nursing for all activities on that unit, and these activities are subject to administrative intervention if necessary.

Now, in order to be successful, it is obvious that the vice-president for nursing must not intervene often. The vice-president must allow experimentation and mistakes to occur, but is kept informed of all decisions, is utilized as a consultant and resource person, and maintains authority for final approval. The management team is not rotated or elected, but appointed by the vice-president for nursing, using specific criteria and qualifications. Then the unit-level nurse-administrator can organize and manage the area as he or she sees fit.

With this approach, the selection process remains decentralized (at the head nurse level), with final approval by the vice-president for nursing.

---

*These titles are used synonymously.

The head nurse may allow staff participation in interviewing and selection, but supply the guidance and ground rules. The final decision may be reached jointly, between the staff and head nurse, with the recommendation and rationale being submitted for approval to the vice-president for nursing. The selection methodology may vary from unit to unit, according to the type of position vacancy, expertise of the staff, and the ability of the staff to reach participative conclusions.

Pros. This approach leaves room for individual differences among nursing units and allows freedom to "do what works." The flexibility allows staff participation, but still maintains ultimate administrative control. Quality is closely monitored, while staff are allowed freedom of expression and some control over their activities. But a system of accountability is well intact that works to maintain standards of care. Although each unit coordinates and collaborates with the other units in its division, decisions flow from the unit coordinator or head nurse. Other than perhaps an assistant vice-president for nursing, who may be responsible for specific areas of the nursing services, there are no intermediate management positions between the unit level and the top.

Cons. As in any system, this approach to selection is only as good as the people in it. If the unit coordinators are not well trained in communication and management practices, or maintain autocratic rule, the results can be devastating. The vice-president for nursing may be *laissez faire* to the point of not knowing what is happening in the units. There must be sound information systems and controls.

Not only can the vice-president for nursing be too uncontrolling, but also too controlling. If the vice-president is unable to relinquish and share control without constant intervention, the system will be a farce. The staff will realize that their unit coordinator has no actual authority. The unit coordinator must be trained, evaluated, then trusted to run the unit competently. The vice-president for nursing must maintain strong leadership by supporting decisions, providing feedback for improvement, and intervening only when absolutely necessary.

Conclusion

Organizing the selection process depends upon the organization and management structure of the nursing department. Although some facilities still exert a strong centralized approach to management, others have begun implementing a participatory approach, including the selection of new employees. There are pros and cons to all methods, and the nurse-administrator must choose the one best suited for the particular organization. The most popular approach may not be realistic or workable with a particular type of nursing staff. A commitment to participative management is fine, but without proper training and development, it will most likely fail. Careful analysis of the needs and abilities of the nurses and the expertise of the management personnel is crucial before delegating authority and organizing responsibilities. But whatever the organization, keep in mind your goals: to enhance patient outcomes and provide an environment that will maximize the potentials, talents, and fulfillment of your human resources. Your organization must be designed to fulfill your goals. Do what works best for *you*.

EQUAL EMPLOYMENT OPPORTUNITY

Interviewers and those involved in the selection and hiring process must be well aware of the legal requirements for equal employment opportunity. Ignorance is no defense. Interview questions pertaining to sex, marital status, and children must be avoided, and jobs should be considered sexless. The federal government publishes *Uniform Guidelines on Employee Selection Procedures,* which delineate regulations and provide a guide for nondiscriminatory hiring practices. Employers should have a copy of this and provide recent updates to interviewers and those responsible for personnel practices.[1]

Executives must be aware of their state laws, regulations, and interpretative guidelines pertaining to equal employment opportunity. There are also scores of federal guidelines and regulations. Shepard and Doudera[2] describe several laws governing equal opportunity in health care employment practices that will assist the executive in understanding the general principles of equal employment opportunity. The following provides a summary of Shepard and Doudera's descriptions.

Civil Rights Act of 1866. This 1866 act prohibits job discrimination based on color, and protects the right of citizens to enforce contracts.

Fourteenth Amendment. This amendment provides equal protection under the law in all actions by the state.

Fifth Amendment. This amendment prohibits the federal government from discrimination.

Equal Pay Act of 1963. This act prohibits wage discrimination on the basis of sex—requires equal pay for equal worth. If working the same or equal jobs under the same or similar conditions in the same establishment, females must be paid as much as males. To prove discrimination, a female must show that wage disparity is not a result of the free market in operation, but the result of compensation depression. She must also prove equal skill, responsibilities, similar conditions, and efforts required between both jobs.

Age Discrimination in Employment Act of 1967 (ADEA). This act bars discrimination in employment practices for those aged 40 to 70.

Rehabilitation Act of 1973 and Vietnam Era Veteran's Readjustment Act of 1974. This act prohibits federal contractors from discrimination on the basis of handicap if the handicapped person is capable of performing the essential functions of the job with reasonable accommodations by the employer. This requirement is also pertinent to any program receiving federal assistance or Department of Labor funding. It also bars pre-employment medical examinations unless exams are part of a routine selection policy.

Title VII of the Civil Rights Act of 1964. Title VII establishes the Equal Employment Opportunity Commission to protect and investigate against discrimination, and bars discrimination for race, color, sex, religion, or national origin in all employee practices. This includes the selection process. Discrimination under Title VII usually takes two forms.

1. Disparate treatment of an employee because of sex, race, national origin, or religion. The employee must prove that
   a. He or she is a minority or a protected class
   b. He or she is qualified for the job or promotion
   c. He or she was rejected
   d. The position remained open and other applicants with the same qualifications were recruited, in order to prove discrimination

   Employers must show reasons for not selecting the applicant. Evidence of affirmative action (discussed later) and a balanced work force helps in the defense.
2. Class action. This concerns disparate treatment of a protected class or a minority. If the work force is not balanced with the availability of minorities in the community, such as qualified women and blacks, it can have a "disparate impact" on that group. The internal work force must have a similar proportion of minorities as compared to the percent of qualified minorities available in the surrounding area. If it does not, even without intent to discriminate, this can be proved. It usually occurs through "neutral" employee practices, that is, lack of affirmative action. Class action can also be proved when employers set restrictive job requirements, such as minimum height and educational qualifications. They must prove that the requirements are a business necessity and needed for job performance. A pre-employment or promotion test must also be validated as being reliable and a business necessity. These restrictions cannot be used for non-job-related purposes.

Religious Accommodation

The Equal Employment Opportunity Commission (EEOC) also requires employers to make reasonable adjustments for employees' religious practices if this does not cause undo hardship to the business. This includes barring pre-employment questions concerning religious absences from work, and the arrangement of interviews when applicants cannot attend due to religious practices.

Affirmative Action

Employers contracting with the government are required to implement Affirmative Action (AA). Otherwise AA is largely a voluntary effort, but one that can provide a defense against charges of discrimination (along with other information to be discussed in the next section). It is a planned program to seek and maintain a work force that is representative of the surrounding labor market and available pool of qualified personnel. The percent of minorities in the employer's work force should be comparable to the percent in the immediate labor area and to the percent who are qualified for the job. Affirmative actions may include recruiting minorities, job posting, and training programs to hire minorities and balance the work force in terms of the surrounding community.

Shepard and Doudera[2] write that employers can prevent discrimination by developing personnel policies and guidelines that provide equal treatment for all employees, and communicating these policies to them. Different employees must be treated the same under the same circumstances. All warnings and personnel actions must be documented: why the action was taken and how the policies were uniformly applied to all employees. All counseling sessions, warnings, evaluations, and attempts to help employees must be documented *prior* to an adverse action. Opportunities for advancement must be made for all employees.

THE APPLICATION PROCESS

The selection process officially begins with the application. Interested persons, either solicited or unsolicited, should be requested to apply formally for a job by completing an application form. A prospective employee who seeks information concerning a job should be requested to complete the application form. Candidates may take the form home to complete and mail in, but "on-the-spot" interviews should be avoided if possible. The prospective employee should agree to arranging an appointment at a later date, even the next day. Time is needed to review the application prior to the interview so that an effective exchange of information can occur; in addition, on-the-spot interviews often are conducted in a hurried session between meetings or engagements, where information required for thorough evaluation of the candidate is not obtained. The application procedure should be systematic, concise, and clear to the applicant.

Screening

Applicant screening usually occurs during the initial application process, and is conducted by nurse-recruiters or the personnel department. Screening can include a preliminary interview or screening of the application for minimum requirements for the job. In some organizations, it involves both procedures.

An example of a screening procedure is when an interested candidate completes a short application form, and a preliminary screening interview is set up. The short application form supplies information so that those screening can determine whether or not the applicant meets minimum requirements for the job. This form saves time in completing and then reviewing an entire application when the prospective employee is not qualified for the job (minimal qualifications should include required licensures, educational requirements, special training, and experience needed for the job). See Figure 7–2.

During the preliminary interview, the applicant is screened for certain behaviors that are defined by the organization as being required for employment. A checklist can be devised as seen in Figure 7–3. This list is completed by the screeners and attached to the short application form, following the interview. At that time the applicant is informed whether or not he or she is eligible for the job. An applicant who is not eligible is given the reasons with suggestions for needed skills or improvements, and perhaps information concerning other job openings. The applicant is also told to communicate any updates or changes in qualifications, in order to be considered for future job openings. The short application form and screening interview are filed for later use.

A candidate who is eligible for the job is given a long application form to complete. At that time, the following selection procedures should be initiated:

1. Applicant is given information concerning the selection process.
2. Applicant is given a job description and explanation of job expectations as developed through the recruitment process (see Appendices 6–1 and 6–2).
3. Applicant is supplied with a personnel handbook and handouts concerning the organization.
4. Applicant is asked to supply official transcripts from previous schools and universities, as well as continuing education transcripts and certificates of attendance.
5. Applicant signs release forms to enable verification of references and previous employment records.
6. Applicant is instructed to bring or mail in the application, and told that he or she will be contacted for an employment interview.

During the initial application and screening process, it is important to treat the prospective employee with courtesy and respect. The applicant should be made to feel important and valued as a human being, because the impression formed of the organization will be taken back into the community. Ensure that secretaries and receptionists are polite and helpful. Many applicants get turned off by condescending secretaries and form a negative opinion of the organization. Each applicant is important, if not for the present, for the future. Make sure that applicants are treated well and that they understand the application and selection procedures. Ensure that the procedures are followed, and that applicants are notified of appointments and results as instructed. An efficient, systematic, and courteous organization will improve your chances of securing qualified employees. Remember that all employees should be treated with the same respect and interest, from the minimum-wage worker to the top-management applicant. All human resources contribute to the successful operations of the organization.

The Long Application Form

Following the screening process, the applicant should be given a long application form to complete. This is to elicit complete and accurate information needed for the job interview and further evaluation of the applicant. This form should be comprehensive but not laborious. Keep in mind that a resume should never substitute for a completed, signed application. Applicants have been known to falsify their credentials.[3] The following items should be considered when evaluating the application form.

Equal Employment Opportunity. Questions on the application form should relate only to a candidate's qualifications and ability to do the job. Equal employment opportunity laws and Federal and state regulations must be upheld. All applicants in the same job classification must be required to give the same information. Questions addressing a particular class, such as blacks or the elderly, should not be asked. If questions focus on a minority group or those aged 40 to 70, you are opening yourself up for discrimination charges. Anything pertaining to race, age, sex, or handicaps should be avoided. After an applicant is hired, needed information concerning sex, age, etc., may be recorded, provided it is not used for evaluation purposes or promotions. Some facilities request these types of data due to affirmative action and fair employment practices. They want to ensure the hiring of appropriate numbers of minorities or handicapped individuals, and therefore need this information.[4] In these instances such requests are justified.

In the same area of thought, personal questions related to marital status, children, and outside activities should also be avoided. It is possible that these questions could later appear to influence hiring. Some employers believe that a single and childless applicant may not be stable and remain with the organization, or that a married but childless applicant will be soon wanting to start a family. Not only do questions in these areas appear discriminatory, but they are also invalid. There is no way to predict a new employee's length of service, and childbearing and raising children during employment has become a common practice that should present no problems.

Do Questions Elicit Needed Information? Questions on the application form should be reviewed for necessity and pertinence. It is a waste of everyone's time to have redundant or unnecessary questions. Decide what information you need to obtain a clear picture of the candidate. Screen all questions for clarity. Just because your facility uses a standard application form does not mean that it cannot be changed.

Agreements. Some applications have an area on the form for agreement to a pre-employment history and physical, a probationary period, and other conditions, such as temporary employment. Most forms have a statement regarding the truth of the information, and subsequent discharge if it is found to be false. Some facilities draw up a contract prior to hiring, delineating the specific conditions of employment, such as the job description and requirements, shifts and hours, and pay scale. If this is the case, it would be unnecessary to include these items on the application form.

Authorization. In order to verify references and check previous employment records, the agency contacted will require a release of responsibility that has been signed by the applicant before releasing any information to you. Many application forms have an area for the applicant to agree to your checking the information on the application form and releasing previous employers from responsibility after providing the needed information. This authorization for release of information is either included on the application form, included on the employee reference form (see page 152), or documented on a separate form that is attached to the reference form. See "Verification Procedures" for more information on employee reference checks.

The Application Form. A variety of standardized application forms are available to health care facilities. You can adopt a pre-existing form or adapt it to meet your needs. Another option is to use a standard application form for all potential employees, with a special attachment that is related to a specific job category, such as registered nurse, aide, etc. This attachment elicits additional information specific to the job. Figure 7–4 displays an example of a standard application form. Figures 7–5 through 7–8 display attachments for a nurse management position, registered nurse, licensed practical nurse, and aide/orderly position. These forms can be used as a guide for designing applications for your own organization.

VERIFICATION PROCEDURES

Verification procedures involve confirming the validity of information on the application, as well as exploring the applicant's previous work habits and employment records. Verification procedures should be initiated immediately following the completion of the long application form. It is important to have all information verified prior to the final selection process, and the procedure can sometimes be lengthy and slow. Even though an applicant may not be selected for the job, selection and placement in other vacancies in the future wili be facilitated if the applicant has already been "checked out."

Despite the importance of obtaining information concerning the applicant's previous work history, it has become exceedingly difficult to elicit any information from previous employers. Due to growing legal problems associated with references, many employers only give favorable references, or simply verify dates of employment. Information concerning work habits, characteristics, interpersonal relationships, attitudes, and expertise has become very difficult to obtain.

Giving and Obtaining Employee References

Bell, Castagnera, and Young[5] explain the legal considerations involved in giving and receiving employee references. Communication concerning prospective employees falls under several laws, including the tort of defamation, which includes libel and slander. Defamation is any communication that is false and can cause harm to one's reputation by inducing poor opinions, loss of confidence or esteem in other persons' minds, and exposure to degradation. Defamation in writing is libel, and through speech is slander. Despite the employee's permission to release information, the employee still has the legal right to sue for defamation of character. Waiving the right to view the previous employee reference does not offer the employer any more protection. Neither does the employee's agreement to release the employer from any responsibility when providing employment information to a prospective employer provide protection. Because the applicant has not seen the information and verified its truth, defamation of character or malice can still be claimed.

Employers must know what is safe to say or write when giving a reference. They must be certain that the information given is true, supported with documentation, and that it is privileged. If it is not true, it can be considered an act of malice (an untrue statement with intent to harm). Privileged information means that the need to hear is more important than a person's individual reputation. Conditional or qualified privilege occurs when a reference is given to a prospective employer, and involves a duty to speak and hear information about a person's performance. This duty to "speak and hear" is more important than the prospective employee's reputation, especially as it pertains to the provision of patient care. If the reference is true and given in good faith by those who were involved in evaluating the employee, and received by those who need "to hear" the information for selection purposes, it is considered privileged. This prevents the exchange of information concerning the applicant from being an invasion of privacy. Bell, Castagnera, and Young give the following guidelines for "defensible" references[5]:

1. Answer inquiries only after checking the validity of the request for information. Do not volunteer additional information.
2. Only communicate employee information to those who have a definite need for the information.
3. Use statements that clarify the need for confidentiality and use of the information. By beginning with "the enclosed is the information you requested for employee selection purposes. This is considered confidential information," you are clarifying your intent.
4. Obtain written consent from the employee for the release of information.
5. Only provide information that relates to work and the employee's performance.
6. Only provide objective, specific information. Avoid descriptions such as "careless," or "has difficulty working with others." Give documented examples of actual behavior, such as "six medication errors in one week;" or "three staff members requested not to work with him."
7. Any personal judgment or opinions should be stated as, "I believe . . ."
8. Any statement with the potential for negative interpretation should be accompanied by the specific incident.
9. Do not answer the question "would you rehire."
10. Do not answer any "off the record" questions.

Employee references are vital components to effective selection. Without honest and accurate information, poor performers are allowed to continue providing patient care. Nurse-administrators are obliged to provide data to prospective employers within the boundaries of the law. Knowledge of what, when, how, and to whom to give references will provide the necessary defense in case of a lawsuit. Figure 7–9 provides an example of an R.N. reference form to be sent to a former employer.

Before concluding the section on verification procedures, attention should be given to verifying educational background, licensure, and other information. Specific procedures should be delineated for confirming licensure, educational degrees, and past accomplishments and experiences. Some organizations require official transcripts to be sent from each educational facility. They use these transcripts to verify not only degrees, but also grade point averages and honors. Continuing education can be verified by requesting an official transcript from the state nurses' association, or by a certificate of attendance. Licensure can be verified by checking with the state board of nursing. Each organization must define its methods for validating this information. Figure 7–10 provides an example of a procedure for checking licensure.

Personal references are difficult to validate. You can call to ensure that the person did write the letter of reference, but you cannot validate the accuracy of the information. Few prospective employees will identify someone for a personal reference who will not give a positive report. Personal references are often worthless, as they are usually from a friend or colleague who will only provide a glowing recommendation.

Listings of publications and research should be verified for accuracy and read for content. Consulting firms can be utilized to verify the application and even check out previous criminal records. For example, The National Verification Service and The Educational Credential Evaluators both investigate applicants' previous records and credentials to uncover fraud.[3]

THE INTERVIEW PROCESS

The next major component of the selection process is employee interviews. This component consists of several steps preceding and following the actual interview. Together, these steps comprise the *interview process,* which leads to the recommendation of candidates for appointment. Figure 7–11 charts the interview process within the total selection process. The following provides a guide and an example for an effective interview process.

Long Application Form Review and Rating

Once the long application form has been completed, it should be reviewed and evaluated. This will serve two purposes. First, it will prepare interviewers for the interview by focusing on specific questions, experiences, or discrepancies on the application. Second, ratings from the evaluation will later be used for comparing and recommending applicants for appointment.

The procedure for application review and rating will vary according to the organizational structure. In a centralized structure, the personnel department, nurse-recruiters, or the nurse-administrator and management team may implement the procedure. In a decentralized (more participative) structure, the head nurse of the area where the new employee will be assigned would rate the application. For simplicity, the examples provided in the remainder of this chapter will focus on the decentralized approach to interviewing and selection.

Application rating involves assigning a numerical weight to each section on the application, in order to facilitate objectivity in evaluating responses. Though it is possible simply to read through applications in order to determine qualifications, prepare interview questions, and compare applicants, the rating system can provide consistency and standardization to this process.

Rating scales must be valid and reliable, and should be fully tested and refined prior to implementation. Determination of the numerical weight of an item on the application will depend on the requirements of the job, as well as on the values and philosophy of the nursing department. A task force can be selected to develop and refine a rating scale for the standard application form, as well as for the specific job-related attachments. The purpose of the rating system is to determine a ranking for all responses on the application, so that each candidate is evaluated by the same criteria. This ensures equal treatment, objectivity in evaluating, and can be utilized as a second screening mechanism as well as in the final selection process. Figure 7–12 provides an example for rating a standard application form. Figure 7–13 provides an example of a rating scale for the nursing management position application attachment. At the bottom of this form is a place for tallying the total scores.

Policies should be developed concerning the use of rating scores. If rating scores are used for a second screening and elimination prior to interviews, what is the point scale for elimination? Also, all information, transcripts, and continuing education verification would have to be complete prior to the interviews, in order to screen applicants further according to their ratings. What about the number of applicants? If one of two applicants has a 10-point lead, would you just interview the one person?

Rating scales can be tricky if not used properly. Even though they are tested for reliability and validity, some degree of subjectivity is always possible in determining a score. Also, applicants may do very well "on paper" and have outstanding qualifications, but not come across well in person. Therefore, the following are recommended when using rating scales:

1. With large number of qualified applicants, use scores from rating scales to screen prior to the interview. Allow a large discrepancy among scores, such as a 25-point lead before eliminating candidates.
2. Always try to interview at least five applicants for maximum comparison and selection results, despite score differences.
3. Use rating scales in conjunction with interviews, to eliminate down to your best applicants (two to three).
4. Receive input from the nurses who will be working with the new employee. After eliminating to the best, similarly rated applicants, obtain feedback from others.
5. Final selection among equally qualified applicants cannot be totally dependent upon application rating scales. The decision is based upon the interview, and the judgment, intuition and input from others, when choosing among similarly rated applicants.
6. Policies must be developed to delineate the weight of the rating score in final selection decisions. If the top scoring applicants (five of ten applicants) are interviewed, decisions regarding the weight of the rating versus the weight of the interviewer's recommendations must be made. The ideal goal is to select the outstanding and highest-rated applicant. More will be discussed under the section concerning recommendations for appointments.

With a large number of applicants, the rating procedure can be time-consuming. The head nurse where the vacancy exists may select a small team of application reviewers and raters. This team can be other management personnel in the hospital (for a more objective view), charge nurses and assistant head nurses on the particular unit, or staff nurses working on the unit. It is ideal to have those involved in the interviewing process also participating in application rating. This would improve their knowledge of the applicants and facilitate an effective information exchange during the interview. If the head nurse knows who the interviewers will be, or has a permanent interview and selection team, this is possible. But usually selection of the interview team will depend upon the number and type of applicants and the appropriate interview methodology. As depicted in the interview process in Figure 7–11, application rating precedes selection of the interview team. Therefore, the head nurse will want to devise a means for assistance and input in rating the applications. Raters must have knowledge and skill in the rating process, and ensure a fair, objective, and consistent rating procedure. Due to this important requirement, the head nurse will often choose raters from the nursing service management team who are experienced in the rating procedure.

Interview Methodology

Following application review and rating, the appropriate method for conducting the interview should be determined. This is not the content of the interview questions, but *how* the questions will be asked. Methodology depends on the number and type of applicants, the needs of the unit, and the involvement and interviewing skill of the staff nurses. An R.N. applying for a position as primary care nurse may be interviewed by a panel of primary care nurses on that unit. But a panel of interviewers would be threatening and inappropriate for an applicant applying as a unit secretary. The nurse-manager on the unit must determine the most appropriate method. The following are some examples of interviewing methodology.

One-to-One Interview. This is the most common interviewing method. The head nurse conducts an extensive interview, then summarizes and evaluates each applicant following the interview. The top-rated applicants are usually asked to come back at a later date and meet the nursing staff on the unit. Sometimes, immediately following the interview, the head nurse invites the applicant to tour the unit and meet the staff. This "informal" introduction is usually prearranged, and the staff is anticipating the visit. The applicant is left for a while to ask questions and talk to the nurses. Later the head nurse receives input from the staff for decision making. Though the interview may formally be "one-to-one," mechanisms are arranged to include the nursing staff's recommendations and input.

With a large number of well-qualified applicants, the nursing staff may be involved in the interview process. Four to five well-trained and qualified nurses may conduct one-to-one interviews with applicants, then compare their ratings and results. Each nurse would conduct an in-depth interview, then be responsible for introducing the applicant to the nursing staff following the interview. It is important that they make notes of input and recommendations from the staff immediately before these comments are forgotten or confused with comments on other applicants. They must also write down their own impressions, a summary of the interview, and complete the appraisal process while it is fresh in their minds.

The nurse-interviewers then get together as a group to discuss the candidates. Although they each interviewed a different applicant, their aim is to discuss strengths and weaknesses and come to a consensus concerning the best-qualified candidate. The use of the application rating scale and objective interview assessment tools will help them in their decisions. Input from the nursing staff is also considered in their recommendations. The head nurse may be involved in interviewing or serve as a resource person during this process. In any event the head nurse facilitates the final decision making and maintains authority to approve or disapprove recommendations.

Two-to-One Interview. This is a variation of the above and involves two interviewers per applicant. These two employees may be a head nurse and assistant head nurse (or charge nurse), head nurse and staff nurse, or two staff nurses. Basically the procedure is the same, but a second person is provided to participate in the interview. This may be a helpful method for nurses new to the interview process. It provides additional input without the threatening feeling that the group interview may cause the applicant. One interviewer may take a more passive, supportive role, while the other interviewer asks most of the prepared questions. The two interviewers aim to provide a supportive and communicative atmosphere, while together gathering data for discussion and evaluation following the interview.

Panel Interview. This method involves several qualified and experienced nurses (managers and/or staff) interviewing an applicant. Questions must be prearranged, with the roles of each participant on the panel delineated. This method requires a group leader to guide questions and answers and precise ground rules such as a certain number of questions per interviewer, or an order to the questioning. Interviewers must be supportive and nonthreatening, and strive to relieve the applicant's nervousness. The panel interview is often implemented for management-level candidates, with the panel consisting of the vice-president for nursing, members of the management team, and staff nurse representatives.

Group Interview. When there are large numbers of equally qualified candidates, group interviews may be conducted as either a means of elimination or of choosing employees for several vacancies. Several vacancies can exist when a new unit is opened or personnel for a pilot program on a particular unit are selected. Group interviews are not appropriate for final decision making for a single vacancy, because it is not possible to collect enough information from each applicant to determine the one who is best qualified. It *is* possible to collect enough information either to screen several applicants or select a number of outstanding candidates.

In a group interview, a number of prospective candidates are gathered together. The procedure and the purpose of the interview are explained. The interviewers (usually three or four) ask a series of predetermined questions. A group leader guides the process and ensures that each applicant has an opportunity to talk during the interview. Applicants are encouraged to discuss and exchange information among themselves, as well as with the interviewers. They are rated according to a predetermined scale on knowledge of issues, communication skills, interaction, assertiveness, and other appropriate characteristics. The highest-rated applicants are then chosen for individual interviews, or several candidates are selected for a number of vacancies. Use of this method will depend upon the degree of preparation, objectivity, and interviewing skills of the interviewers. Rating scales would have to be simple and brief, as detailed and lengthy information cannot be obtained in a group setting.

Interviews may be conducted using one or a combination of these methods. Managers may want to experiment and determine the method most effective in selecting successful and well-adjusted new employees.

Selection and Preparation of Interviewers

Those involved in the interview process must be carefully chosen and well trained in the art of interviewing. Whether conducting a one-to-one, two-to-one, panel, or group interview, the same skills and characteristics are required. When selecting interviewers, look for those with supportive attitudes who can communicate effectively with others. In addition, look for:

1. Nurses with varied backgrounds and experiences, to provide more input for decision making and broaden the interpretation of information
2. Nurses who can reach a consensus with others
3. Nurses who can uphold confidentiality
4. Nurses who can be objective
5. Nurses with the ability to observe and interpret verbal and nonverbal behavior
6. Nurses capable of relaxed and easy conversation
7. Nurses knowledgeable about organizational goals, philosophy, and the job vacancy
8. Nurses aware of the needs of the unit where the vacancy exists
9. Nurses who are interested in participating

Preparing interviewers for the interview involves two parts: providing needed information about the job and the applicant, and training in the art of interviewing. Because the preparation process can be time-consuming, the nurse-manager must look carefully at the pool of potential interviewers. If there are many interested and qualified nurses who wish to take part in this process, regular classes on interviewing techniques and skills should be arranged. This way, if the interview "team" is rotated, or if job vacancies are rare, the nurse-interviewers will have had some basic training in the interview process. Then, prior to the interview, a short refresher period can be offered to review the principles and techniques of interviewing. The following are some areas to cover in a basic training program.

Equal Employment Opportunity Laws and Regulations. As discussed earlier in this chapter, interviewers must be well aware of EEO laws and avoid discriminatory questions. The organization should develop an interviewing handbook containing regulations, "dos" and "don'ts" of interviewing, and policies concerning nondiscriminatory employment practices. Equal Employment Opportunity is an essential part of any interview training program.

Communicative Atmosphere. The objective of the interview is to allow an exchange of information from *both* parties. In order to accomplish this, a relaxed and nonthreatening environment must be established by interviewers. A training program might discuss the following ways to promote a communicative environment.

Establish Rapport. At the beginning of the interview, aim to establish rapport. A pleasant greeting, introductions, and small talk will help to relax the applicant. Arranging informal seating (not behind a desk), offering a cup of coffee, and showing friendly interest in the applicant as a person is also helpful.

Explain Procedures. An explanation of the interview and selection procedures is important to the applicant. A brief discussion of what to expect during the interview, the system for scoring applications and rating interviews, and the time frame for hearing results will answer immediate concerns. Let the applicant know that you will allow time for any unanswered questions at the end.

Questions. Don't ask too many "why" questions. These types of questions can be threatening to the applicant and put him or her on the defensive. Reword questions to get the desired information. For example, "I see you worked three months in your last job. Could you tell me about this?" This line of questioning is less threatening than "Why did you leave your last job after only three months?"

Interviewing Styles. Training programs should also include various styles of interviewing to obtain different results. The *tightly controlled interview* occurs when interviewers ask a number of specific questions to elicit factual information. The scope of the applicant's comments and answers is narrow. The *loosely controlled interview* is just the opposite of this. The applicant controls the interview by talking about himself or herself, past experiences, other jobs, etc. Interviewers may learn much about the applicant, but this type of interview is very time consuming. All needed information may not be obtained by allowing the applicant to control the line of conversation.

The *guided interview* allows the applicant to talk freely, but keeps the discussion on track, and directs it to certain subjects. The questions are planned and allow elaboration and explanations by the applicant. In turn, the applicant also has an opportunity to discuss concerns and questions. Interviewers should be trained in the skill of conducting a *guided interview.*

Types of Questions. The training program should focus on the types of questions to ask during the interview. A variety of questions may be asked to elicit desired information. The following are some "dos" and "don'ts" for questioning:

1. Do ask for clarification. "I'm unsure of your exact meaning on your application. Could you explain this to me?"
2. Do allow a pause after a question, to give time for thought. Tell the applicant to take a moment and think over the answer.
3. Do refocus the conversation. "You mentioned your rotation through Baptist Hospital's burn unit. What did you think about the primary nursing on that unit?"
4. Do rephrase your questions. When the applicant does not provide information to your satisfaction, state your question in a different manner so that the applicant understands what you are asking.
5. Do not ask leading questions. "You know we have primary nursing in our hospital. How do you feel about primary care?" This question has a built-in answer. The applicant will surely tell you what you want to hear. If you want honesty, listen and observe comments and reactions throughout the course of conversation. Asking leading questions will most likely not elicit any true information.
6. Do not ask loaded questions that could backfire on the applicant. "How did you feel about your last supervisor?" Questions of this sort will rarely elicit an honest answer, as a negative response could reflect poorly on the applicant. You might ask instead, "What were the strengths and weaknesses of your last supervisor?"

Obstacles to Effective Interviewing

The interview training program should also focus on obstacles to effective interviewing. Some of these are as follows:

Constant Interruptions. Arrange privacy for the interview, away from the telephone. Letting the applicant know you have "held all calls" shows you are interested in him or her. Constant interruptions will break the flow of conversation and prevent a good exchange of information.

Condescending or Authoritative Attitude. If you "look down" on the applicant, not only will the applicant not open up—he or she will not want to work for you. This attitude places the applicant in a compromised position. Always display an attitude of respect, warmth, and concern.

Not Listening. Nothing is more frustrating than for you to ask a question the applicant has already answered. The applicant will know you were not paying attention. Listen to what the applicant says and *does not say.* Be aware of what is left out.

Expressing Criticism or Judgment. When an applicant is explaining past behavior or experiences, never express surprise or judgment. This will shut off communication, or the applicant will only tell you what he or she thinks you want to hear. Save opinions for the evaluation process, and just focus on getting information.

Beware of the Snow Job. Some applicants are exceptional at interviewing and can say all the "right things." Be wary of the one with perfect answers and clichés. Try to delve beneath the surface and perceive the person underneath.

Avoid Snap Decisions and Early Judgments. Sometimes an applicant may look like someone you know or have a characteristic that causes you to label him or her as a certain type of person. From that point on you may keep a certain impression. Do not draw conclusions from subjective likes or dislikes. Formulating an opinion early in the interview can block objectivity and effective exploration of information. Use a consistent line of questioning with all applicants, and avoid a decision until the process has been completed.

Avoid Prejudgment. If you have heard about or know the applicant, you probably have formed an opinion. If you cannot be objective, you should not participate in the interview process. Always avoid listening to gossip and subjective opinions prior to the interview. Information used for evaluation purposes should only be obtained through the appropriate channels, i.e., work references and other verification procedures.

Observation of Nonverbal Behavior. Interviewers must learn not only to listen to what is said, but how it is said. This includes the quality of the voice and changes in tone or loudness. Also watch facial expressions, hand movement, mannerisms, and body movement. Though you expect some nervousness, watch for unusual talkativeness, agitation, lack of eye contact, and other clues to behavior. Gather all possible information so that the person best suited for the job can be selected.

Objectivity. As stated earlier, the objective is to elicit the same types of information from each candidate, and have a standard means for interpreting the information. This involves a large degree of objectivity—that is, as much as is humanly possible. By developing an understanding of human behavior, sharpening the senses of perception, and avoiding communication pitfalls, a more effective interview can take place. A supportive atmosphere will enhance communication and create a favorable image for your facility. This is an important recruitment tool for the future.

Preparing for the Interview

Needed Information. In addition to training for the interview process, there is certain information the interviewer will need to prepare for the interview. This information should be obtained several days in advance of the interview and should include:

1. The job description and specific information related to the job (see Appendices 6–1 and 6–2).
2. The short and long application forms, with completed preliminary screening form (Figures 7–2 through 7–4) and rated application form (Figure 7–12).
3. The appropriate position attachment (Figures 7–5 through 7–8) completed by the applicant, and the completed rating of the attachment (Figure 7–13).
4. Any work references, letters of recommendation, etc.
5. If all information has not been validated from previous employers or educational facilities, final ratings are postponed until a later date. (All information must be received and evaluated for the applicant to be eligible for selection, however). The interviewer can still conduct the interview pending receipt of transcripts, etc. Of course, if application ratings are utilized for screening purposes, information must be complete before elimination of any applicants.

Interviewers should receive the information, review it carefully, and make notes and questions for the interview. If more than one nurse will be conducting interviews, they should get together and discuss the line of questioning, procedure, group leader, and other appropriate concerns. Time limitations should also be agreed upon.

Preparation for Interviews and Development of Questions and Evaluation Tools

As stated earlier, interviewers must strive for objective, consistent gathering of information, with a standard means for interpreting this information. During their preparation period, they should meet to discuss goals, philosophy, and strategies for interviewing. They should agree upon the ground rules as a group. Individually, they should review all appropriate materials, mark questions and clarification needs on the application and rating forms, and note special areas to explore with the applicant. In addition, they can use standard interview checklists or formats to further ensure uniformity of questioning. Interview guides can be developed with a list to follow during the interview, to ensure that all needed areas are covered. Figure 7–14 displays an example of an interview guide. The interviewer can follow this line of questioning, then write comments and notes on the lines provided. Later these notes assist in the evaluation process. It is important not to rely on memory, but to take careful notes. At the close of the interview, the summary and additional observations should be recorded immediately.

Figure 7–15 is a guide to collecting information concerning the applicant's characteristics, values, and behaviors. During discussion of work experiences and other subjects, the interviewer constantly observes and listens for deeper information. Specific questioning can be geared to collect this information, and be prepared in advance. In general, this guide concerns impressions formulated during the interview, and does involve subjectivity. But keep in mind that *all* information, including rating scales and input from others, is used in the decision-making process. Impressions of the applicant can be important tools when choosing between two equally rated candidates.

Interviewers can develop other types of tools to assist in data collection. Tests are available that measure motivation, problem-solving skills, and other characteristics. Sentence-completion questions, written testing, case studies to analyze hypothetical situations, and other evaluation methodology may be used. Actual demonstration of clinical skills in a lab or real-life situation may be used to measure clinical competency. Evaluation tools can increase the objectivity of decision making, but must be validated and tested for reliability. Each method must have specific and measurable evaluation criteria.

The use of tests and evaluation tools will depend on the sophistication of the facility and the job vacancy, as well as the philosophy of the nursing service. Tests must also be job-related, provide necessary information for selection of a candidate, and be nondiscriminatory.

If tests are used, keep in mind that they should never be the sole basis for selection. They are simply tools to assist in the decision-making process. Used in combination, all tools contribute to the effectiveness of the decision. Remember, the final decision is always based upon *human judgment.* Testing can be a threatening experience for many individuals. They may not respond well under observation, or may simply not do well on tests. The degree of nervousness and *need for a job* can interfere with their true abilities. This must be considered when using this evaluation methodology.

Summary of Interviews and Evaluation of Applicants

After the interviews are conducted, the interviewer should document all thoughts, notes, and comments on the interview guides. Then the evaluation process begins. As seen at the bottom of Figure 7–15, there is a space for summaries of strengths, weaknesses, and recommendations. This is a tool for evaluation that is used in the following example. If a two-to-one, panel, or group interview was conducted, interviewers discuss and complete this tool together. Otherwise, the interviewer should review all notes, documentation, and comments on the interview, and come to some conclusions. The conclusion, based upon the interview, will be whether the applicant is outstanding, highly recommended, recommended, or not recommended for the position. Rationale for this conclusion must be stated, with reference to specific items on the interview guide.

In evaluating applicants and determining recommendations, interviewers should be careful to avoid the same type of pitfalls that can occur during the interview process. They must avoid being overly lenient or strict, but try to be fair and objective. Some interviewers avoid extremes, and always rate applicants "middle of the road." Others may feel sorry for a candidate who is in great need of a job, so give him or her a higher recommendation. If an applicant is outstanding in one area, some raters tend to evaluate that applicant as outstanding in all areas. Nurse-managers must work with the interviewers to overcome these types of obstacles, and only allow recommendations that are based upon sound and thorough documentation. All decisions must be supported by facts and an explanation of interpretations. Although the interpretation is a human judgment, all efforts must be taken to maintain objectivity. This takes training, monitoring by management, and willingness by interviewers to improve their skills.

RECOMMENDATIONS FOR APPOINTMENT

This component of the selection process involves the actual selection of the best-qualified candidate for the position. It extends from the interview process and is based upon the judgment, interpretation, and data collected by the interviewers, as well as all other available information on the applicant. This component is the decision-making step to matching the right candidate to the job.

Recommendation of an applicant for appointment may occur through various mechanisms. If a panel or several people have conducted interviews, the final decision may be reached by total group consensus of the interviewers. This means that all applicants are discussed, strengths and weaknesses are explored, and one candidate is agreed upon by every interviewer. This method can be very effective. If the decision is based upon group consensus or one interviewer's recommendations, it must still be guided by input from the nurses who will work with the new employee, and by a selection policy. An example of a selection policy and procedure is shown in Figure 7–16.

The interviewers may select the new employee, or the nurse-manager may form a selection team to make the recommendation. This team could include interviewers and two to three other people such as the head nurse, nurse-recruiter, and another nurse-manager. If management conducted the interviews, staff nurses from the unit could be included on the selection team. Either way, the head nurse and nurse-recruiter must be involved and provide direction and assistance throughout the entire process. The nursing staff should participate either in the interview process or in the selection decision. Staff input will facilitate the acceptance and adjustment of the new employee.

Although the selection policy (Fig. 7–16) guides decision making for selecting a candidate, it cannot make the decision. When several equally qualified candidates must be eliminated, the selection team must call upon deep insight into human behavior. They must be aware of the culture and personality of the unit and look for a candidate who can not only fit this culture, but grow and contribute to the organization.

The team must call into play the intuitive and creative thought processes, and allow intuition to take a part in the decision. Up until this point, the process has been as analytical and objective as possible. But when numbers and ratings can no longer contribute to the decision, the skills of perception and intuition must enter in. The organization that practices, trains, and encourages creative thought will have personnel who are in tune to its intuitive abilities. These people will be ready and able to call on their deeper perceptions to assist in the final decision.

NO QUALIFIED CANDIDATES FOR APPOINTMENT

If the selection team determines that no qualified candidate is available to fill the position, several steps can be taken. The nurse-recruiters and the nurse-manager can reassess the pool of candidates to determine the status of candidates who were eliminated due to low application rating scores or who were not interviewed due to a large number of applicants. Another series of interviews may be set up for these applicants.

If no qualified applicants are available, the recruitment search may be reactivated. A training program may be developed due to the lack of qualified candidates. In some cases of small numbers of interested and "trainable" internal candidates, a program may be developed to train outside applicants who lack certain skills. Or the nurse-manager may choose to appoint a person temporarily to the position, who may enter the training program or be eligible for permanent appointment following a trial period.

Lastly, the nurse-manager can decide to leave the vacancy or alter the position. Although this decision should have been made during the planning and recruitment process, the expense in training and lack of qualified internal or external candidates may cause this to become the only solution.

APPROVAL MECHANISMS

As stated earlier, in a decentralized approach to management, the nursing staff participates in decision making. The staff is involved in screening, interviewing, and selecting new employees, but the head nurse maintains final approval for recommending a candidate for appointment and is accountable for all activities on the unit. The head nurse must monitor and evaluate the selection process, correct any problems or deficiencies, and ensure that the interviewers are objective and that the best-qualified candidate was selected by a fair and systematic process. The head nurse is accountable to the vice-president for nursing, who can approve or disapprove the final decision.

Management must take great care to allow freedom and participation while avoiding unnecessary interference. The nurses must know their responsibilities, expectations, and ground rules. The structure should be provided, then freedom to be creative should be allowed within that structure; mistakes must also be allowed. The nurses must know also that they must strive for constant improvement and maintain standards and policies. They must know that their actions, based upon sound rationale, will be supported. However, deviations from standards and policies, or actions in conflict with the basic goals and philosophy of the nursing department, should not be tolerated.

All nurse-managers must learn the art of participative management. Any interference or disapproval of the nurses' decisions must be followed with valid explanations. At times an unpopular decision will be made due to necessity. By opening communication, allowing the nurses to ventilate their feelings and explain their opposition, and always being "aboveboard" and open, the nurse-manager can gain their respect and trust. The key to remember is that human resources are the most valuable element in the success of the organization. Communicate and practice this belief.

AGREEMENT ON TERMS OF EMPLOYMENT

After a candidate has been selected for appointment and approved through the appropriate mechanism, a contract should be signed delineating the terms of employment. By this time the nurse-manager should know whether the candidate is willing to accept the position. On some occasions, however, applicants have received other job offers or have changed their minds. They may have been turned off by the interviewers or some other element of the organization. Reasons for declining an offer of employment can be investigated and documented on the bottom of the interview guide (see Fig. 7–15). Then the nurse-recruiter is notified, and the selection process is reactivated. The selection team reviews the pool of applicants' ratings and interview recommendations and recommends another candidate.

If the applicant accepts the position, a contract is drawn up with the agreed-on terms of employment, and both the nurse-manager and the applicant sign. This signifies the hiring of the new employee, and an orientation date is set. Contracts will vary according to the needs of the applicant and the facility. An example of a contract agreement is provided in Figure 7–17.

NOTIFICATION OF OTHER APPLICANTS

Once the contract is signed, those applicants not chosen should be notified immediately. They can be contacted by phone or letter, and given the opportunity to come in and discuss other possibilities with the nurse-recruiter. Reasons for not being selected, and recommendations for continuing education, additional skills training, or other improvements should be given. A list of other vacancies or future job openings for which they are qualified can also be supplied. All efforts must be made to project an appreciation for their time and interest and show respect and concern for them as individuals. Contact should be maintained with qualified applicants as a means of recruitment for the future.

CONCLUSION

The selection process is a crucial part of any successful organization. Policies and procedures should be developed and managed according to the needs of the organization and the needs of the work force. Prospective employees want to know about not only the job responsibilities, but also their degree of involvement, independence, and decision making within the organization. They must be allowed to meet and talk to staff nurses on the prospective unit and interact with employees. On the other hand, employees should participate in decisions regarding their peers. Because they know the needs of the unit and must work with the new employee, they should be allowed to have some say in the selection process. This participation will contribute to improving morale, professionalism, accountability, and acceptance of the new employee. It will also help to decrease turnover.

Selection of internal employees for promotion or a different position can also follow these procedures. Evaluation and ratings may include additional criteria, such as seniority, scores on performance appraisals, and participation within the organization. Otherwise, the selection process is similar.

Although the focus of this chapter has been on participative selection of the staff nurse, a nurse-management position can also be filled in a similar fashion. The decision to allow staff nurses to select their manager will depend upon the degree of professionalism and the needs of the unit. But their input and involvement is still important, if only as consultants to the selection team. As with any process, the outcome is dependent upon those involved. Flexible, creative thinkers who maintain high standards are necessary to effective selection outcomes. And, as in all personnel processes, a high regard for the human resource must be upheld.

The nursing staff should be included in the evaluation of the selection process. When selected candidates turn down a job offer, an assessment should be made of reasons, and problem areas should be identified and corrected. If a decision is made to leave a position vacant, staff nurses must be involved in how to redistribute the work, change the position, and how to compensate nurses absorbing these responsibilities. If a candidate terminates employment within the first year, reasons should be determined as to the role of selection in this turnover. Although other personnel processes play a big role in retention, selection should be evaluated to ensure that the right person was chosen for the right job. If selection processes were effective, then the orientation procedures should be investigated and evaluated.

The outcome of selection will greatly depend upon the adjustment of the new employee in the new job. Orientation processes are a crucial link in retaining new employees. When the right candidate has been selected for the right job, he or she must then be provided the tools and assistance to achieve desired competencies and become a part of the organization. Without this assistance, a potentially creative individual can become frustrated, dissatisfied, and terminate employment. Successful selection is dependent upon the adjustment of the new employee into this new role.

REFERENCES

1. Poteet, G. W. The employment interview—Avoiding discriminatory questioning. *JONA*, 1984, *14*(4), 38–42.
2. Shepard, I. M., & Doudera, A. E. *Health care labor law*. Ann Arbor, Michigan: Health Administration Press, University of Michigan, 1981, pp. 179–214.
3. Poteet, G. W., & Pardue, S. F. Falsifying credentials: A dilemma in the faculty appointment process (Unpublished manuscript, University of Texas School of Nursing, University of Texas Medical Branch, Galveston, 1985), pp. 1–14.
4. Koen, C. M. Application forms: Keep them easy and legal. *Personnel Journal*, 1984, *63*(5), 26–29.
5. Bell, J. C., Castagnera, J., & Young, J. P. Employment references: Do you know the law? *Personnel Journal*, 1984, *63*(2), 32–36.

SUGGESTED READING

Anonymous. Evaluating employment applications. *Personnel Journal*, 1984, *63*(1), 22, 24.

Battle, E. H., Bragg, S., Delaney, J., et al. Developing a rating interview guide. *JONA*, 1985, *15*(10), 39–45.

Bayne, R., & Fletcher, C. Selecting the selectors. *Personnel Management*, 1983, *15*(6), 42–44.

Bloom, R., & Prien, E. P. A guide to job-related interviewing. *Personnel Administration*, 1983, *28*(10), 81–86, 112.

Bray, K. A. The interview process. *Critical Care Nurse*, 1984, *4*(3), 65–67.

Brinckerhoff, J. H. The job interview as a marketing tool. *Marketing Communications*, 1983, *8*(12), 74–75.

Campbell, A. Hiring for results—Interviews that select winners. *Business Quarterly*, 1983, *48*(4), 57–61.

Campion, M. Personnel selection for physically demanding jobs: Review and recommendations. *Personnel Psychology*, 1983, *36*(3), 527–550.

Daum, J. W. Interviewer training: The key to an innovative selection process that works. *Training*, 1983, *20*(12), 62–63.

Day, C. M. Recruiting and interviewing. *Hospital Forum*, 1983, *26*(1), 43–46.

Drake, J. D. Interviewing for managers: A complete guide to employment interviewing. New York: AMACOM, 1982.

Ertl, N. Choosing successful managers: Participative selection can help. *JONA*, 1984, *14*(4), 27–33.

Hough, L. M. An evaluation of three "alternative" selection procedures. *Personnel Psychology*, 1983, *36*(2), 261–276.

Johnson, E. P., Wagner, D. H., & Sweeney, J. P. Identifying the right nurse manager. *JONA*, 1984, *14*(11), 24–30.

Kohl, J. P. Personnel decisions: How to avoid discrimination charges. *Cornell Hotel and Restaurant Administration Quarterly*, 1983, *24*(3), 86–92.

Korn, L. Selecting chief executives—Their relationship with a corporation. *Vital Speeches*, 1984, *50*(7), 204–207.

Lawsche, C. H. A simplified approach to the evaluation of fairness in employee selection procedures. *Personnel Psychology*, 1983, *36*(3), 601–608.

Lorber, L. Z. Basic advice on avoiding employment-at-will troubles. *Personnel Administration*, 1984, *29*(1), 59–62.

Merrit-Haston, R., & Wexley, K. N. Educational requirements: Legality and validity. *Personnel Psychology*, 1983, *36*(4), 743–753.

Mumford, M. D. Social comparison theory and the evaluation of peer evaluations: A review and some applied implications. *Personnel Psychology*, 1983, *36*(4), 867–881.

Niehoff, M. S. Assessment centers: Decision-making information from non-test-based methods. *Small Group Behavior*, 1983, *14*(3), 353–358.

Parker, R. S. How do superiors judge you? *Security Management*, 1984, *28*(4), 88–92.

Riley, J. R. Successful salespeople have experience in other fields. *Rough Notes*, 1984, *127*(2), 16, 40–41.

Sadek, K. E., Hall, R. W., & Tomeski, A. E. *Leadership and Organization Development Journal*, 1983, *4*(4), 10–16.

Scott, S. Finding the right person. *Personnel Journal*, 1983, *62*(11), 894.

Silver, M. B. Picking promotable people. *Hospital Forum*, 1982, *26*(6), 45–49.

Snodgrass, G., & Wheeler, R. W. A research-based sequential job interview training model. *Journal of College Student Personnel*, 1983, *24*(5), 449–454.

Souder, W. E., & Leksich, A. M. Assessment centers are evolving toward a bright future. *The Personnel Administrator*, 1983, *28*(11), 80.

Spang, S. Business besieged by bogus resumes. *Business and Society Review*, 1984, *48*, 39–40.

Sullivan, E. J., Decker, P. J., & Hailstone, S. Assessment center technology: Selecting head nurses. *JONA, 1985, 15*(5), 13–18.

Wolf, M. Hiring people who do good research. *Research Management*, 1984, *27*(1), 8–9.

Wouder, B. D., & Keleman, K. S. Increasing the value of reference information. *Personnel Administrator*, 1984, *29*(3), 98–103.

Zedeck, S. Interviewer validity and reliability: An individual analysis approach. *Personnel Psychology*, 1983, *36*(2), 355–370.

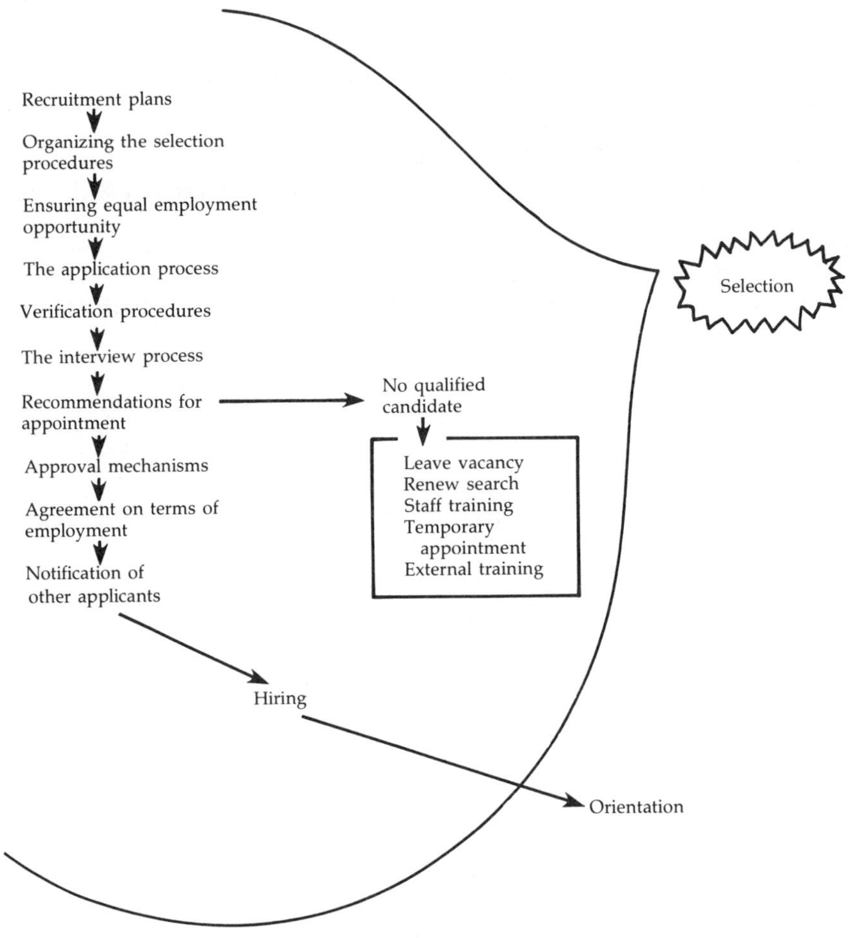

Figure 7–1. Components of the selection process.

(Please print)

Full name ____________________ Date ______ Home phone ________
Address ______________________________ Work phone ________
Position desired ____________________ Licensure/certification ________
Highest academic degree held ____________________ Specialized training and skills ____________________
Summary of past five working years' experiences pertinent to the job
____
____
____
____
Signature ____________________

Figure 7–2. Short application form for screening.

Applicant's name____________________ Position____________________

Required behaviors: Must all be checked "yes" to be eligible for the job.

1. On time for the interview, or provides sufficient rationale for being late. yes________ no________
2. Appearance is neat, clean, and well groomed. yes________ no________
3. Is able to communicate. Speaks so can be understood; affect is appropriate with conversation; understands and responds appropriately to questions. yes________ no________
4. Has congenial attitude. Is not hostile or abrasive. yes________ no________
5. Appears interested in the job. Is attentive. yes________ no________

Meets minimum requirements for employment according to short application form provided: yes________ no________

If any "no's," explain____

Additional comments____

Signature of interviewer____________________________ Date:______

Evaluation of short application form (Must all be checked "yes")

Holds required licensure/certification	yes________	no________
Holds required educational degrees	yes________	no________
Has required training/skills	yes________	no________
Has required job experiences	yes________	no________
Meets minimum requirements for employment	yes________	no________

If any "no's," explain____

Additional comments____

Signature of screener____________________________ Date:______

Figure 7–3. Preliminary interview and screening evaluation form.

Date______
Full name____
Address_________________ Phone_________________ or________________
Desired position________________________ Other positions for which you may be qualified____________________ Social Security number________________
U.S. citizen: yes no. If no, type of visa________________ Immigration no.________
Desire full-time [ ] part-time [ ]. Describe days and shifts available to work, and if part-time, number of days/week____

____

____

Date available to begin work________________ Have you applied here before? yes no
If yes, when?__________________ Have you ever been employed here before? yes no
If yes, when?______ Were you known by a different name in a previous job that we will need for verification of this information? yes no
If yes, give name______________________ How long have you been a resident of this city?______ Do we now employ any of your relatives? yes no If yes, list names________

____

____

Do you have any health-related conditions that could interfere with your ability to carry out the functions of the job for which you have applied? yes no
If yes, please explain____

____

____

What languages do you speak and write fluently?____________________________
Are you 18 years of age or older? (legal age of employment) yes no
Have you ever been convicted of a crime? yes no. If yes, where, when, and nature of conviction____

____

____

Are any felony charges presently pending against you? yes no. Military record: Have you served in the armed forces? yes no. If yes, branch__________ Dates of active service______ Person to notify in case of emergency__________________________
phone________________________________ How were you referred to our hospital?

____

____

If presently employed, may we contact your current employer for a reference? yes no

Professional Licenses or Certifications:____________________________________

____

Type____
Organization, or state issued____
Date issued____
Number____
Exp. date____

*Information on these forms will be verified for accuracy.

Figure 7–4A. Standard application form: front.

Education

List all schools and colleges attended, including technical, business, and military schools and training. (Official transcripts required.)

School	Dates	Academic Degree or Certification	Major subjects studied
Name__________ Address__________			
Name__________ Address__________			
Name__________ Address__________			
Name__________ Address__________			

Employment History

Begin with your current or last employer and trace the past ten years of work experience, or since school. Attach additional sheets if needed.

Employer name and address __________ Phone _____ Dates of employment __________ Salary at start _____ Salary at termination _____ Supervisor __________ Position and responsibilities __________ Days/week _____ Reason for leaving __________

Employer name and address __________ Phone _____ Dates of employment __________ Salary at start _____ Salary at termination _____ Supervisor __________ Position and responsibilities __________ Days/week _____ Reason for leaving __________

Employer name and address __________ Phone _____ Dates of employment __________ Salary at start _____ Salary at termination _____ Supervisor __________ Position and responsibilities __________ Days/week _____ Reason for leaving __________

Employer name and address __________ Phone _____ Dates of employment __________ Salary at start _____ Salary at termination _____ Supervisor __________ Position and responsibilities __________ Days/week _____ Reason for leaving __________

Employer name and address __________ Phone _____ Dates of employment __________ Salary at start _____ Salary at termination _____ Supervisor __________ Position and responsibilities __________ Days/week _____ Reason for leaving __________

Figure 7–4B. Standard application form: back.

1. Why did you apply for this position?

2. Briefly describe your philosophy concerning human resource management.

3. Any previous involvement in research? Explain.

4. Publications:

5. Awards/honors:

6. Continuing education related to this position (verification of attendance required):

7. Seminar/workshop presentations:

8. Participation in professional organizations:

9. Community service involvement:

10. Professional growth and development goals:

11. "I have expertise in the following:"

	Yes	**Somewhat**	**No**
Nursing standards of care			
Problem solving			
Patient care planning			
Quality assurance and control			
Creative planning			
Effecting planned change			
Risk management			
Employee interviews and selection			
Performance appraisals			
Conflict resolution			
Budgeting			
Progressive discipline			
Communication and interpersonal skills			
Scheduling			
Counseling			
Patient acuity systems			
Management information systems			
Delegation			

I certify that the above information on this application is true, and agree that any concealed or false information is grounds for my immediate discharge.

Signature ______________________ Date ______________________

Figure 7–5. Attachment for nursing management position.

1. Reason for applying for this position:
2. Briefly describe your philosophy of nursing and patient care.
3. Describe your professional growth and development goals.
4. Any experience in research? Explain.
5. Participation in professional organizations:
6. Community service and involvement:
7. Honors/awards:
8. Special scheduling preferences, such as 12-hour shifts, weekends only, etc.
9. Expanded skills and training, i.e., advanced cardiac life support, hemodynamic monitoring, certification in chemotherapy, expertise in working with computers, and other job-related CE (verification required):
10. Any special talents that could contribute to creative patient care?
11. "I have expertise in the following:"

	Yes	Somewhat	No
Implementing nursing standards of care			
Quality assurance			
Nursing process			
Patient care planning			
Documentation			
Discharge planning			
Patient teaching			
Problem solving			
Patient assessment			
Planning and effecting change			
Committee participation and group work			
Delegating and coordinating care			
Total patient care			
24-hour accountability			

I certify that the above information on this application is true, and agree that any concealed or false information is grounds for my immediate discharge.
Signature ________________________ Date ________________________

Figure 7–6. Attachment for a registered nurse position.

1. Reason for applying for this position:
2. Briefly describe any special training, continuing education, or experiences that help to qualify you for this position.
3. What are your feelings about providing total patient care under the supervision of an R.N.?
4. Describe your career and/or learning goals.
5. Participation in nursing organizations:
6. Participation in community organizations and services:
7. Honors/awards:
8. Any special talents that could contribute to creative patient care?
9. Other advanced training in expanded practice, i.e., inserting IVs and NG tubes, working with computers or cardiac monitors, etc.:
10. "I have experience and/or training in the following:"

	Yes	**Somewhat**	**No**
Total patient care			
Patient assessment			
Patient care planning			
Documentation			
Problem solving			
Committee participation and group work			
Patient orientation			
Patient teaching			
Discharge planning			

I certify that the above information on this application is true, and agree that any concealed or false information is grounds for my immediate discharge.
Signature ______________________ Date ______________________

Figure 7–7. Attachment for a licensed practical nurse position.

1. What special training, continuing education, or experiences have you had that help to qualify you for this position?

2. Any special career or educational plans for the next 5 years? Explain.

3. Honors/awards:

4. Special equipment you operate with skill:

5. Any additional talents that could contribute to patient care?

6. "I have experience/training in the following:"

	Yes	**Somewhat**	**No**
Baths and skin care			
Oral hygiene			
Intake and output			
Walking patients			
Specimen collection			
Positioning patients			
Vital signs			
Enemas			
Weighing patients			
Lifting patients			
Patient admissions			
Patient discharges			
Transporting patients			
Handwashing			
Feeding patients			
Patient observation			

I certify that the above information on this application is true, and agree that any concealed or false information is grounds for my immediate discharge.

Signature ______________________ Date ______________________

Figure 7–8. Attachment for an aide/orderly position.

Dear ____________________,

____________________ (applicant's name), Social Security number ________________ has applied for the position of ____________________ at our hospital. To thoroughly evaluate his/her qualifications, we need information from previous employers. This information is strictly confidential and used for employee selection only. Thank you for your time and assistance.

Sincerely,

____

Jane Doe, Director of Nursing
University Hospital

Authorization for Release of Information: I have agreed to this reference check and release you from any liability in providing information concerning my work, work habits, and employment while at ____.

________________________ ________

Applicant's Signature Date

Please complete the following and return in the stamped, self-addressed envelope

Name of Facility ________________ Employee's name and SS# ______________

Dates of employment______to______ Full-time [ ] Part-time [ ] ______________ hours/week

Position and responsibilities ____

____

Immediate supervisor ________________ Reason for leaving ______________

________________________________ Starting and ending salaries ____________

Please check the following and provide rationale below for any excellent, below average or unacceptable ratings. Additional comments are welcomed.

	Excellent	**Above average**	**Below average**	**Unacceptable**
Attendance and dependability				
Patient rapport				
Motivation for self-improvement				
Interpersonal relations (ability to work with others)				
Clinical skills/expertise				
Committee participation and organizational involvement				
Attitude/tolerance to change				

Rationale ____

____

____

Additional strengths/weaknesses/comments ______________________________

____

Rater's signature ________________ Position ________________ Date ______

Figure 7–9. Sample R.N. employment reference form.

Policy

All nurses employed at ________________ will maintain a current Alabama license, as administered by the Alabama Board of Nursing.

Persons not properly licensed will not be allowed to practice nursing. This includes nurse-anesthetists.

Procedure

New employees. Will present their Alabama license to the administrative secretary for nursing when submitting an application for employment.

Re-registration. Each nurse is responsible for maintaining a current Alabama license. Each nurse will present his/her new renewal card to the administrative secretary prior to the expiration of the current license.

New graduates. Must present a current Alabama temporary permit to practice in the state of Alabama with a specific expiration date. Following state board examinations, the permanent license must be presented to the administrative secretary prior to the expiration of the temporary permit. If the new graduate fails state boards, he or she is reduced to aide status until completion and evidence of passing boards. All efforts will be made to provide employment during this interim.

Graduates of foreign nurse training programs. Must present a current Alabama registration or current temporary permit to practice in the state of Alabama, with a specific expiration date.

Out-of-state graduates. Must present a current Alabama registration or a current Alabama temporary permit to practice nursing in the state of Alabama, with a specific expiration date.

Outside agencies. Nurses employed by outside agencies must present a current Alabama Registration, or a temporary permit, with a specific expiration date.

The Administrative Secretary for Nursing will:

1. Inspect the license or renewal card for each nurse, to verify the correct name, expiration date, and its authenticity.
2. Record the registration number and renewal number from the card on a licensure list. This list maintains all nurses employed in the institution, with their license numbers and expiration dates. Names are recorded on this list *only* following inspection and verification of authenticity of license.
3. Licenses of new nurses (not currently employed in the institution) are verified by contacting the Alabama Board of Nursing.
4. The licensure list is reviewed monthly by the Administrative Secretary for expirations. When a permanent license is presented, the new number and expiration date are recorded to the side.
5. At the end of each "licensure year," renewal cards must be presented prior to the expiration date on the old license.

Figure 7–10. Sample procedure for verifying licensure.

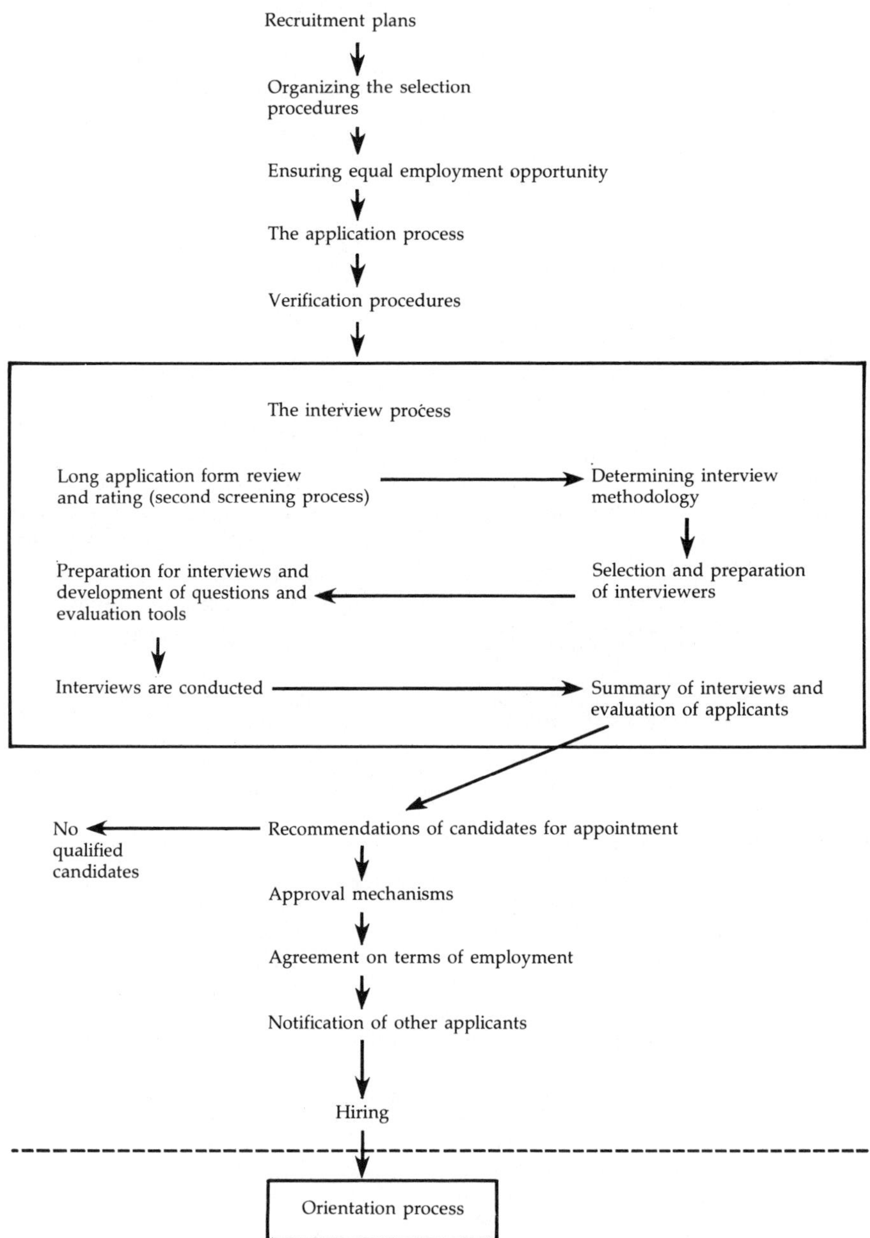

Figure 7–11. The interview process within the total selection process.

Applicant's name ________________

1. General: The application form is Complete ___ Legible ___ Neat ___ Consistent information ___

(award 1 point for each) ______

(total possible points = 4) Total

2. Employment

Work experience directly related to the job vacancy:

Full-time: award 0.5 points times number of months worked ________

Part time: award 0.1 points per average days worked each week, times number of months worked. (If worked 3 days/week for 6 months—3 × 0.1 × 6 months = 1.8 points) ________

Additional work experience *indirectly related** to job vacancy-

Full time: award 0.25 points times number of months worked ________

Part time: award 0.05 point/days worked each week times months worked ________

3. Education: High school graduate or GED (must have for employment) ________ yes

Certification in job vacancy by accredited program. Nurses include clinical certification through ANA or accredited specialty organization. Award 3 points ________

Certification in related field through accredited program. Award 1.5 points ________

Other formal CE *related to job vacancy* (use transcripts to calculate credit). This *excludes* minimum degree requirements. Award *0.1 point per semester hour* completed over minimum requirements. (If Associate Degree ________ or Diploma in Nursing required, but applicant has a B.S.N., award 6 points) ________

4. Academic Achievement

For completion of educational program leading to the *minimum degree* requirements (high school, A.D., Diploma B.S.N. or M.S.N.)

If overall grade point average 3.5–4.0 award 5 points ________

If grade point average between 3.0–3.4 award 3 points ________

For completion of additional *educational degrees related to the job*. GPA 3.5–4.0 award 2.5 points; for 3.0–3.4 award 1.5 points ________

Previous employer references: verifies *accuracy* of information on application (required for employment) ________ yes

Educational transcripts: verifies accuracy of information on application (required for employment) ________ yes

Licensure verification (required for employment) ________ yes

Is legal age to work (18 years or older) ________ yes

U.S. citizen or has work permit/visa ________ yes

If previously employed here, performance evaluations satisfactory. ________ yes

Total points ______ Meets all requirements (yes items) ________________

*Criteria should be predetermined and standardized.

Figure 7–12. Rating the standard application form.

1. Why did you apply for this position?
   - **U** (Unsatisfactory): Poor sentence structure, spelling, and writing skills; "need a job;" lack of planning or thought about the facility and personal goals. 0 points:________
   - **S** (Satisfactory): Proper grammar, spelling, and sentence structure; congruence of position opening with personal/career goals; displays preplanning and thought concerning the future. 1 point:________
   - **A** (Above Average): Includes all of "S," plus matching of personal talents, experiences with job opening, opportunities for personal growth and contribution to the organization. 2 points:________
   - **E** (Excellent): All in "A," plus creative, innovative approach, scholarly writing style. 3 points:________
2. Briefly describe your philosophy concerning human resource management.
   - **U** Poor sentence structure, spelling, and writing skills; lack of thought; theory X attitude (workers are unmotivated and lazy). 0 points:________
   - **S** Regard for each worker's worth; statement of management style; for example, favors decentralized versus centralized approach; favors employee input and participation; open-door policy, etc. 1 point:________
   - **A** Provides rationale for philosophy, such as to maximize productivity and job satisfaction; relates philosophy to outcome. Includes all of "S." 2 points:________
   - **E** Includes all of "A;" cites need for creativity and innovation and management's role in fostering these things; uses skill in writing. 3 points:________
3. Previous involvement in research:
   - None 0 points________
   - Assisted in implementing research 2 points________
   - Assisted in developing and implementing a research project 3 points________
   - Developed, initiated, implemented, and evaluated two or more research projects. 4 points________
4. Publications: Award 1 point for every publication in a job-related, recognized journal or magazine. ________
5. Awards/honors: Outstanding employee, scholarships, or awards for outstanding achievement; civic awards, selection to honorary societies, appointment to special professional or civic boards and committees, professional recognition awards. Award 2 points each ________

Figure 7–13. Nursing management position attachment rating scale.

6. Continuing education related to this position: Award 1 point for every CEU (10 contact hour) directly related to this job. Verify with certificates of attendance or transcripts from professional organizations. ________
7. Seminar/workshop presentations: Award 0.5 points for every hour presented (prepared and presented the seminar or presentation). Include only past 5 years. Maximum points allowed = 10 points. ________
8. Participation in professional organizations:
   0.1 point for every professional membership ________
   add
   0.5 points for each year held an office or chaired a committee. Include only past 5 years. ________
9. Community service involvement: Award 0.1 point for each hour of participation in community education, prevention, screening programs, health fairs, and other health-related public service. ________
10. Professional growth and development goals:
    U Nonspecific, such as "to be the best nurse I can be," etc. 0 points________
    S Identifies learning needs, areas in need of growth 1 point________
    A Gives specific plans such as working toward B.S.N., taking a course in computers, certification, with projected time and pace 2 points________
    E Includes creative contributions, innovative thought, plans for political involvement, networking, publishing, and ideas for how this will contribute to the nursing profession and the organization. 3 points________
11. I have expertise in the following: yes 0.5 somewhat 0.2 no 0 points
    (refer to attachment)
    Total number of "yes" ________ times 0.5 = ________
    Total number of "somewhat" ________ times 0.2 = ________

Totals from questions 1–11 = ________

Total from numbers 1–4 of standard application form = + ________

and meets all minimum requirements (yes items on standard form) Total Score = ________

____

Application rating completed by:________ ________

________ ________

________ ________

________ ________

signatures date

Figure 7–13. *(continued)*

Date ______________________

Applicant's name ______________________

Interviewer ______________________

1. Greetings and introductions
2. Purpose of interview and explanation of selection process
3. Small talk to ease nervousness and establish rapport
4. Reference to application—start with page 1 of application and clarify questions, problems, preferences, health-related problems, date can begin working, and areas in need of clarification. ______________________
5. Employment history—expand on experiences, responsibilities, and expertise the applicant thinks makes him or her qualified for the job. ______________________

   Further clarification of reasons for leaving, lapses in employment. ______________________

   Allow discussion of growth and progressive development in previous positions, i.e., promotions, career ladder advancement, increases in salary, increased responsibilities during employment. ______________________
6. Position attachment—clarify questions and discuss. Include types of experiences, training, and discussion of areas of expertise—attempt to validate self-appraisal. ______________________
7. Explore attitude towards patients—what is a "good patient," their rights, involvement of family, and other patient needs. ______________________
8. Employee references—praise outstanding references, inquire about problem areas, and allow explanation by applicant. ______________________
9. Review job description—request applicant's questions/concerns and determine willingness to carry out responsibilities. ______________________
10. Review specific information about the job and unit—allow applicant to explain why he or she meets these qualifications. Discuss strengths and weaknesses of the job. ______________________
11. Discuss salary and scheduling—questions/problems. ______________________
12. Additional questions specific to the job, or applicant's qualifications. ______________________
13. Allow questions by the applicant. ______________________
14. Close interview—state appreciation of time and interest, enjoyment in meeting and talking with applicant, praise and recognition of talents and accomplishments. Let the applicant know when he or she will hear from you. If any questions, whom to call. Thank the applicant again.
15. Additional notes. ______________________

Figure 7–14. The interview guide.

What is your impression of the applicant's

1. Confidence and self-esteem________
2. Ability to accept change/flexibility________
3. Ability to cope with stress and frustration________
4. Interaction and communication skills________
5. Self-motivation for growth and improvement________
6. Stamina to perform duties________
7. Potential for creativeness and innovative contributions________
8. Problem-solving abilities________
9. Potential for a cultural fit on the unit and in the organization________
10. Additional comments and notes________

Summary of Special Strengths | *Summary of Special Weaknesses*

Recommendations based upon interview (outstanding, highly recommended, recommended, or not recommended) with rationale________

Application rating score______
Selected for position: yes no Date______
Rationale________

If not selected, follow-up actions and recommendations________

If selected, administrative approval obtained________

Position accepted by applicant: yes no. If no, rationale________

Figure 7–15. Guide to collecting information concerning characteristics, behavior, and values. (Printed on reverse side of the interview guide, Figure 7–14.)

Position vacancies are filled by the best-qualified candidates. These candidates are identified and recommended for appointment according to precise and objective procedures.

Applicants are recruited according to recruitment planning and the recruitment philosophy (see Table 6–1).

Candidates are first screened by the nurse-recruiter, using specific criteria for *minimum job requirements* (Fig. 7–3).

Those applicants eliminated in the initial screening process are provided rationale and suggestions for improvement or other job opportunities.

Selection processes and all employment practices are monitored to ensure equal employment opportunities for all current and prospective employees.

Application review, interviews, and recommendations for appointment occur at the unit level where the vacancy exists.

The head nurse is responsible for these activities, but the nursing staff on that unit is actively involved in screening, interviewing, and recommending candidates for appointment.

Applicant's previous work experiences, education, and information on the application are verified following the applicant's permission. Educational transcripts and continuing education certificates are also required for validation purposes.

Valid licensure of nurses is ensured through strict procedures (Fig. 7–10). All information must be validated before being eligible for selection.

Information on the candidate's application is rated according to a valid and reliable rating system. Then the total score is tabulated. This rating system includes experiences, education, and all activities that contribute to the candidate's qualifications (Figs. 7–12 and 7–13).

Applicant interviews are conducted on the unit level. Interview questions are discussed and preplanned by interviewers to facilitate the standardization of collection of information. Interview guides are utilized (Figs. 7–14 and 7–15) to ensure consistency of data collection.

Interviewers are provided training in the skill of interviewing in order to increase the objectivity and uniformity of interviews.

Following interviews, interview guides are completed, and strengths and weaknesses of the applicant are summarized.

Interviewers rate candidates according to four categories: outstanding, highly recommended, recommended, and not recommended, based upon the results of the interview process.

Candidates are selected for appointment according to a combination of their application rating scores and the recommendations of the interviewers. Decision making is based on the following guidelines:

1. A candidate with an "outstanding" recommendation and who has the highest application score is selected for the job if he or she is the only outstanding candidate.
2. If more than one candidate is "outstanding," the outstanding one with a score leading by more *than 10 points* is selected.
3. If the above candidates' scores are within 10 points of one another, they are considered equally qualified and subject to selection by one of the following methods:
   a. Complete group consensus by the selection and interview team.
   b. Undergoing a second interview with the vice-president for nursing or management team (other than the ones involved in the previous interview). Selection is then based upon group consensus.

Figure 7–16. Sample selection policy and procedure.

4. If there is only one "outstanding" candidate, and his or her application score is within 20 points of the highest score, that candidate is selected.
5. If the above outstanding candidate is *not* within 20 points of the highest score, he or she is put in the "highly recommended" procedure that follows.
6. If one candidate is "highly recommended," and also has the highest application score, that candidate is selected.
7. If that candidate does not have a score of within 20 points of the highest score, he or she is put in the "recommended" procedure. If his or her score is within 20 points of the highest score, that candidate is selected.
8. If more than one candidate is "highly recommended," the one with a score that leads by *greater* than 10 points is selected.
9. If the "highly recommended" candidate scores are all within a 10-point spread, they are considered equally qualified and selected by the procedure outlined in 3 (a) and (b).
10. If no candidates are rated as "outstanding" or as "highly recommended," those rated as "recommended" follow the same procedure as described in 1–3. In addition:
    a. If "information specific to the job" (see Appendix 6–2) specifies the need for an outstanding or highly recommended candidate, interviewers must notify recruiters of *no qualified candidates*.
    b. If only one candidate is evaluated as "recommended," interviewers have the option of reactivating the search. Although there is a qualified candidate, the procedure for "no qualified candidate" is followed. This candidate could still be considered eligible for the job.
11. Candidates determined to be "not recommended" cannot be eligible for selection. Following selection decisions, the remainder of the interview guide is completed (Fig. 7–15). If decisions result in "no qualified candidate," the following may occur:
    a. Nurse-recruiters are notified.
    b. Decision is made to renew recruitment efforts, train personnel to fill position, appoint a temporary replacement, leave vacancy, or alter the position.

Following selection of a candidate, the recommendation for appointment is approved by the head nurse on the unit and the vice-president for nursing. Any disapproval must be supported with valid rationale.

Following approval, the candidate is notified of the results, and must agree to the terms of employment. A contract is signed, and the new employee is scheduled to begin the orientation period.

Other applicants are then notified of the results, and given rationale, suggestions, and recommendations for improvement. They are also counseled concerning other or future job opportunities for which they may be qualified.

All efforts are taken to speed the selection process. Unnecessary delays can result in frustration and loss of qualified applicants. The initial screening, application rating, and interviews should be completed within a week. Results from interviews and final selection decisions should occur within two days. Applicants should be notified of the decision within four days of the interview. The entire procedure, from application to hiring, should occur within a two-week period. By establishing policies, procedures, and guides, this is possible. Any need for additional time should be communicated to the applicants, along with a progress report.

Figure 7–16. *(continued)*

I have read and agree to perform the responsibilities in the ________________ job description.

I understand the additional expectations for the job described in the "specific information concerning the job," attached to the job description.

I agree to the salary of ______ and shift differential of ______. I understand that I will be evaluated in three months, and eligible for a 3% raise if satisfactory at that time.

I understand that following my three months' evaluation, I will receive a yearly evaluation from that date, at which time I will be eligible for a 3% or 5% raise. These raises will be based upon my performance evaluation, of which I have been given a copy, along with the evaluation rating scale.

I understand that my first three months are probationary, where either I or the organization may terminate this agreement without advanced notice, with stated reasons. If performance evaluation and orientation procedures show satisfactory performance, I will become a permanent employee at the end of three months.

I agree to work ______ hours/week during orientation (first two weeks of orientation), then ______ hours/week and ______ shift on a permanent basis. I understand that during the four-week orientation period my schedule and shifts may vary to provide me with the experiences I need to complete orientation. I understand that I will work every other weekend.

I understand that prior to my first day of work I must undergo a complete history and physical through employee health, including a CBC, RPR, and TB skin test, and be free of communicable diseases. This must be updated yearly.

I understand that during times of emergencies I may be called upon to temporarily change my hours or schedule. I am willing to do this.

I understand that following my orientation I will be assigned to ________ unit, and must work ________ months on that unit before requesting a transfer.

I have received a personnel handbook and will abide by the policies and procedures in that handbook.

My day to begin work is ______.

We also mutually agree to ____

____

____

Signature of New Employee ________________________________ Date ______
Signature of Nurse Manager ________________________________ Date ______

Figure 7–17. Sample agreement on terms of employment.

8 The Orientation Process

Orientation is the process of assisting a new employee to adjust to new roles and responsibilities within the organization. It involves providing needed information and support so the new employee can become socialized to the new environment, fostering the "cultural fit." This socialization must be interactive between the new employee and organizational personnel (most critically on the specific unit), and must be geared to the ultimate goals of both the individual and the organization. As the individual works toward personal and career goals, he or she is able to achieve a greater sense of well-being and satisfaction. This satisfaction can lead to creative contributions and productivity, thus enhancing organizational success. The orientation process begins with the adjustment phase, then initiates the growth and development of the new employee toward mutually beneficial results. Then the growth and development processes are continued and fostered through the personnel processes of performance evaluation and staff development.

All organizations have a culture that evolves over a period of time; this culture consists of accepted habits, customary practices and procedures, values, and a general personality that is established by the group. Specific units have their own unique cultures. The orientation process aims to teach and guide the individual so that he or she can fit into this culture. The recruitment and selection processes have already selected the optimal match for the unit's needs and culture. Orientation must now provide the employee with the tools, support, and knowledge actually to work within this culture. The object is not to ensure conformity by the new employee, but to facilitate a complement or fit that results in optimum creativity and productivity. New employees must be allowed to maintain individuality and freedom of expression while becoming part of a team. The socialization into a new position concerns gaining needed knowledge, skills, and behavior to perform the job expectations, as well as to function creatively and independently within the team. A carefully recruited and selected employee will possess the values, characteristics, and personality that can serve to complement other unit personnel and achieve unit goals. An effective orientation process will further ensure a complementary match between the new employee and the position, assess the individual's knowledge and skills, and initiate procedures to integrate the immediate and long-term needs of the employee and the organization.

The orientation process is a crucial link to successful recruitment and selection; it can ensure that a new employee is secure, competent to perform patient care, and satisfied and challenged within the organization. Stevens states that turnover often occurs due to inadequate orientation procedures and lack of readiness to perform duties.[1] If orientation is inadequate and leads to frustrated or unhappy employees, recruitment and selection processes will have been in vain. Effective orientation can greatly reduce the cost of recruitment, selection, and turnover by facilitating the retention and satisfaction of new employees.

The nurse-administrator is highly interested in maintaining effective orientation procedures—not only because the Joint Commission on Accreditation of Hospitals requires that orientation be based upon individual needs and provide documented instruction to correct deficiencies prior to providing patient care,[2] but also because orientation is critical to the retention and optimum contribution of employees. Although orientation procedures are usually delegated to staff development personnel, the nurse-administrator provides continual support, assistance, and feedback to ensure that the processes achieve optimum results and management personnel work collaboratively with instructional personnel to ensure the successful orientation of new employees.

A PHILOSOPHICAL BASE FOR THE ORIENTATION PROCESS

An effective and successful orientation process depends on thoroughly planned and organized processes that are also flexible and responsive to change. Certain underlying principles and concepts can serve as a guide in planning procedures and methodology.

An employee's prior learning and life experience are intimately related to adjustment and socialization into the new role. Orientation must be based on these experiences and the employee's learning needs, and consider the individual holistically. Assuming new responsibilities, relocation, and working in a new environment can cause anxieties and concerns that may affect physical and emotional well being, as well as mental readiness to learn. Orientation must be designed to assess individual needs, knowledge, and experiences and provide guidance, counseling, and support based on the assessment.

Orientation procedures must be flexible and alter methodology and content as needed. They must be designed to keep pace with change by revising objectives, developing new competency requirements, reprioritizing learning activities, and continually updating learning materials and resources. As the changing work force is more independent and self-directing, orientation processes become more self-directing and self-paced. Also, as the changing work force requires more involvement in organizational decision making, new employees are involved in assessing and planning their own orientation, and their judgment and expertise is used throughout the orientation process.

Staff development personnel should work closely with recruiters and selectors to ensure that the orientation is continuous with previous processes. Information provided to new employees during initial recruitment and selection should be both consistent and used as a base during the orientation, to ensure continuity. The philosophy and goals of the organization should be practiced and evident to the new employee. Evidence of a commitment to human resources, administrative openness, and support will help satisfy emotional needs for security and minimize anxiety, frustration, and confusion due to preconceived ideas about the organization. The orientation process should provide a realistic picture of organizational expectations, roles, and behaviors to promote trust and stability.

Because employees often encounter problems during their initial employment, orientators should use these problems and conflicts for teaching. Employees are assisted in viewing problems as opportunities and challenges and as a means for learning. Preceptors, support groups, and staff development instructors help the employee to identify problems and to use these problems as opportunities for growth and learning. Special contracts may be devised between employees and their preceptors as a means for developing strategies to overcome conflict. Learning is problem oriented, situational, and applied to the work setting. Orientation uses problem solving to foster the adjustment and socialization process.

The goal of orientation is to attain competency and develop a creative mind-set for continued growth and innovative contributions. Creativity and innovation are the ultimate goals for a successful and vital organization. Orientation begins the development of a creative attitude. New employees are allowed freedom to discuss thoughts and suggestions and choose their direction for orientation. They are used as a source of new ideas based on their unique experiences and knowledge. During orientation the new employee is included in creative planning sessions and problem-solving groups in order to foster intuitive skills early on. The employee's experience of freedom and independence during the initial encounter with the organization helps to stimulate creativity and innovative thinking.

Finally, the new employee's goals are integrated with organizational goals to facilitate optimum personal satisfaction and organizational contribution. High expectations for excellence, reward and reinforcement for learning, mutual respect and freedom in learning, self-evaluation, and open communication all begin in the orientation process. In addition, preceptors and staff development instructors play a big part in creating an attitude for creativity. Performance evaluation, counseling and coaching, and staff development processes take over from the initial orientation process, and foster continual change, improvement, and evolution.

COMPONENTS OF AN EFFECTIVE ORIENTATION PROCESS

As a result of environmental change, certain strategies and methodologies have evolved that can affect the success of the orientation process. Competency-based education, self-directed learning, performance-based evaluation, role models and mentors, and peer group support may not be new, but due to changing environmental demands, organizational requirements, and human resource needs, they have become instrumental in determining effective socialization into the new system. Although the use of these methodologies does not ensure success, and although they are not the only means for effective orientation, they are important components of the orientation process. The nurse-administrator should consider their merits and usefulness, and can adapt those elements that are appropriate for the particular organizational needs. The remainder of this chapter will be devoted to discussion of each of these methodologies and their relation to a successful orientation process. An appendix is provided, presenting samples and examples of forms, checklists, and various guides that may be useful for orientation procedures.

COMPETENCY-BASED EDUCATION

The chief goal of orientation is to begin socialization of the individual into the new environment. Effective socialization results in developing a commitment to the organization and obtaining appropriate competencies.[3] Achievement of competency must come first. Only after an employee has a sense of mastery of required skills and behaviors can he or she begin to identify with the organization; only after securing positive interactions and interpersonal competence can he or she feel a part of the environment and become committed to it. From this commitment flows growth and development and the striving for self-actualization. Effective socialization is the impetus for future growth, but it all depends on competence.[3]

Competence can be viewed from two perspectives during the orientation process. One is the *perception* of competence by the individual. The feeling of mastery, achievement, and capable functioning in the system results in well-being and inner gratification for the new employee. This is necessary for self-image, confidence, and motivation to stay and grow with the organization. As discussed in Chapter 11, the perception of competence is necessary for job satisfaction and successful growth and development. It is achieved through positive reinforcement, psychic income, guidance and support, and attaining *actual* competence.

Actual competence is the state of being appropriately qualified, able and fit, and having the capacity to achieve a goal. It begins with recruitment and selection of qualified people who have the potential for meeting the expectations of the job. Orientation processes must then ensure that minimum-level competencies are attained for implementing new roles. The processes of performance evaluation, coaching, and counseling serve to maintain competencies and guide continued growth and development.

The concept of competency based education (CBE) has grown in popularity over the past several years, and is proving to be a cost-effective means for ensuring minimum-level competency for new employees. It involves analyzing prospective desired outcomes for a role or behavior, and then basing the curriculum and learning experience on these outcomes. Learning is evaluated according to achievement of these outcomes or demonstrating the required behaviors of the particular role. Competency based education calls for problem-oriented and realistic education and learning by doing, as well as in a classroom. It stresses what is useful and what one can do—using knowledge, not just acquiring it. It calls for increased accountability by faculty and management for defining outcomes, interactive teaching, increased observation of the learner, and a wide variety of assessment methods. With CBE, the below-average performer is not allowed to go unnoticed.[4] The competencies must be achieved—there is no alternative. A learner who is unable to achieve competencies is offered special guidance and coaching, and allowed additional time to study and learn the required behaviors. Continued inability to perform, however, would result in dismissal from the system.

Several conditions have led to the popularity of CBE; changing attitudes about education and life-style is one. With increased lifespans, financial resources, and leisure time, many people are returning to school later in life. Others are interested in acquiring new skills or knowledge. An attitude of lifelong learning and the increase in adult learners with various backgrounds has influenced the development of flexible teaching methods, credit for and basing educational activities on experience and prior learning, and more independent, interactive learning. Growth and developments in high technology have also made this possible.[5]

The CBE concept has also been influenced by society's demand for competence and the need for employees to develop a variety of competencies to keep pace with change. Technical competence is no longer enough;

competence is now needed in ethics, psychology, sociology, communication—caring, humane competence. Moreover, the demand for cost-effective services and reduced expenditures has resulted in a need for efficient, effective, and cost-effective education.[4] The focus of CBE is on performance, self-paced learning, and individualized learning. It zeroes in on required or essential outcomes for role performance, and allows freedom and flexibility for the adult learner in achieving these outcomes; CBE can also be a cost-effective learning mode for adults.

Although desired competencies can be general, knowledge-related, or performance-oriented, most CBE programs tend to be behavioristic, relating to well-defined functions and skills, versus humanistic or more cognitive and generic programs. Educators and managers determine what is really needed and wanted in a particular role, and then validate this assessment with experts and outside data. Course content is designed with learning methodologies, and then learners are assessed to determine who requires assistance and who already has the required competencies. Self-assessment is important and integrated into the CBE system. The content is then completed, with feedback, guidance, and practice, followed by evaluation. The learning is self-paced and individualized, putting the responsibility for learning on the student's shoulders. Instructors provide ongoing assistance.[4]

The staff development department works closely with management to help nurses achieve the level of competency necessary to reach the desired outcomes in patient care and achieve the goals of the nursing department. The CBE system must also include a means for validating the staff's competence.[6] This competency must be obtained through the most efficient and effective means with the available resources; CBE helps to achieve this by identifying the most frequently performed critical functions, prioritizing these functions, and establishing them as desired outcomes or competencies with specific criteria for evaluation. Then self-instruction learning modules can be developed, saving up to 50 percent of staff development costs, as well as saving time away from patients. In addition, the learner is assessed prior to teaching, thus avoiding unnecessary teaching, and performance can be objectively measured.[7]

Mastery of skills is the key, not simply attendance at classes and inservices. Evaluation should be on application of knowledge, not just obtainment of knowledge. An orientation process that does not achieve competency according to established standards will have higher costs and be ineffective, eventually affecting all personnel processes and patient care. With CBE, standards and required activities for patient outcomes are defined, knowledge and skills needed to obtain these competencies are identified, behavioral objectives with criteria are established, and educational material is developed to help the learner meet the criteria. Finally, knowledge and performance are evaluated and compared to the performance evaluation on the clinical unit to ensure validity of both the educational content and the evaluation.[8]

The CBE system is especially useful for orientation programs and highly technical skills; however, its uses are being expanded into all aspects of nursing. With the need for extensive training of new graduate nurses, staff development personnel have had to devote growing time and resources to the orientation process. The traditional orientation procedures, with lectures, buddy systems, written tests, subjective evaluation of performance and uniform procedures for all new employees have proved to be expensive and time-consuming. All orientees are taught the same information, regardless of need, and evaluation of the transfer of learning to the clinical unit is often unreliable or incomplete.[9] The CBE system is performance based. It can eliminate waste in the training process because it is *results oriented*. Because learning is self-paced, CBE fits any time frame, decreases time spent away from patient care, and allows instructors to focus on the application of learning.[10]

While CBE may be utilized for advanced skills and training, in the orientation process it is focused on *minimum-level competencies* to ensure safe practice on a particular clinical unit. Managers work with staff nurses to determine minimum level requirements for competent functioning on the unit. These standards are determined by identifying what a competent practitioner *does*, not what he or she knows.[9] Specific criteria are identified to achieve each competency standard, along with resources and learning options and the means for evaluation. Because the criteria reflect minimum-level competency, *the evaluation must be passed with 100 percent accuracy*. Anything less dictates restudying of materials and reevaluation.[11] Standards and job descriptions already in use in the organization can be used in CBE. Specific, behavioral-outcome criteria can be developed as a means for achieving and evaluating the standards and job descriptions.

With CBE, the time schedule for completing orientation is flexible and based on the learner's needs. The goal is mastery of competencies, and time frames may only be set for maximum allowable time affordable by the organization.[12] Examples from a competency based orientation program are presented in Appendices 8–1, 8–2, and 8–3.

SELF-DIRECTED LEARNING

Integrated into the concept of CBE is self-directed learning. At the beginning of orientation the new nurse reviews the competencies and assesses his or her own learning needs. The nurse may forego the learning modules and proceed directly to the evaluation phase by taking a test and/or demonstrating a procedure. No time is spent relearning what is already known.

In addition to the self assessment and demonstration of learning, achievement of competencies is self-paced. By following directions in a learning module and using available resources, learning is done independently. Nurses also work in groups and with their preceptors to obtain the needed skills and prepare for evaluation. Individual contracting may be used between nurse and preceptor to delineate special clinical experiences and guidance required prior to evaluation. A learning resource center may be available with audiovisual resources and library materials. Staff development instructors also provide support, guidance, and expertise in attaining required competencies.

Self-paced learning involves the learner taking responsibility for attaining the needed competencies. The learner may control one or more of the following variables:

1. Identification of learning needs
2. Choosing the subject and content of learning experience
3. Delineating own learning objectives
4. Choosing own learning resources
5. Choosing own learning environment
6. Determining learning pace and time period
7. Determining the means for evaluation and documentation

The staff development instructor acts as a facilitator to guide the individual in becoming independent and in *learning how to learn.* In addition to attaining competencies, self-directed learning aims to foster the commitment for lifelong learning.[13]

The self-directed learning experience should contain certain elements. These include[13]:

1. The standard, competency statement, or focus of the experience
2. The specific learning objectives
3. The selection of learning resources
4. The content of the learning experience
5. Needed consultation and guidance
6. Method for evaluation
7. Method for documentation of results

Self-directed learning is also addressed in Chapter 12, "Staff Development."

PERFORMANCE-BASED EVALUATION

It was stated earlier that a system must be provided for evaluating the staff's competence. While written tests may measure the acquisition of knowledge, a means must be provided to determine the application of knowledge in clinical practice. Orientation processes must be geared to ensuring the competence of new employees. So evaluation methods should be performance-based. Following a learning experience, staff development instructors and managers can utilize criterion-referenced tools to evaluate performance.[10] The criteria would relate specifically to the criteria in the required competency or standard and could be checked off as the nurse properly performs the procedure. Checklists could also be developed to evaluate the required criteria for documentation in nurses' notes, care plans, and patient assessments. Simulated clinical experiences may provide a means for practice as well as evaluation. A skills laboratory duplicating the clinical setting can allow the nurse to demonstrate competencies, such as medication administration or intravenous therapy, using a model. The nurse can be evaluated by a criterion-referenced checklist prior to providing patient care, and may then be evaluated again by the supervisor or preceptor on the unit.[14] Other techniques such as role playing, in-basket problem solving, and a pre-established performance evaluation checklist can also be used for evaluation purposes. The evaluator must be trained in the evaluation process, and the tools must be tested for reliability and validity. If qualitative evaluation is made through question-answer interviews or in-basket problem solving, the questions, answers, and process must be standardized for all involved. The performance evaluation system should provide a means for follow-up evaluation and ensuring the maintenance of competencies.

As part of the evaluation process, it is important that practice time be provided and adequate support and feedback be given to the learner. Preceptors, supervisors, and staff development instructors continually assess the employee's stress level, self-confidence, and psychological adjustment to the new environment. Evaluation of performance should be ongoing, with continual interaction and communication. Some nurses will demonstrate competencies immediately and without problems. But for those with numerous learning needs and/or lack of experience, continued guidance and support is necessary.

ROLE MODELS AND MENTORS

Successful orientation is greatly facilitated by the development and utilization of role models or mentors. A supportive resource person with expertise in the clinical area can provide guidance, counseling, and needed "inside" information to the orientee. This close working relationship facilitates the successful transition into the new role. It also helps create a positive attitude toward the organization. Close working relationships based on mutual respect and sharing can blossom into mentor–mentee relationships. Relationships of this kind can be instrumental in developing commitment to lifelong learning, creativity, and excellence.

Management personnel and staff development instructors serve as role models for excellence; their actions and behaviors are closely observed by new employees, and can leave lasting impressions that affect attitudes and behaviors. The nurse-administrator must not tolerate anything less than excellence in appearance, behaviors, and performance, in order to set the standard for all employees.

In addition to role modeling by administrative and educational staff, systems can be devised to identify and train specific staff members to serve as role models and, hopefully, mentors to new employees. This person interacts closely with the new employee on a one-to-one basis and serves as support and facilitator to the employee. If a good match can be made, a long-term mentoring relationship may develop. The use of preceptors in an orientation program can be an effective means for developing role models and ensuring a good cultural fit between the orientee and the unit personnel.

PRECEPTORS

The identification of role models and the appropriate training of the preceptor is critical to successful relationships and outcomes. Preceptors must possess certain characteristics in order to successfully facilitate the socialization process and promote a positive development and attitude by the new nurse. Specific criteria for selecting preceptors should be developed. The following are required characteristics that will facilitate developing these criteria:

1. Clinical expertise in the specified area
2. Professional attitude, practices, and role model
3. Commitment to organizational and unit objectives
4. Sound interpersonal relationships with unit personnel
5. Effective communication skills
6. Desire and ability to form close, sharing relationships
7. Desire and ability to teach and counsel
8. Keen perception of human nature
9. In tune with intuitive and creative thoughts
10. Ability to assess learning needs and facilitate self-directed learning

Although there is no perfect person, the nurse-administrator should maintain high standards in choosing a preceptor. When assigning a new employee to this person, the administrator has placed a "stamp of approval" on the preceptor's behaviors and performance. The new employee will look to this person as an example of what administration expects.

Interested nurses who have these characteristics should be sought out for involvement in the preceptor program. There are often a number of excellent choices who have talent and resources that are not being tapped. These unrecognized people may desire a means for self-expression, and when given the opportunity, begin to offer many kinds of contributions to the organization. A preceptor program may be one means to facilitate the growth, development, and creativity of current, experienced staff nurses. These nurses may not have had the right opportunity to "shine," and when recognized, begin to flourish.

Training the Preceptors

Regular preceptor training programs should be developed and offered by the staff development personnel. Experienced people from other fields or organizations may be brought in to share their knowledge and expertise in the preceptor process. Basic class content could include:

Definition and Exploration of the Preceptor Role. The preceptor is a person who befriends and guides a new nurse. This nurse may be a new graduate, a nurse returning from an extended leave of absence, or a nurse moving into a new role, such as from a transfer, promotion, or simply a new employee. There are no rules that govern the relationship; it must evolve from mutual willingness and an interest to learn. The preceptor facilitates attaining competencies and behaviors required to fit into the new role; works with the employee to determine appropriate schedules, assignments, learning experiences, and a course of study; evaluates the orientee's performance and progress, provides suggestions and feedback for improvement, and facilitates the orientee's self-assessment and evaluation skills. The preceptor serves as a role model for professional behavior, expert clinician, and guidance counselor. The preceptor opens communication, develops a trusting relationship, and provides direction for growth, problem solving, and behavior modification.

The preceptor relationship may vary in degrees. A preceptor may simply be a "buddy" who provides the orientee with needed information during the first few weeks of employment. The orientee may not require additional assistance and may not desire it. On the other hand, a preceptor and orientee may develop a mentoring relationship where a bond is formed between individuals. In this case, the preceptor teaches, guides, and supports, while learning more about himself or herself and about work in the process. By teaching, the preceptor also learns new skills of perception, communication, and creativity. The orientee seeks the help and guidance of the preceptor, emulates the preceptor's characteristics and practices, and grows personally and professionally. There is no real way to predict or preplan this mentoring relationship, but the stage can be set to foster potential mentoring.

Goals. Another component of the preceptor training program concerns the goals of the preceptorship. The program strives to develop satisfied, well-adjusted new employees who have a positive attitude and will strive to grow and develop with the organization. The initial goal is for role adjustment—learning how to function, developing needed competencies, and learning policies and procedures. The long-term goal is to learn the unwritten rules and practices, become socialized into the new environment, and create a good cultural fit.

Besides competency and commitment, socialization involves developing individuality, creative thought, and intuitive skills. It is necessary that the work environment support and encourage individuality, freedom of thought, and creativity. In keeping with the organization's philosophy and objectives, creative and productive human resources are the ultimate goal. The preceptorship strives to initiate the creative attitude and promote the socialization process.

Orientation Policies and Procedures. Preceptors must know the policies and procedures of the orientation process, including objectives and required competencies, learning material and options, evaluation methods and checklists, and other means for documentation. They should be able to answer questions concerning hospital policies and procedures, or know appropriate resource people to contact. They must be well versed in the ins and outs of the organization, so that they can implement orientation procedures.

Training. Training should be offered in teaching the adult. Principles involved in adult learning and techniques for facilitating learning should be offered. The need for self-assessment, participation in learning, building on experience, and self-evaluation of learning are important for effective orientation. The anxiety of a new role and environment, insecurities or lack of confidence, and previous experiences can interfere with learning and adustment. Preceptors must be taught to assess barriers to learning and the appropriate interventions and strategies to overcome obstacles.

Performance Evaluation and Reinforcement of Learning. Preceptors may be insecure about providing constructive feedback and evaluating performance. They must be trained in objective and consistent evaluation techniques and in the use of evaluation tools. They must also learn the importance of continual feedback and positive reinforcement in learning and building the new employee's confidence.

Preceptors must understand the relationship between standards of practice, job descriptions, and performance evaluations, and how competency based education fits into this system. They will assist the new nurse to adapt to the formal evaluation system and to carry out the job expectations satisfactorily.

Communication, Role Modeling, and Mentoring. Preceptors should be instructed in the skills of communication and ways to enhance perception, openness, and the exchange of ideas. They should understand the principles of role adaptation and transition and the part they play as role models. The mentoring process should be explored and discussed. This understanding can make the preceptor more receptive to potential mentoring relationships.

Fostering Mentoring Relationships

Preceptors are the key to success for a new employee's well-being and socialization. Therefore, the stage must be set to foster positive preceptor relationships and, it is hoped, mentorships. Preceptors must be allowed the time to implement their roles. If they are working with a new employee, they should not receive a full patient load, especially in the first 1 to 2 weeks. The first week they need to be free to cover competencies, checklists, and other procedures. The second week they will be demonstrating skills and providing special learning experiences on the unit. Gradually they will increase their patient load together until finally the orientee is able to provide independent patient care. The time required for orientation will vary according to the needs of the new nurse, and flexibility in scheduling and assignments is essential. Preceptors work closely with the head nurse to determine time needed for teaching, patient load, special learning experiences, and schedules. At first, assignments may be made only a day in advance, or may remain flexible contingent upon nursing procedures and learning experiences. Additional staff may have to cover temporarily during the initial orientation process when the preceptor is spending more time with the new employee. This flexibility will pay off in the long run, as a well-trained and productive new employee emerges.

Assistance and support must be provided for the preceptor. When unsure, confronted with problems, or simply in need of advice, the preceptor must have the support of hospital personnel and available resources. The assistance of head nurses, staff development personnel, and unit nurses is required for effective orientation. Everyone shares in the responsibility for orientation and continued learning. Preceptor support groups may also be formed to discuss concerns and problem solving.

Administration must recognize the contribution of preceptors and encourage the mentoring of new nurses. Development of sharing relations and preceptor skills should be written into career development objectives for promotions, monetary raises, or some sort of recognition and honors. Outstanding mentoring or role-modeling behaviors should be rewarded, either through existing promotional channels or by developing new mechanisms. Preceptors may be awarded a salary increase for accepting the role. Administration must provide incentives to encourage these types of behaviors, as well as the tools, environment, and encouragement to take risks and accept new challenges.

PEER GROUP SUPPORT

Another important component to orientation is the use of peer group support. While support and guidance is offered through preceptors, role models, and other interactions during the orientation process, peer group support offers a special means for "group coaching and counseling" of the new employee. The purpose of group support is ultimately to enhance the socialization process. Its specific objectives include conflict resolution concerning work-related problems and issues, establishing an identity within the organization through group purpose and cohesiveness, and facilitating creativity and innovation.

Peer group support can be organized and planned in conjunction with counseling and coaching processes (see Chapter 10), or can be a flexible technique utilized on a contingency basis. If in-house counseling services exist or a specialist is available in interpersonal relations or group process, peer support can be arranged through these existing channels. Staff development personnel and nurse-managers can be alert to arising conflicts and stresses, and arrange for group support sessions as the need indicates. New nurses may be told of this process and given the option of participating or forming a peer support group. Lastly, peer group support may be organized as a permanent part of the orientation process and included in the goals and objectives for every new nurse. The exact use of peer group support will depend on the needs of the new employees, the environment and conditions at the time of employment, and the needs of the organization. The benefits from the group process can be lasting for both the employee and the organization.

Conflict Resolution

Problems, issues, and concerns related to role adjustment, new work environment, new relationships, and patient care can cause anxiety, frustration, and conflict for the new employee. This not only affects job performance and ability to learn, but it can also influence the employee's decision to remain with the organization. Peer support groups can be formed, consisting of new employees and a group leader-role model, to identify and resolve these conflicts. The group can generate alternatives for dealing with problems, recommend solutions to management for problem solving, and discuss feelings about these conflicts. Individuals are allowed to freely verbalize concerns, and the group objective is to determine constructive means for conflict resolution. An experienced group leader ensures that the group's desired outcomes are clear and the experience is a positive, constructive, and rewarding one for the participants. The results can be problem solving and conflict resolution through a group effort and personal satisfaction of needs for security, support, and belonging.

Establishing Organizational Commitment

Group problem solving and interaction can also have another important effect on the new employee. The experience of sharing ideas and concerns can lead to a feeling of cohesiveness, establishing an identity with the new organization, and developing a commitment to the new role. By becoming involved personally and seeing positive results from this interaction, the new employee can begin to identify with the new environment and feel a part of things. Rather than simply following the procedure in an orientation manual and working independently, the new employee has an opportunity from the beginning to contribute ideas for problem solving and help others in their adjustment to their new roles. The group leader serves as a role model, communicating administration's commitment to human resources and the importance of each individual to organizational functioning. Group learning can occur through exchange of ideas, and the concept of team work and commitment to one another is fostered and strengthened early on. If executed properly, the peer support group experience can play an important part in the socialization process.

Facilitating Creativity and Innovation

Orientation support groups can be an early means for stimulating intuitive thinking and fostering the creative attitude. Techniques for problem solving can be taught that include brainstorming and other mechanisms for generating new ideas. The new employee is a fresh source of ideas whose input is sought from the very beginning. Group ideas are presented to administration for further refinement and testing. New employees can learn the importance of creativity and group work and are exposed to the use of imagination and divergent thinking in the very beginning while they are still open to new experience. This way they can be socialized into the organizational culture and readily take part in creative innovations. Though, of course, this technique is not always 100 percent successful, it can establish the attitude and mind-set that is so vital to organizational success.

Groups of new nurses assigned to various clinical specialties can contribute to effective outcomes by sharing divergent background experiences and knowledge for problem solving and conflict resolution. New employees can meet weekly for an hour with the group leader in a quiet, confidential room throughout the orientation experience. Groups can be organized after the first month and meet regularly for a specific period of time, or they can be organized for a specific problem or need and meet daily for a week or two. The exact arrangements, purpose, and time period are flexible and open. Managers and staff development personnel can experiment with various strategies and approaches and even vary their approach with each new group. If the goal is chiefly problem solving and stress reduction, the approach will be different from creativity training and generation of new ideas. The goals of the support group process should be clearly defined; then strategies should be planned as part of the orientation process to achieve these goals. In some cases groups can be quite effective, and may continue to meet after completion of the orientation period.

ADDITIONAL APPROACHES AND AIDS

Before concluding this chapter on orientation, mention should be made of some additional approaches and aids to the orientation process. In many facilities the use of internships, externships, and student practicums have proved effective in reducing turnover and smoothing the transition period.

Internships

Rowland and Rowland[15] describe the internship as bridging the gap for new graduates into their new roles. New graduates with less than six months' experience are selected according to academic standing and willingness to participate. The program may last from 10 weeks to 1 year, and often involves a commitment by the new graduate to remain for one year with the organization. The content of the program involves orientation, leadership, role adjustment, problem solving, clinical skills, and counseling. The results can be a decrease in frustration and turnover, and increase in satisfaction, skill level, and improved patient care.

Strauser[16] describes a program in Florida where post-baccalaureate graduates pay tuition to the university and complete a nine-month internship with a selected hospital. The hospital pays a stipend, and the intern works with both university instructors and hospital personnel. The intern receives academic credit (4 hours) to use toward a master's degree. The internship results in a better-prepared graduate who is oriented and experienced when he or she becomes a full-time employee. Some internship programs allow graduates to choose participation in a year-long program at a reduced salary.

Other studies show that internships must be approached cautiously prior to implementation. They may not be more effective than preceptorships, and are often more expensive. The key to orientation is to provide needed instruction, good evaluations, informal discussion groups, and a preceptor for guidance and support.[17]

Externships

These are helpful not only as a recruitment tool, but also as a means to decrease orientation needs and reduce turnover. Nursing students are selected to work in hospitals, receive minimum wage compensation, and complete special course work and clinical rotations.[18] They work with a professional role model, obtain skills and knowledge in various clinical areas, and gain confidence and improved self-image as nurses.[19] Stidger states that a precise plan for screening and training students is necessary. Questions such as how they should be screened, areas they can work, types of skills they may perform, and length of time from graduation should be agreed upon. Programs may vary from one semester to one year, from part-time to full-time. Compensation may be minimum wage or mileage and meals. Evaluation and progress reports are essential to the process.[20]

Student Practicums

Students in many nursing programs are now offered a practicum in their last semester, where they work with a preceptor in their chosen clinical specialty. The preceptors are usually nurses with affiliations or close ties with the university, trained in evaluation and teaching. The student gains academic credit and obtains skills and experience as a clinician. Practicums are very helpful recruitment tools to hospitals, as students often return to work where they feel comfortable and secure. In addition, orientation needs are greatly reduced, as new graduates are already familiar with the organization, personnel, and have begun role transformation.

CONCLUSION

Orientation is an important process for any employee assuming a new role or a role change. New employees as well as those being promoted, transferred, or returning from an extended leave of absence require orientation to assist them in the transition. To be effective, a program must be pertinent to the needs of the employee and the organization, and be flexible enough to allow self-direction in learning. It should be performance-based and provide needed support and guidance during the adjustment phase.

Self-assessment and ongoing evaluation are the key. An experienced and skillful nurse will speed through the objectives, demonstrating competence in performance of skills. A new graduate may require extensive guidance, practice, instruction, and demonstration prior to evaluation of performance. The orientation process is geared to setting standards of expectations, facilitating achievement of those expectations, and providing a means to evaluate this achievement. It also allows a mechanism for the organization and the employee to determine whether an appropriate and complementary match has been made.

Orientation prepares the new employee for required competencies and is instrumental to effective socialization. Then, from the initial adjustment, performance and behaviors are guided for continued growth and development. Performance evaluation is continuous with orientation and builds upon the learning experiences and competencies gained through the orientation process. And so this leads us to Chapter 9.

REFERENCES

1. Stevens, B. *The nurse as executive* (2nd ed.). Wakefield, Mass.: Nursing Resources, Inc., 1980, p. 25, 332, 333.
2. Joint Commission on Accreditation of Hospitals. *Accreditation manual for hospitals.* Chicago: JCAH, 1983, p. 115.

3. Hardy, M. E., & Conway, M. E. *Role theory: Perspectives for health professsionals.* E. Norwalk, Conn.: Appleton-Century-Crofts, 1978, p. 55, 78.
4. Grant, G., Elbow, P., Ewens, T., et al. *On competence: A critical analysis of competence-based reforms in higher education.* San Francisco: Jossey-Bass, 1979, pp. 1–66, 95–137.
5. Nickse, R., & McClure, L. (Eds.). *Competency-based education: Beyond minimum competency testing.* New York: Teachers College, Columbia Univ., 1981, pp. 220–222.
6. Del Bueno, D. J. What can nursing service expect from the inservice department? In Journal of Nursing Administration, *Staff development* (Vol. II). Wakefield, Mass.: Contemporary Publishers, Inc., 1977, pp. 44–45.
7. Del Bueno, D. J. The cost of competency. In Journal of Nursing Administration, *Staff development* (Vol. II). Wakefield, Mass.: Contemporary Publishers, Inc., 1977, pp. 10–11.
8. Cantor, M. M. Certifying competencies of personnel. In Journal of Nursing Administration, *Staff development* (Vol. II). Wakefield, Mass.: Contemporary Publishers, Inc., 1977, pp. 8–9.
9. Del Bueno, D. J., & Altano, R. Competency-based education: No magic feather. *Nursing Management,* 1984, *15*(4), 48–53.
10. Boyer, C. M. Performance-based staff development: The cost-effective alternative. *Nurse Educator,* 1981, *6*(5), 12–15.
11. Ghiglieri, S., Woods, S. A., & Moyer, K. Toward a competency-based safe practice. *Nursing Management,* 1983, *14*(3), 16–19.
12. Del Bueno, D. J., Barker, F., & Christmeyer, C. Implementing a competency-based orientation program. *JONA,* 1981, *11*(2), 24–29.
13. Cooper, S. S. *The practice of continuing education in nursing.* Rockville, Maryland: Aspen, 1983, pp. 147–149, 153.
14. Vendura, N. Pharmacology program produces results. *JONA,* 1979, *9*(9), 34–39.
15. Rowland, H. S., & Rowland, B. L. *Nursing administration handbook.* Germantown, Maryland: Aspen, 1980, pp. 236–238.
16. Strauser, C. J. An internship with academic credit. *AJN,* 1979, *79*(6), 1071–1072.
17. Dear, M. R., Celentano, D. D., Weisman, C. S., & Keen, M. F. Evaluating a hospital nursing internship. *JONA,* 1982, *12*(11), 16–20.
18. Harkins, S. B., Schamback, A. V., & Brodie, K. J. Summer externs: Easing the transition. *Nursing Management,* 1983, *14*(7), 37–39.
19. Allison, S. E., Anderson, B., Balmat, C. S., et al. Externship programs: The Mississippi model. *Nursing Outlook,* 1984, *32*(4), 207–209.
20. Stidger, R. W. *The competence game: How to find, use and keep competent employees.* New York: Thomond Press, 1980, p. 9.
21. Jernigan, D. K., & Young, A. P. *Standards, job descriptions and performance evaluations for nursing practice.* E. Norwalk, Conn.: Appleton-Centory-Crofts, 1983, pp. 107–140.

SUGGESTED READING

Adams, S. Self-study for independent learning. *The Journal of Continuing Education in Nursing,* 1971, *2*(3), 27–31.

Althaus, J. N., Hardyck, N. M., Pierce, P. B., & Rodgers, M. S. *Nursing decentralization: The El Camino experience.* Rockville, Maryland: Aspen, 1981, pp. 103–129.

Bille, P. A. *Staff development: A systems approach.* Thorofare, New Jersey: Charles B. Slack, Inc., 1982.

Chickerella, B. G., & Lutz, W. J. Professional nurturance: Preceptorships for undergraduate nursing students. *AJN,* 1981, *81*(1), 107–109.

Clough, J. A. Developing and implementing orientation to a critical care unit. *Focus AACN,* 1982, *9*(5), 24–29.

Darling, L. Mentoring types and life cycles. *JONA,* 1984, *14*(11), 43–44.

Detrick, R. L. Helping employees make the transition from classroom to workplace. *Supervisory Management,* 1983, *28*(10), 40–42.

Dew, J. R. Redesigning orientations. *Personnel Administration,* 1983, *29*(7), 28.

Fagan, M., & Fagan, P. Mentoring among nurses. *Nursing and Health Care,* 1983, *4*(2), 77–82.

Farrell, J. Orienting the float team to orthopedic patient care. *Orthopedic Nurse,* 1982, *1*(5), 42.

Feldman, D. A socialization process that helps new recruits succeed. *Personnel,* 1980, *57*(2).

Ford, R. Reducing nursing staff stress through scheduling, orientation and continuing education. *Nursing Clinics of North America,* 1983, *18*(3), 597–601.

Freeman, A. Staff development program for critical care nurses. . . . The competency based education model. *Critical Care Nurse,* 1983, *3*(2), 86–92.

Gast, M. R., & Patinka, P. J. Imprinting the young employee. *Business Horizons,* 1983, *26*(7), 11–13.

Hillelsohn, M. J. How to think about CBT. *Training and Development Journal,* 1984, *35*(12), 42–44.

Jones, D. F. Developing a new employee orientation program. *Personnel Journal,* 1984, *63*(3), 86–87.

Ignatavicius, D. D. Clinical competence of new graduates: A study to measure performance. *Journal of Continuing Education in Nursing,* 1983, *14*(4), 17–20.

Kalminski, S. OR orientation to meet the needs of both the entry level and the experienced medical staff. *Today's OR Nurse,* 1983, *5*(5), 24–25, 28–29.

Knowles, M. *Self-directed learning: A guide for learners and teachers.* New York: Association Press, 1975, pp. 34–37.

Lee, G., & Raleigh, E. D. A half-way house for the new graduate. *Nursing Management,* 1983, *14*(1), 43–49.

Luke, R. D. Professionalism, accountability and peer review. *Health Services Research,* 1982, *17,* 113–123.

May, L. Clinical preceptors for new nurses. *AJN,* 1980, *80*(10), 1824–1826.

Matz, L. Initiation rites, corporate style. *Training,* 1983, *20*(11), 67–70.

McGarrell, E. J. An orientation system that builds productivity. *Personnel,* 1983, *60,* 32–41.

McIntyre, E. Clinical evaluation of a new critical care nurse. *Focus AACN,* 1982, *9*(5), 3–6.

Mills, E., Harris, R. J., & Brische, H. R. Internships in an instant bureaucracy: Some organizational lessons. *Journal of Applied Behavioral Science,* 1983, *19*(4), 483–495.

Moorhouse, C. New graduates: The preceptor plan. *Australian Nurses Journal,* 1983, *12*(9), 44–46.

National League For Nurses. Nurse intern program. *Nursing And Health Care,* 1984, *5*(3), 136–138.

National League For Nurses. *Competencies of graduates of nursing programs.* NLN Publ 1982, #14-1905, pp. 1–19.

Pascale, R. Fitting new employees into the company culture. *Fortune*, 1984, *109*, 28–30.

Ramsborg, G. C. Evaluation of clinical performance. . . . Student Progress, Part 1. *The American Association of Nurse Anesthetists Journal*, 1983, *51*(1), 55–62.

Ramsborg, G. C. Evaluation of clinical performance, Part 2. *The American Association of Nurse Anesthetists Journal, 1983, 51*(2), 167–174.

Snyder, D. J. New baccalaureate graduates: Perceptions of organizational conflict. *Nursing Research*, 1982, *31*(5), 300–303.

Scott, B. Competency based learning: A literature review. *International Journal of Nursing Studies*, 1982, *19*(3), 119–124.

Sovie, M. D. Fostering professional nursing careers in hospitals: The role of staff development, Part 1. *JONA*, Dec. 1982, pp. 5–10.

Stowe, W. M. Placement and recruitment personnel: How well do they communicate? *Journal of College Placement*, 1983, *43*(4), 60.

Stredl, D. R. Administrative turnover. . . . total nursing turnover, (TNT) = dynamite. *Nursing Management*, 1982, *13*(11), 24–26, 38.

Ulschak, F. L. Coming on board and staying. . . . Staffing turnover is a problem that has long plagued OR supervisors. *AORN Journal*, 1983, *38*(1), 51–56.

Varney, M. An educational curriculum based on the clinical levels concept. *Journal of Neurosurgical Nursing*, 1983, *15*(3), 169–173.

Winscott, D. P. Therapy for organizational tunnel vision. *Supervisory Management*, 1982, *27*, 8–11.

APPENDICES

The following appendices are provided as examples for establishing and documenting orientation procedures. This is only a guide, and many of the examples are incomplete. Appendix 8–1 shows an example of competency requirements established for an ICU or CCU unit. Each competency has subcompetencies that delineate exact criteria for evaluation (not included, but Appendix 8–3 shows an example). Appendix 8–2 is a skills inventory for self-assessment and documentation of competencies. This is a list of requirements for that particular unit, and each skill corresponds with a subcompetency that delineates the exact criteria for implementing that skill. Appendix 8–3 is an example of a learning module for a subcompetency. The subcompetency 63 can be identified on the skills inventory (Appendix 8–2), and as part of the competency statement under "Implementation" on Appendix 8–1. Appendices 8–4 and 8–5 are simply checklists used by the preceptor to ensure that certain information has been covered. These checklists can be used in scavenger hunts or for self-evaluation by the new employee to see if he or she has obtained this information by the end of the orientation period. They are used as tools for covering required information, such as personnel policies.

APPENDIX 8–1

Intensive and Coronary Care Nurse Competencies[21]

The following are the required ICU and CCU competencies and are derived from the Standards of Intensive and Coronary Care Nursing Practice. These competencies are included in the ICU/CCU Nurse Job Description and in the Performance Evaluation System. Refer to attached subcompetencies as indicated for implementation of nursing procedures, and to specific learning modules and evaluation requirements.

I. *Assessment* (learning modules A-2 and A-3)
  A. Assesses the health status of an assigned patient as outlined in the nursing standards
    1. Completes a comprehensive patient history and physical including:
      a. Patient interview:
        Chief complaint
        History of present illness
        Allergies
        Medications
        Past medical–surgical history
        Family history
        Cultural, environmental, and socioeconomic conditions
        Activities of daily living
        Personal habits
        Food and fluid preferences
        Appetite and weight changes
        Sleep and rest patterns
        Fatigue and activity tolerance
        Available and accessible human, community, and material resources
      b. Psychological assessment:
        Emotional status
        Patterns of coping
        Concerns during hospitalization
      c. Physical assessment:
        Personal hygiene and grooming
        Nutritional status
        Pain
        Vital signs
          Physical status including (see subcompetencies listed under Patient Assessment):
          Head, ears, eyes, nose, throat
          Heart
          Respiratory system
          Vascular system

Skin
Gastrointestinal system
Musculoskeletal system
Mental/neurological system
Genitourinary system

d. Perception of illness:
Understanding of disease process or illness
Understanding of reasons for hospitalization
Desired outcome from hospitalization

B. Collects data from available sources
1. Patient
2. Family
3. Significant other
4. Health care providers
5. Individuals or agencies in the community

C. Collects data by using scientific methodology
1. Interview
2. Observation
3. Inspection
4. Auscultation
5. Palpation
6. Percussion

D. Interprets and assesses records and reports
1. ECG
2. Radiology studies
3. Hematology studies
4. Chemistry studies
5. Coagulation studies
6. Urinalysis
7. Serial cardiac enzymes
8. Previous records
9. Arterial blood gases

E. Recognizes and assesses alterations in health status; records and communicates this to members of the health care team

F. Organizes assessment data so they are
1. Accurate
2. Complete
3. Accessible
4. Confidential

G. Communicates data in an orderly fashion
1. Records data
2. Updates data
3. Reports pertinent information to members of health care team

II. *Planning* (learning modules AB-4)
   A. Completes a written nursing care plan for an assigned patient
      1. Identifies the patient's present/potential problems from the patient assessment:
         Determines patient's health status
         Compares health status to norms
         Prioritizes problems according to impact on health status
      2. Formulates desired outcomes specific to the patient problems/needs and established norms
      3. Ensures that desired outcomes are mutually agreed upon by the patient, family (when appropriate), and nurse
      4. Formulates desired outcomes that are specific, measurable within a certain time frame, and consistent with other health providers' expectations
      3. Incorporates home health care into desired outcomes: Includes support systems, health information, and resources that will enable the patient to identify and accept necessary modifications in lifestyle. Includes patient learning of
         a. Disease process and complications
         b. Medications
         c. Diet
         d. Exercise/activity pattern
         e. Self-care techniques and materials
         f. Available support systems and resources

III. *Implementation*
   A. Takes immediate action in response to an emergency situation (learning module C-1 and 2)
      1. Acts rapidly and effectively
      2. Manages self, patients, and other employees
      3. Takes charge during cardiac arrest until physician arrives
      4. Provides a calm, reassuring atmosphere
      5. Communicates effectively with family members to reduce stress
   B. Locates, cares for, and operates ICU or CCU equipment including (learning module C-6)
      1. Monitors
      2. Defibrillation equipment
      3. Crash carts and contents of carts
      4. Trays (such as for trachs, CVP—see attached list)
      5. Temporary and permanent pacemakers
      6. Ventilators
   C. Formulates nursing prescriptions on an assigned patient that delineate actions to be taken. Prescribed actions are included in the written nursing care plan and (learning modules AB-5)
      1. Are specific to the patient problem and expected outcome

2. Are based on current scientific knowledge
3. Are based on principles of patient teaching as appropriate
4. Are based on principles of psychosocial interactions as appropriate
5. Are based on environmental factors influencing the patient's health as appropriate
6. Include human, material, and community resources
7. Include keeping patient knowledgeable of health status and total health care plan

D. Implements the actions delineated in the nursing prescriptions. (Refer to attached subcompetencies 1 through 67 on the skills inventory.) Actions implemented:
1. Actively involve the patient and family
2. Are consistent with nursing prescriptions
3. Are based on current scientific knowledge
4. Are flexible and individualized for each patient
5. Include principles of safety
6. Include principles of infection control
7. Are consistent with hospital policies and procedures
8. Are documented according to established policies and procedures

IV. *Evaluation* (learning module AB-6)

A. Evaluates the outcome of nursing actions on the assigned patient for further assessment and planning
1. Collects data concerning the patient's health status
2. Compares data to specific desired outcomes
3. Evaluates with patient (as appropriate) the achievement of desired outcomes

B. Reassesses the nursing care plan of an assigned patient following evaluation of desired outcomes
1. Reassesses the patient's problems and health status
2. Reassesses nursing plans
3. Reassesses nursing prescriptions
4. Reassesses nursing actions for effectiveness in achieving desired outcomes

C. Revises plans on the assigned patient as directed by the outcomes and reassessment
1. Determines new patient's present or potential problems
2. Formulates and revises desired outcomes
3. Revises nursing prescriptions
4. Revises nursing actions to be implemented in accordance with new plans and prescriptions
5. Evaluates outcome of nursing actions
6. Documents changes in plan of care and outcomes

APPENDIX 8–2

Intensive and Coronary Care Nurse Skills Inventory

The following is a list of the required skills and procedures for ICU/CCU. The nurse must assess his or her ability to perform each of these procedures competently. A list of subcompetencies is attached that further delineates the exact required performance and refers to specific learning modules for each subcompetency. Following self-assessment the nurse determines his or her learning needs in consultation with the preceptor. Together they plan learning experiences and the nurse completes the appropriate learning modules. At the end of each learning module is the method of evaluation of the particular competency. The nurse may proceed directly to the evaluation or be evaluated after having completed the learning experiences. The time period and method for learning is flexible and individualized, as is the exact time for evaluation. When the evaluation has been completed with 100 percent accuracy, the evaluator documents his or her initials and the date in the appropriate space below. There may be several initials if evaluation occurs by post-test, in skills lab, and on the clinical unit.

Name ______________________________ Date ______
Preceptor ______________________________

Responsibility, Skill, Procedure	I am competent performing	Demonstrated competence (evaluator's initials and date)	Comments
1. Patient assessment (according to required competencies and subcompetencies attached)			
2. Patient care planning			
3. Patient admission			
4. Transcribing physician's orders			
5. Documentation procedures and policies			
6. Standing orders			
7. Attaching patient to monitor			
8. Oxygen therapy			
9. Intravenous therapy			
10. Intravenous medications			
11. Administering blood			
12. Initiating and providing hyperalimentation			
13. Caring for patients on the hypo/hyperthermia units			
14. Injections—Intramuscular, subcutaneous, and intradermal			
15. Administering insulin			
16. Care of the patient on isolation			
17. Cultures—nose, throat, and wound			
18. CVP insertion and care			
19. Insertion and care of nasogastric tube			

Responsibility, Skill, Procedure	I am competent performing	Demonstrated competence (evaluator's initials and date)	Comments
20. Chest tube insertion and care			
21. Obtaining and interpreting blood gases			
22. Inserting urinary catheters			
23. Administering enemas			
24. Urine checks for diabetics			
25. Decubitus care			
26. Rotating tourniquets			
27. Care of the patient with multiple traumas			
28. Care of the patient with burns			
29. Administration of emergency drugs (see attached list of subcompetencies)			
30. Intracranial pressure monitoring			
31. Care of the surgical patient (see list of subcompetencies)			
32. Neurologic assessment and documentation			
33. 24-hour urine collection			
34. Assisting with lumbar punctures			
35. Assisting with paracentesis			
36. Assisting with thoracentesis			
37. Assisting with cutdowns			
38. Collection of specimens			
39. Care of the ostomy patient			

Responsibility, Skill, Procedure	I am competent performing	Demonstrated competence (evaluator's initials and date)	Comments
40. Tube feedings—NG and gastrostomy			
41. NG irrigations			
42. Reality orientation			
43. Use of restraints			
44. Transfer of patients			
45. Initiates emergency actions according to competency and subcompetency statements			
46. Locates, cares for, and operates ICU/CCU equipment			
47. Formulates nursing prescriptions for care planning according to ICU/CCU competency statements			
48. Demonstrates proper body mechanics			
49. Arterial line insertions and monitoring			
50. Swan-ganz insertion and reading			
51. Cardiac output determination			
52. Patient teaching and documentation of learning			
53. Placement of endotracheal tube			
54. Suctioning			
55. Administering narcotics			
56. Routine cardiac medications (see attached subcompetencies)			
57. Troubleshooting monitors			
58. Care of patient on ventilators			

Responsibility, Skill, Procedure	I am competent performing	Demonstrated competence (evaluator's initials and date)	Comments
59. Use of doppler			
60. Tracheostomy care			
61. Defibrillation			
62. Cardioversion			
63. Temporary pacemakers			
64. Permanent pacemakers			
65. Care and observation of the cardiac patient			
66. Hazard checks			
67. Care of the dying patient			

Initials	Signature
________	______________________________
________	______________________________
________	______________________________
________	______________________________
________	______________________________
________	______________________________

APPENDIX 8–3

Learning Module NS 63

Competency: Implements the actions delineated in the nursing prescriptions
Subcompetency: #63 Temporary pacemakers
By the end of this learning module the nurse will comply with established policies and procedures for insertion and care of the temporary pacemaker, as evidenced by:

Criteria	Learning Experience	Evaluation
1. Explaining procedure to patient 2. Obtaining baseline ECG 3. Maintaining patient IV 4. Preparing emergency equipment and crash cart 5. Checking pacemaker for new battery and proper functioning 6. Maintaining sterile technique during insertion 7. Checking vital signs and ECG throughout procedure 8. Turning pacemaker on upon request 9. Adjusting rate and MA on request 10. Obtaining stimulation threshold and sensitivity on request 11. Securing electrode on patient 12. Performing site care 13. Checking vital signs, pacer beats, muscle stimulation, and patient level of consciousness to determine response to pacemaker 14. Documenting pacer setting and procedure in nurses' notes 15. Checking pacer setting every shift 16. Checking site for redness, swelling, and performing site care every day 17. Checking ECG for pacing and documenting the strip every shift	Videotape N23—Care of the patient during insertion of a temporary pacemaker Nursing Policy #N28—Infection control Nursing Procedure #40—Insertion of a temporary pacemaker Nursing Procedure #41—Care of the patient with a temporary pacemaker Practice and simulation in skills lab Tuesdays and Thursdays 7AM until 11PM with assistance from staff development personnel	Demonstrate criteria during simulation in skills lab with 100% accuracy (evaluator can be staff development or personnel preceptor) Completion of attached written test with 100% accuracy

APPENDIX 8–4

General Orientation Checklist

Use this checklist as a guide for covering needed information and becoming oriented to new surroundings.

Disaster zone numbers ______
Addressograph operation ______
Stationery supplies ______
Requisition forms ______
Patient charts ______
Old charts—how to find ______
Telephone directories ______
Bulletin boards ______
Suggestion boxes ______
Time cards ______
Assignment sheets ______
Patient call system ______
Crash carts ______
Telephones ______
Physician's boxes ______
Kardexes ______
Paging system ______
Treatment rooms ______
Location of equipment for treatments ______
Other available equipment (IV, dressings, B/P cuff and stethoscope, ophthalmoscope, flashlight, etc) ______
Utility rooms—clean and soiled ______
Contents of utility rooms ______
Central supplies ______
IV fluids ______
IV supplies ______
Charge tickets ______
Requisitions—location and procedure ______
Ice machines ______
Refrigerators ______
Patient nourishments ______
Waiting rooms ______
Classrooms ______
Conference rooms ______
Educational resources for patients ______
Learning resource center ______

Charting
Procedure for charting ______
TRP sheet ______
Errors in charting ______
Flagging for allergies ______
Flagging for drug stopping and re-ordering ______
Daily kardex checks ______
Physician color codes ______

Reports and other forms
Master assignment sheet ______
Individual assignment sheets ______
X-ray and lab schedules ______
Census sheet ______
24-hr condition sheet ______
Patient classification system and sheets ______
Incident reports ______
Maintenance requests ______
Dietary checklist ______
Consent forms ______
Autopsy permits ______

Patient policies
Admission procedures ______
Discharge procedures ______
Transfers ______
Release against orders ______
Visiting regulations ______

Absent without leave ______
Care and loss of valuables ______

Patient's room

Operation of bed ______
Bathroom equipment ______
Emergency lights ______
Call system from room ______
Oxygen and suction outlets ______
TV and radio operation ______
Heating/cooling system ______
Bedside table and over-bed tray operation ______
Side rails—operation ______
Restraints—policies, types, how obtained ______
Patient orientation procedure ______

General location and layout

Rooms (number, location, type) ______
Exits ______
Linen closets ______
Linen carts ______
Night pharmacy ______
Storage rooms and equipment (IV poles, scales, wheelchairs, stretchers) ______
Fire extinguishers and alarms ______
Oxygen cut-off valves ______
Zone numbers ______
Employee restrooms ______
Employee lockers and closets ______

Organization of unit

Unit objectives and plans ______
Types of patients ______
Capacity, census, accommodations ______
Time schedules and assignments ______
Schedule request procedures ______
Authority and decision making ______
Resource people ______
Primary nursing care system ______

Clarification of roles

Head nurse ______
Charge nurse ______
Primary care nurse ______
LPN ______
Nursing assistant ______
Orderly ______
Unit secretary ______

References and resources

Nursing texts and journals ______
Physician Desk Reference ______
Medical dictionary ______
Policy manuals ______
Procedure manuals ______
Fire and disaster manuals ______
Diet manual ______
Isolation and infection control manual ______
Lab and radiology manuals ______
Care planning guides—how to use ______
Patient education guides and audiovisual resources and handouts—how to use ______
Standardized discharge planning guides—

how to use in discharge plans ______

Medication area

Medicine carts ______
Medicine trays, cups, alcohol syringes, etc. ______
Medicine refrigerator ______
Narcotic drawers ______
Narcotic keys ______
Narcotic book and sign out sheets ______
Narcotic count and procedures ______

Policies and procedures for medications

Doctor's orders, verbal, phone, and written ______
Transcribing orders ______
Charting medications on med record and nurses' notes ______
Narcotic replacement ______
Requisitioning and refilling meds ______
Obtaining meds after hours ______
Use of kardex ______
Crediting medications ______
Medication errors ______
Medications brought from home ______
Medications to be sent home with patient ______

Introductions to personnel

On unit ______
Department heads ______
General tour and introduction to hospital employees ______
Review of nursing standards ______
Explanation of standards, job descriptions, and performance evaluations ______
Explanation of nursing committees, task forces, and staff involvement ______
Code 9 procedure—crash cart contents, locations, operation of monitors ______
Standards, job descriptions, and performance evaluations ______

APPENDIX 8–5

Checklist for Personnel Policies and General Hospital Information

Use this checklist as a guide for covering needed information.

_____ Philosophy and background of hospital
_____ Names and positions of administrative team
_____ Hospital organizational chart and chain of command
_____ Hospital goals and objectives
_____ Commitment to creativity
_____ Participative management

Personnel policies:
    _____ Vacations
    _____ Holidays
    _____ Sick days
    _____ Pay periods
    _____ Meals
    _____ Breaks
    _____ Leave of absence
    _____ Insurance
    _____ Pension plan
    _____ Christmas savings plan
    _____ Time cards
    _____ Progressive discipline procedures
    _____ Grievance procedures
    _____ Equal employment opportunity organization

Hospital policies:
    _____ Health requirements
    _____ Dress code
    _____ Conduct
    _____ Visiting control and regulations
    _____ Incident reports
    _____ Smoking regulations
    _____ Travel policy
    _____ In-service requirements
    _____ Internal recruitment protocols
    _____ Selection—internal and external
    _____ Personnel inventory
    _____ Orientation procedure
    _____ Performance evaluations and merit raise systems
    _____ Staff development opportunities and facilities

_____ Employee suggestion boxes
_____ Employee gain sharing

Fire and disaster plans:
- _____ Code blue flash—fire
- _____ Code two—internal disaster
- _____ Code three—external disaster
- _____ Code four—bomb threat (never paged)
- _____ Bomb threat information sheet

_____ Pastoral and religious services
_____ Volunteer services
_____ Community services
_____ Hospital information systems
_____ Quality assurance

9 The Performance Evaluation Process

We all need to know how we are doing in our work. This need may simply concern security: "Am I doing well enough to keep my job?" It may involve security and self-esteem: "Am I doing a *good* job?" Or it may include security, self-esteem, and achievement: "How can I do better? How can I excel?" In turn, the organization needs to know about the employee. Is the employee performing at his or her best? Is he or she developing and using talents and potentials? Are personal and career needs being met? What environmental climate and support will facilitate growth and development? The performance evaluation process serves to satisfy this "need to know." It not only searches for and provides answers, but it also functions to guide changes in employee or organizational behavior that will maximize potential and promote organizational success.

What exactly is performance evaluation? Basically, it is drawing a conclusion about the nature and character of an individual's work. It is estimating the value or degree of excellence of both the process and outcome of an employee's implementation of roles and responsibilities. But effective performance evaluation draws upon principles of communication, leadership, adult education, and intuition to accomplish a multitude of purposes. It is a process of human resource management that aims to

- Assess the past and present performance of employees and communicate this assessment to them
- Compare this information to organizational plans, to ensure a match

- Receive information from employees concerning their personal goals, needs, and plans
- Improve employee performance and maximize potentials through counseling, mutual goal setting, self-evaluation, and development strategies
- Recognize achievements and creative contributions; link achievements to reward systems such as clinical ladder progression, bonus systems, merit raises, and job promotions
- Be used for management and personnel decisions concerning staffing, planning, and the other personnel processes
- Be a link to improving retention and productivity; be a basis for staff development
- Assist in removing unsatisfactory employees
- Be one means for promoting change

The performance evaluation is also a means for monitoring the organization's response to change. As discussed in previous chapters, many changes are affecting health care workers and the nature of their work, and continually stressing the organization. Management in turn must continually assess and predict the impact of these changes, and must alter systems and plans to restore equilibrium. As environmental change affects the health care system, mechanisms must be used to alter personnel processes, administrative functions, organizational structures, and policies and procedures, to balance the forces of change. As change affects human resources, needs and behaviors will also change, as will the work environment. Management must continually make responsive changes in order to restore stability.

The performance evaluation can reflect equilibrium and successful responses to change. When collective performance is outstanding or above expected standards, the organization is functioning at its best and responding well to human needs, but when collective performance is within minimal standards or below standards, there is a problem that management must find and correct. When several employees are practicing at substandard levels, there is a breakdown in human resource management and the response to change. Were these employees not adequately selected and prepared for the job? Is the training or development program not assisting employees to maintain clinical excellence? Are efforts at retention and job satisfaction failing, allowing low morale and productivity? Are disciplinary measures ineffective, allowing unsatisfactory workers to remain in the system? Or is the performance evaluation itself not valid and effective?

In addition to monitoring response to change and providing evidence of a breakdown in human resource management, the performance evaluation also contributes to quality assurance. As will be discussed later, standards of practice are developed to reflect and measure quality patient care. The performance evaluation stems directly from the standards, and therefore reflects the implementation of these standards. It provides one means to determine whether these standards are being maintained. In combination with audits, research, observation, and other monitoring techniques, it can be an important tool in ensuring quality. By monitoring the level of performance and correcting deficiencies, the evaluation can help to maintain quality practice.

The performance evaluation is also an instrument for implementing organizational plans. Standards and job descriptions are developed to promote progress toward goals and plans, and the performance evaluation determines the degree of adherence to standards and job descriptions. In addition, the performance evaluation involves setting individual goals and objectives for enhancing creativity and skills in the organization. These personal objectives are correlated with organizational plans, thus enhancing their attainment. The function of the performance evaluation is to set goals and monitor performance, so that it complements and facilitates the achievement of organizational objectives; it can be seen as a tool for facilitating progress towards these overall objectives.

Of course, a satisfied, fulfilled, and productive worker also promotes the achievement of organizational plans. Only people can make things work. If the organization consists of people enjoying their work and taking pride in their performance, the results facilitate organizational success. Therefore the performance evaluation also aims to foster retention, job satisfaction, and productivity. By promoting growth, development, and well-being, the organization can prosper and achieve its goals.

Management must be aware of results and personal goals indicated on the performance evaluation. These results should be compared to nursing and organizational objectives. Incongruencies and gaps should be identified, and strategies planned to correct deviations from overall plans. All employees must be working in some way to achieve the goals and aims of the organization. It is up to management to assist and guide the development and achievement of personal employee goals that will contribute to the whole.

For example, one organizational objective may be to involve the family in patient education and health care. Nursing plans may include patient/family counseling sessions, group classes, and development of family care plans. Individual nurses' goals and objectives should complement these plans, and are reflected on the performance evaluation. An objective for the future may involve studying family theory, enhancing communication and teaching skills, or developing specific tools to assess and teach the family aspects of health care. As the nurse strives to achieve personal goals and objectives, the nurse is also working toward organizational objectives.

The process of performance evaluation, therefore, is more than appraising the employee's work. It serves a variety of purposes, all aimed at ensuring organizational viability. This chapter will explore principles and techniques required for effective performance evaluation. The point to keep in mind is that no matter what tools or techniques are used, effective performance evaluation is up to the manager. The management team must possess skills, abilities, and insight into human behavior, or this process is doomed to failure.

A PHILOSOPHY FOR PERFORMANCE EVALUATION

The focus of performance evaluation is on growth and development. Only following the failure of all efforts to counsel, support, and assist the employee in maintaining minimal standards does the process become punitive; otherwise, it is a learning tool. If used in this manner, performance evaluation can be seen as rewarding and satisfying by both managers and employees. If a genuine concern for employee well-being and growth is communicated, a sense of trust can be developed between management and employees. This is the crucial element in an effective performance evaluation system. It is necessary to formulate *and practice* a philosophy for the performance evaluation process. The following is an example of such a philosophy.

> Performance evaluation is intimately linked to job satisfaction, productivity, retention and, ultimately, system viability. It is a process that begins where orientation leaves off—at the end of adjustment and beginning of growth and development. At this point employees have been matched with the job and culture, have been oriented and assisted in "fitting in," and have developed initial objectives and plans to begin their growth and development within the organization. Performance evaluation serves to continually provide feedback concerning performance and guide improvements, thus directing the employee's development.
>
> Performance evaluation focuses on total development of the individual and organization, not isolated tasks or parts. It identifies the effect of continual change on this development. It aims to promote the development of tools, insight, and attitudes necessary to grow with the changing times. The performance evaluation reinforces the need for flexibility, creativity, and innovation, and links with staff development processes to further develop these tools for change.
>
> Employee involvement through the entire process of performance evaluation is crucial to effective development. Participation in planning, policy and procedure development, self-evaluation, and evaluation of the process can ensure involvement and promote growth. Principles of adult learning are also used to aid this growth and development.
>
> The focus of performance evaluation is to develop trust. Each individual is valued as contributing to the success of the organization. The performance evaluation is the process of mutual sharing of ideas, concerns, and needs for the future for each role within the organization. The top priority is for the individual's well-being and fulfillment of creative potential. Management and the individual work together to achieve these

goals. Each one mutually alters behaviors in order to promote an environment of trust and growth.

The organization is committed to lifelong learning. The performance evaluation is a learning process; it is a time to reflect on inner strengths and weaknesses, and learn about oneself. It is a time to identify the important role each person plays in the future of the organization, and plan ways to develop inner skills and abilities. It is a time to map out the future course of learning, in order for the employee to develop fully as an individual and as part of the organization.

ORGANIZING THE PERFORMANCE EVALUATION PROCESS

In organizing and planning this personnel process, certain principles should be followed to ensure successful results. The following are some principles to consider in organizing performance evaluation, and developing policies and procedures.

Performance evaluation should:

- Be based on policies, procedures, and tools that are developed and agreed upon by both management and staff
- Minimize bias and subjectivity, and be based on valid and reliable tools
- Be derived from standards of practice and job descriptions
- Be used to identify needs and set specific, measurable objectives for self-development
- Provide a means for recognition and reward for performance exceeding minimum standards
- Be implemented by a manager trained in evaluating performance, who continually observes and supervises the employee's performance
- Be based upon behavior and productivity, not personality
- Be based upon self-evaluation and employee input. Final decisions reflect this employee input.
- Be based upon ongoing observation and feedback, not sporadic observation or incidents. Should be a continual process of communication, resulting in a final summary of performance
- Should identify both strengths and weaknesses and reflect the employee's average performance. Results should be based upon consistent behavior and provide assistance for improvement
- Be used by management and employees as a communication tool. It is a time to formally communicate and make improvements

The questions that must be answered in organizing and planning for performance evaluation include: Who will evaluate whom? When? How frequently? How will employees be evaluated? What is the desired outcome of the evaluation? The answers to these questions must be clearly

Policy

All employees are evaluated by their immediate supervisors. Head nurses evaluate the employees on their units, with assistance and input from assistant head nurses. Directors of nurses evaluate the head nurses in their jurisdiction, and they in turn are evaluated by the vice-president for nursing.

Evaluations are completed annually and filed in the employee's records. A six-month evaluation interview is also conducted to communicate strengths, weaknesses, and areas in need of improvement. This report is utilized in the annual evaluation.

Annual evaluations are completed 12 months following the completion of the orientation period. All new employees receive an evaluation following their first 90 days with the organization. Annual review begins from that point.

Standards, job descriptions, performance evaluation, and criteria for evaluation will be accessible to employees at all times.

Self-evaluation and self-objectives are a part of the performance evaluation. The objectives are mutually evaluated and recorded at the six-month and annual evaluation sessions. Throughout the year communication is ongoing between managers and employees concerning performance and progress towards objectives. The employee's growth, development, creative contributions, and perception of progress must be included in the evaluation results.

Signatures on the evaluation and six-month report form indicate understanding of the information on the form. A completed form must contain the signatures of the employee, the nurse-manager, and the vice-president for nursing.

Managers must document suggestions for improvement, guides for growth and development, and specific approaches to gaining needed skills. Creative innovations are also the focus for development.

Performance evaluation ratings, achievement of self-objectives, and recommendations by nurse-managers will feed into incentive programs for salary increases, promotions, or development for new or different positions. This information will also be added to the employee's personnel inventory data for later use by recruitment and selection personnel.

All employees are rated as *unsatisfactory* (does not meet job expectations), *satisfactory* (meets job expectations), *above average* (exceeds job expectations), or *excellent* (outstanding performance).

Any performance areas evaluated as *unsatisfactory* or *excellent* must be accompanied by specific documented rationale. Any specific strengths, weaknesses, or recommendations in performance should be explained under the appropriate item.

Employees unable to agree to evaluation decisions may initiate the appeals proceedings. Rationale and documentation must be provided to justify the appeals proceedings.

Employees are expected to score *satisfactory* in order to meet job expectations and maintain standards of practice. An *unsatisfactory* total rating results in the employee being placed on probation for three months. During that time the employee is assisted in achieving satisfactory performance. At completion of three months, the employee is re-evaluated. A *satisfactory* rating removes the employee from probation, and he or she reverts to the annual performance evaluation. An *unsatisfactory* rating results in dismissal.

New employees must receive a *satisfactory* evaluation following their three months' probationary period. An *unsatisfactory* score results in dismissal. A *satisfactory* results in their

Figure 9–1. Sample policy for performance evaluations.

removal from probation (some contractual agreements with unions do not allow a probationary period).

Employees placed on probation are counseled by the vice-president for nursing. Any employee dismissed for *unsatisfactory* performance is provided an exit interview by the vice-president for nursing.

An employee evaluated as *unsatisfactory* in a performance area during the six-month interview, and again *unsatisfactory* in the same area at the annual evaluation period, is placed on probation. Any employee rated as *unsatisfactory* in a performance area during the annual evaluation, and again as *unsatisfactory* in that area at the six-month interview, is placed on probation. After a three-month period of counseling and assistance, the employee must raise that performance area to *satisfactory*. An employee who is unable to perform *satisfactorily* is dismissed.

Employees are encouraged to participate in the evaluation process. Their self-evaluation should be submitted at least three days prior to the annual evaluation, and the supporting data be used in the final rating. The purpose of the evaluation is to determine quality of performance and set goals for the future. A consensus should be reached by the manager and employee, based upon factual evidence and information.

Figure 9–1. *(continued)*

understood by all personnel, and documented in policies and procedures. A specific performance evaluation policy can answer many of these questions, and set the ground rules for both managers and employees. Figure 9–1 is an example of a policy for performance evaluations.

This evaluation process is an ideal example. Few organizations would have the luxury of such heavy time emphasis on this one process as presented in this chapter. The reader should alter and revise these various policies, processes, and procedures to fit the unique organizational setting. For example, this in-depth approach may not be necessary every year. A simpler version, such as a brief summary evaluation, may be more appropriate and acceptable every other year, especially for outstanding performers. The performance evaluation forms may be shortened and consolidated. There are many alternatives to the systems presented here. This process is offered as a guide and example only, to assist in developing and implementing effective performance evaluation systems.

STANDARDS, JOB DESCRIPTIONS, AND PERFORMANCE EVALUATIONS

It is necessary that the staff and management develop and agree upon what is to be evaluated, or *what is the desired outcome.* Aside from personal objectives for growth and development, the minimum level of expectations should be defined. This is the acceptable level of performance for keeping one's job. Employees must be evaluated on what they have "contracted" to perform in the organization, or the job description. In turn, job descriptions must be based upon the standards of practice defined by the institution as representing quality. Appendix 9–1 provides an example of standards of practice developed for medical–surgical nursing practice. A medical–surgical registered nurse performance evaluation is shown in Appendix 9–2. This evaluation form was directly drawn from the medical–surgical registered nurse job description shown in Appendix 6–1. It can be seen, by comparing these three items, that satisfactory outcome on the performance evaluation would signify compliance with the expectations agreed upon in the job description, and compliance with standards of practice.

With any evaluation, there are levels of expectation and levels of performance. Some scale or means to determine the quality or level of performance must be devised. The staff and management must be clear as to criteria for unsatisfactory, satisfactory, above average, and excellent performance. The staff must know how they can obtain a specific performance rating, and management must understand how to determine this rating.

One means for determining a measurement of performance is for the staff and management to define specific criteria for unsatisfactory, satisfactory, above average, and excellent performance for each component on the performance evaluation. This can be a time-consuming process, but once developed will ensure a more effective and fair evaluation system. If the staff and management agree to specific levels of achievement, then the system will be accepted as worthwhile. In addition, the criteria in the *above average* and *excellent* ratings provide direction for improvement, growth, and development.

Each nursing unit can form a committee of staff and management to develop these criteria. The critiera can be very specific and outcome-related, or simply provide general guidelines, allowing individual freedom and interpretation. If the latter is the case, each unit must understand the intent and goals of each criterion, and provide direction in its achievement. Appendix 9–3 provides an example of a medical–surgical registered nurse performance evaluation with evaluation criteria.

Of course, the directions for completing tools and forms must be understood and accessible. Directions should be provided on each form, and scoring should also be clear (see Appendix 9–4 for scoring procedure).

There are many means for evaluating performance other than the one presented in Appendix 9–2. Essay reports, testing, management-by-objectives (MBO), as well as a multitude of various evaluation forms may be used. The six-month interview and evaluation form shown in Appendix 9–5 could be used every other year as the standard evaluation tool. The approach presented in this chapter was chosen because it is based upon the nursing process (assess, plan, implement, evaluate) and satisfies the Joint Commission on Accreditation of Hospitals Standards related to standards, job descriptions, and performance evaluations.

VALIDITY AND RELIABILITY

It is important that whatever methods or tools are used in the performance evaluation, they be valid and reliable. The staff and management should work together to test their tools prior to implementation. The performance evaluation form or instrument must measure the expected behaviors as defined in the job description. The various criteria must actually reflect unsatisfactory, satisfactory, above average, or excellent performance. Through direct observation and data collection from charts and care planning, nurses can validate performance against the performance evaluation scores. In addition, the management team must be consistent and implement the tool in a similar fashion. For instance, a particular employee should receive a similar scoring on the evaluation regardless of which supervisor completed it. Management must be trained in performance evaluation and follow procedures specifically. Through trial practices, feedback from staff, and monitoring by the nurse-executive, reliability of scores can be monitored and ensured. Reliability and validity should be tested at regular intervals, to reflect consistency with changes in the work and work environment.

PREPARING FOR THE PERFORMANCE EVALUATION

The biggest challenge is in implementing the performance evaluation. Skills in communication, adult education, and intuitive thinking are needed to foster participation and a positive response by the employee. The following discussion will assist in preparing for an effective evaluation process.

Data Collection and Documentation

The crucial component in the evaluation process is the collection of accurate and consistent information about the employee that reflects his or her performance. This collection must be systematic and ongoing. In addition, the employee must be told of problem areas or praised for strengths during the day-to-day work routine. There should be no surprises at the evaluation interview. As managers collect information, they must also communicate their findings, so that employees receive feedback concerning their performance.

The nurse-manager should prepare a notebook specifically for evaluations. Each section in the notebook concerns a specific employee. The manager should develop a timetable to observe certain behaviors and performance areas for all employees on the unit. For example, two days each month may be set aside for assessing the performance criteria under *Assessment* (see Appendix 9–3). The manager reviews patient interview forms, listens in on shift reports, reviews nurses' notes, and observes during patient care. Although the manager continually assesses and documents information pertaining to assessment items throughout the year, some time is set aside specifically for auditing this performance. The next month the manager concentrates on *Planning*, then *Implemention* and *Evaluation*. Then the cycle begins again.

When collecting information about performance, the manager needs guides or checklists to ensure all areas have been assessed. The performance evaluation form may be used as a guide. In the notebook each employee has a form, which is documented with notes and facts throughout the year. At the completion of the year, incidents and evaluation have virtually been done. Also, discrepancies in performance or areas not thoroughly assessed can be focused upon. These forms should be reviewed three months prior to the annual evaluation date, to allow time for focusing on specific behaviors not previously assessed.

Information should also be collected throughout the manager's daily routine, such as during patient rounds and committee work. Nursing care that detects and prevents complications and decreases length of stay should be recorded in the daily log or notebook. Patient interviews that reflect continuity in patient education, family participation, and creative interventions should be credited and documented for the nurses involved. And these nurses should be recognized and praised at that time.

By continually assessing performance throughout all interactions, the manager will stay in tune with what is happening on the unit. The manager will assess problems, determine quality of care, and recognize strengths, progress, and growth of the staff. The manager will also be alert to areas in need of immediate change, and can intervene early rather than after events have turned into a disaster.

Although the manager constantly evaluates performance, every incident that is written in the daily notebook is not necessarily recorded on the annual evaluation form. This information is used for assessing *repetitive* and *ongoing* behaviors. A one-time mistake or incident may be jotted down in the notebook, but only if it *continues* to occur despite counseling or specific instruction does it affect the final evaluation rating. Conversely, positive behavior exhibited on one or a few occasions may be used in the annual evaluation. By relating an employee's ability to excel to this demonstration of positive behavior, the manager can provide a guideline and direction for future behavior. This approach focuses on the *positive*, rather than the negative, as a mechanism for improvement.

There are times when one incident is so severe that it warrants immediate suspension or dismissal. Such incidents should be identified in the employee handbook or policies. Stealing medications, chemical abuse or intoxication on the job, physical or mental abuse of patients, and other such incidents are an example. This will be further addressed in the following chapter.

The documentation of incidents concerning positive performance or critical problems should be consistent. Incidents should be recorded as soon as they occur. That which was directly observed by the manager or reported to the manager must be specified. The facts should be presented with the outcome or results. Any corrective action or communication with the employee should be documented. No judgment or opinions are recorded, only the facts. The names of any employees involved should also be recorded, along with the time, date, and location of the incident. If the occurrence was considered a positive contribution to the organization or a severe incident that could warrant disciplinary action, it should be documented on a form and signed by the employee. An example of such a form is provided in Appendix 9–6. This form is used for both positive recognition and proof of warning and reprimand. It can be used for any unusual occurrence that justifies formal communication with the employee.

Rating the Employee

Following the continual data collection and prior to the interview, the employee's performance must be rated on the performance evaluation form. During this process objectivity must be maintained to the extent that is humanly possible. Certain guidelines can be followed to help overcome bias and errors in ratings. These are:

1. Review daily log and documentation, and past employee self-objectives. Avoid reviewing previous ratings before completing the evaluation, for this may sway your decisions.
2. Reflect on the employee's strengths and weaknesses for each area of performance. Concentrate on one trait at a time, not overall performance.
3. Focus on typical behavior, not just recent or one-time events.
4. Base decisions on facts from your data collection.
5. Focus on significant behavior, not trivial incidents or personality.
6. Do not use the evaluation process for discipline or to discuss negative behaviors only. Always bring out strengths and improvements.
7. Be thoroughly familiar with all aspects of the job, policies, procedures, etc.
8. Utilize the employee's self-evaluation. Review each rating and consider the employee's documentation and rationale. Make notes and questions to be discussed in the interview.
9. Avoid typical rating errors, such as the following:
   a. Avoid the tendency to be overly strict or lenient.
   b. Avoid the tendency to rate all employees as average.
   c. Avoid rating an employee according to your general attitude or impression of that employee.
   d. Avoid letting one excellent or deficient quality influence the rating of all other qualities.

e. Avoid giving similar ratings for qualities or behaviors that seem similar or logically related.
f. Avoid high ratings in order to prevent confrontation or interruption in employment or because you believe other managers rate high. These problems must be addressed with top administration, and must not enter into the rating process.
g. Avoid rating employees according to their job status, such as higher for professional employees and lower for minimum-wage workers.
h. Compare employees to others in their job status and according to their job descriptions. Do not expect professional performance from nonprofessional employees.

By being aware of these errors, you can attempt to overcome them and maintain objectivity for each performance area.

Self-evaluation

Another important source of information for the performance evaluation is the employee himself or herself. The employee's evaluation of achievement of objectives, level of performance, and supporting rationale must be included in the evaluation.

Employees should be taught and required to perform self-evaluations. The simplest self-evaluation tool is to use the performance evaluation form itself and the criteria for evaluation. The time to provide in-servicing on self-evaluation is when the forms are first developed. After that time, the manager works with the employee on a one-to-one basis, to develop skills and insight into self-evaluation.

Employees should collect information concerning their performance of various areas on the evaluation, and document this information throughout the year. They discuss their progress toward objectives and self-evaluation of performance during the six-month interview with the manager. They receive validation and suggestions concerning their perceptions and assessment, and use this to alter or continue their performance. Prior to their annual evaluation, they submit their completed self-evaluation form to the manager. Their progress and assessment should have been discussed throughout the year. The manager uses this information in finalizing the evaluation results. During the interview, any discrepancies in interpretation are discussed. If sufficient evidence has been documented to justify a certain rating, there should be little problem in reaching a consensus. For instance, if an employee rates himself or herself as *excellent* under item 4, "promotes harmonious relationships and favorable attitudes among the health team," and the manager rates the employee as *above average,* the employee must provide justification for the self-rating. This employee has organized and implemented group discussion meetings after hospital hours in order to resolve differences among physicians and nurses concerning patient care decisions. The manager was aware of the employee's role in resolving physician-relation problems, but did not realize the extent of this involvement. Documentation of this effort to restore harmony and a good working environment justified the manager's changing the employee's rating to an *excellent*.

The inclusion of the self-evaluation assists employees in many ways. When the manager and employee discuss differences and reach a consensus, they both must reflect on their perceptions and interpretations. The employee learns to continually assess and improve his or her performance, if for no other reason than to justify a high rating on evaluation. The employee realizes that his or her perceptions and judgment do count but must be accompanied by sound rationale. This forces employees to become more objective in self-evaluation. An employee who rates himself or herself highly with no documentation quickly learns that the manager makes no alterations or compromise in the evaluation results. The employee who spends time and effort to complete an objective self-evaluation, however, learns that the manager readily receives input and is eager to improve ratings based on his or her rationale. The employee who is interested and involved in growth and development reaps the rewards.

The manager uses the self-evaluation not only as input into evaluation results, but also as a learning tool. The manager works with the employee to compare his or her perceptions to the manager's own, resulting in deeper insight, sharper perceptive abilities, and improved communication. The experience can enhance understanding and strengthen the relationship for mutual growth and development.

No situation is perfect, and there are times when the performance evaluation experience results in disagreement and unsatisfactory communication. The nurse-administrator must work to ensure that management provides the optimum environment to foster positive relationships and results. If the employee refuses to cooperate, then the relationship will switch from mutual growth and development to a more autocratic, controlling one on the manager's part. Unfortunately, all employees are not professional or desire improvement and positive relationships. It is up to the manager to identify ineffective employees, work to guide and help them meet expectations, then rid the system of those unwilling to participate. This is essential if the organization is to remain viable.

Managers must be in tune with employees who underrate themselves. Although self-evaluations are used for the performance evaluation process, managers must be cautious as to their effect on the outcome. An employee who is skillful at documentation and self-assessment and has good writing skills should not receive a higher rating than an equally good performer who was not able to "influence" the final decision. In addition, an employee whose self-rating is lower than it should be must be assisted in seeing his or her strengths and receiving an appropriate rating. The self-evaluation is an important source of information for the manager. It not only provides input concerning performance, but important insight into the nature, characteristics, and needs of the employee. It is used by management both as a learning tool and as a reinforcer of management decisions. But in the end, management must still make the decision, which must be *based on the facts*. The self-evaluation may assist in the decision, but it cannot be the sole basis for the decision.

Performance Evaluation Depends on Effective Management

Ineffective managers must be identified and dismissed if unable to perform satisfactorily. Unsatisfactory relationships or communication are often due to poor management. This cannot be tolerated if the system is to be viable and successful. Poor evaluation results and unsatisfactory manager–employee relations can indicate this ineffective performance and dictate investigation. The appeals process can also assist in identifying management problems (this will be presented later in the chapter). The nurse-administrator must assist and guide the management team in achieving excellence, but expect and accept nothing less. The success of the entire operation depends upon this.

Skill in performance evaluation cannot be learned in one class, but must be obtained through continual management development programs. Communication, leadership, interpersonal relations, and counseling skills—crucial to the performance evaluation process—are necessary for the effectiveness of all personnel processes. These skills must be continually practiced and developed through management training. In order to implement this personnel process successfully, management personnel must be trained and continually evaluated on their ability to execute these skills expertly.

Management Guidebook

Specific information and techniques for rating, interviewing, and other performance evaluation procedures can be summarized and compiled in a guidebook for the management personnel. This book could provide a handy reference for preparing and implementing the evaluation process. The material in this chapter could be used to compile such a handbook. The following are a few items that might be included in this guide:

- Purpose of performance evaluation
- Philosophy for the performance evaluation process
- Performance evaluation policy
- Relationship of standards, job descriptions, and performance evaluation
- Validity and reliability
- Writing and evaluating behavioral objectives
- Organizational plans and objectives
- Using employee self-evaluation

- Collecting data for performance evaluation
- Reinforcing positive behavior
- Using criteria for evaluation
- Counseling, coaching, and disciplinary measures for unsatisfactory behaviors
- Principles of adult education
- Rating the employee
- Conducting the interview

This guidebook can be used in conjunction with ongoing management development to promote an effective performance evaluation process.

SELF-OBJECTIVES

Planning, implementing, and evaluating self-objectives are a part of the performance evaluation process. For example, under II in Appendix 9–2, item 2 "Plans and develops self-objectives," integrates this important process into the performance evaluation itself. Various levels of achievement are identified in the criteria, ranging from documenting self-objectives on annual evaluation to revising objectives on a regular basis. An area is provided for documenting self-objectives on the last page of the evaluation form. Revisions, achievement of objectives, and new self-objectives should be written and attached to the self-evaluation form by the employee.

During the evaluation interview, the manager and employee discuss achievement or lack of achievement of objectives, needed changes, and development of new objectives. Throughout the year the nurse will discuss objectives with the manager while working toward goals. The six-month evaluation is simply a time to discuss progress formally and ensure that the employee is on the right course. The manager should provide assistance in meeting objectives, such as by consulting staff development personnel and providing time and resources to accomplish the objectives.

While objectives must be written, they should be done so as simply as possible. Elaborate requirements will focus more attention on the wording than the desired outcome. They may also be threatening to many employees and discourage optimum participation. Objectives should contain what is to be accomplished (the desired outcome) in measurable terms. They should contain a timetable for completion and review. Specifics pertaining to method or plan for attaining objectives, resources needed, and other support should be discussed. Freedom and flexibility, however, must be provided in the process. Employees are encouraged to use creative techniques and ideas to achieve objectives and should not be held to rigid plans. Objectives must be followed and reviewed when designated. Managers must make notes to meet with employees at three-month intervals and to follow up on progress.

In evaluating objectives, inability to achieve outcomes should result in reassessment. What prevented the achievement of the objectives? How can the strategies be improved? Was the objective realistic? Did unforeseen circumstances prevent its completion? The object is not to focus on failure, but on ways to improve. If the employee shows the *effort* to improve and achieve the objective, then the employee should be praised, regardless of the outcome. Although a successful outcome is the goal, learning and development while striving toward the objective is the true focus. Through this growth and development, and assistance by management in improving techniques and strategies, the employee will benefit in many ways, as will the organization.

Managers should assist employees in developing these objectives, and ensure that the objectives are a challenge to the employee. Routine tasks and responsibilities are not considered appropriate for self-objectives. Rather, problem solving, leadership skills, professional development, creative change, and research should be the focus. These objectives should also be linked to career development or other recognition systems, as should the performance evaluation rating.

CONDUCTING THE PERFORMANCE EVALUATION INTERVIEW

Employees are aware when their performance evaluations are due, but they should be given prior notice to prepare for the interview. An appointment should be made at least a week in advance, and their self-evaluation should be completed and submitted at least three days before the interview. The interview should not follow completion of the 11P.M. to 7A.M. shift or an unusually stressful day. If there is evidence that the employee is extremely fatigued, the appointment should be postponed to a later time.

During the interview you should communicate your belief in the philosophy and worth of the evaluation process. This communication will reflect on the employee's attitude and acceptance and facilitate focusing on growth and development. Maintain confidentiality and provide privacy. Choose a location that is free from interruptions, comfortable, and relaxing. Employees must know that you care about them enough to devote 100 percent of your attention to them during this interview. They must also know that they can trust you to keep the discussion confidential and make sure it will not be overheard.

Begin by being open, friendly, and supportive. Explain the purpose of the evaluation process, and that you have reviewed the self-evaluation. You may want to begin the discussion by going over the self-evaluation, making comments, asking for clarification, and discussing strengths. Allow the employee to do much of the talking and to identify his or her own areas of weaknesses. Some employees will respond readily, and others will remain silent. Opening communication will depend on knowledge of each employee's unique personality and needs, as well as on the employee's confidence in the employer–employee relationship. Your ability to strengthen this relationship and open communication will improve with experience and development of intuitive skills. Constantly observe body language as well as verbal behavior in order to alter and improve your communication skills. In the long run, by maintaining confidentiality, working to help employees grow and improve, and genuinely caring for their well being and satisfaction, you will bring them to trust you and respect your decisions. This will not occur by what you say, but by what you do throughout the day-to-day routine.

Following discussion of the self-evaluation, you should begin your performance review. You can either review each item in sequence, or first discuss strengths and then weaknesses. The exact format will depend on the employee's needs and your preference. While reviewing items, compare self-evaluation ratings and discuss any discrepancies. Review documentation and rationale to justify the individual rating. Focus on strengths and praise special talents or good performance. Identify weaknesses, and allow the employee to elaborate and discuss need for improvement. Questioning the employee about your observation without drawing conclusions may open the way for the employee to provide the conclusion. Offer suggestions for improvement.

During the performance review, discuss ways to improve satisfactory performance to *above average* or *excellent* performance levels. By completion of the review of all items on the form, a consensus should be reached on the final rating. Review previous self-objectives, and include the present evaluation and priorities for improvement in the development of new or different objectives.

It must be anticipated that you may receive a variety of responses from the employee during this interview. As stated earlier, much will depend upon your objective documentation of facts, and the employee's effort and honesty in the self-evaluation procedure. And, of course, the ineffective or unsatisfactory employee will most likely deny or resist identification of poor performance. It is important for you as the manager to realize that you *are* dealing with human beings. They have faults, weaknesses, want to feel special, desire that salary increase, and do not want to feel like failures. You must maintain compassion and understanding of human nature throughout this interview process. Allow employees to ventilate anger, frustration, and disagreement. Listen to their arguments and rationale, and never display anger, impatience, or take their comments personally. If, following discussion, you see no justification for changing your ratings, maintain your decision. Never allow yourself to enter into an argument. Explain that you understand how they feel, but go back to the facts and the need to maintain hospital standards. Stick to significant factors such as quality patient care, employee growth and contribution to the organization, and standards of practice. If they attempt to discuss what other employees have done or insignificant circumstances, remind them that this is *their* performance review. Remind them that you are together to discuss their strengths and weaknesses and how they can improve their performance and job satisfaction. Let them know that you want to help them, but that it must be for the good of the organization and the patients. It may be impossible to get a full consensus on all areas of the evaluation. But if you can make the employee understand your reasoning and agree to implement your suggestions, this may be the best that you can do. If continual feedback has been provided throughout the year, there should be no surprises. The employee may just not want to admit his or her weakness or fault.

If an employee totally disagrees with your ratings and is not open to communication, you may want to give him or her a day or two to reflect on the evaluation. Ask the employee to think about your comments and meet with you again at a designated time. If the employee continues to disagree, he or she should be informed that the decision may be appealed. Management must be open about this alternative action, and freely communicate this option to the employee. Employees then sign their understanding of the evaluation, and may write personal comments and opinions on the form, under their signatures.

Most employees will be receptive and open to suggestions. There are rarely extreme confrontations or problems during the interview, so managers must not fear this evaluation process. In most cases the evaluation interview is a time of mutual sharing, growth, and enthusiasm for the future. Following the performance evaluation, a date should be set for follow-up and review of achievement toward self-objectives.

THE APPEALS PROCESS

Whenever there are human beings involved in reaching a consensus that affects rewards and self-esteem, there is room for disagreement. An appeals process must be built into the personnel processes to identify biases and human error, and demonstrate management's concern for fairness to all. If the organization is unionized, this appeals process is part of the agreed-upon grievance procedures. A nonunionized organization can formulate a grievance procedure to handle all personnel problems, or organize an appeals process specifically for performance evaluation disagreements. Policies and procedures must be specific and clear to all employees. Whichever mechanism is chosen, the procedure must be seen as fair and nonbiased.

An appeal may simply follow the traditional grievance process of appealing higher on the administrative hierarchy. If the head nurse has completed the performance evaluation, the employee has a specific number of days to write an official grievance to the supervisor or director who is immediately over the head nurse. Then this supervisor has a set number of days to take action. The action would involve reviewing the information, perhaps setting up a meeting with the head nurse and employee, and reaching a decision. If the employee does not agree to the decision, the next highest-ranking manager would be approached in the same manner, and so on.

An employee must state the rationale for this appeal and any evidence to support a contrary decision. It is obvious that in the case of performance evaluation, supervisors not directly observing the employee's performance would have difficulty evaluating his or her abilities. They must rely mostly on the facts presented, and judge the fairness of the procedure. It is evident once again that documentation is of the utmost importance. It is also important that the head nurse or other manager's authority not be usurped unless justified.

The appeals process can be used as a control process to monitor and correct management ineffectiveness. If through the grievance procedure a management problem is identified, corrective action is taken immediately. Conversely, fair and effective management decisions must be supported, despite employee disagreement. Fair hearings and judgments will communicate the intent to correct improper management practices, as well as to maintain standards of practice. Employees will learn that it is useless to file a grievance based upon a personal grudge or unjustified reasoning.

Appeal or Grievance Board

In some organizations, the appeal process may be channeled to a board or committee who hears the grievance and determines a verdict. This board should consist of various members who can remain neutral and come to an impartial decision. Management and staff representatives should sit on the board, but anyone who feels unable to remain neutral in a certain instance should dismiss himself or herself from the hearing.

Decisions of whether to allow the employee's colleagues to remain in the hearing would depend on the level of professionalism of the staff. A peer who must work with this employee following the appeal may feel a great deal of stress from the process. As emotions rise, a great amount of almost superhuman professionalism is required not to allow tension and conflict to affect the working relationship.

Board members may be elected or appointed, and may be rotated. But criteria must be developed for eligibility in order to ensure that members meet needed standards.

The board may first review the employee's grievance, and determine whether an appeal proceeding is justified. If the complaint or grievance appears unwarranted or based simply on anger, the board may vote to deny an appeal. If an appeal is allowed, it would consist of an investigation, hearing, and a decision based on majority vote. Some boards may require a group consensus prior to issuing a decision. If a consensus is not reached, a new board may be temporarily formed and re-hear the appeal. Failure to reach a consensus the second time might dictate a decision by the vice-president for nursing or an outside arbitrator. See Chapter 10, "Grievance Procedures."

A decision in management's favor would require the employee to accept the performance evaluation and work on the documented needs and weaknesses. Failure to do so would result in more severe disciplinary measures (see next chapter). A decision in the employee's favor would dictate top administration's evaluation of the particular manager involved. Special training or counseling may be needed, or the incident may justify meetings with the entire management team to discuss problems in implementing policies and procedures. A manager who demonstrates unfair employment practices may be closely monitored, suspended, placed on probation, or demoted. The particular situation and circumstances would determine the action.

PEER REVIEW

As discussed in Chapter 7 on selection, staff members may be involved in varying degrees of participative management. The degree of their participation will depend on the nature of the organization, its structure, and the characteristics of the staff. The performance evaluation process can involve the use of peer review, such as in the review of evaluation results for determining promotions and selection for new or different positions.

Use of peer review for the evaluation process must be approached cautiously. Although it may be effective for determining advancement on the clinical ladder, it is difficult to monitor and maintain minimum standards on a daily basis. Working staff members are busy with patient care and do not have time to continually collect data and assess one another's performance. The continual feedback and assessments that are needed for effective performance evaluation can only be done by a manager selected, trained, and provided with the time to implement these processes. Peer review often is dependent on the employee's written self-appraisal and progress toward self-objectives. A group of peers may be making decisions based upon writing skills and little observation or proof to validate what the employee says he or she has accomplished. In addition, there is "good old human nature." People find loopholes in systems, or the evaluators may be pressured to promote a friend or colleague, or not consider the good of the whole organization.

A staff of professionals working together toward growth and development would find peer review a rewarding experience. If there is an attitude of learning from one another and concern for the progress of the organization, constructive criticism may be received readily and eagerly. This is the ideal situation, and peer evaluation can only be effective when in this ideal setting. If salary or promotion is tied to evaluation results, even an ideal situation may find employees giving ratings similar to what they received, or everyone receiving high ratings.

Peer review is basically concerned with maintaining standards of care and evaluating patient outcomes. If a staff nurse displays unprofessional conduct or incompetency, a system should be provided for review by peers. But the regular process of performance evaluation is beyond the realm of peer review. It is a management responsibility that must be controlled, corrected, and monitored continually. Peer evaluations may be used in the performance evaluation process. A mechanism for peer involvement and input concerning contributions, progress, and interpersonal relations could be useful to managers and rewarding for employees. But its connection to final decisions must be controlled to ensure that friendship and personalities do not influence performance ratings.

EVALUATION OF THE TOTAL PROCESS

The nurse-administrator must use information systems and checks and balances to monitor and control the performance evaluation process. Spur-of-the-moment audits should be implemented by top administration to determine whether nursing care actually reflects the ratings on the performance evaluation. If a particular unit has mainly *above average* ratings on care planning, a quick audit of the criteria for care planning would validate this rating. Managers must know that they are being monitored and the nurse-administrator reviews and signs every evaluation. Performance evaluation scores can be reviewed as a whole for nursing service. Average ratings can be determined in each performance area to determine future needs for staff development or management intervention. Consistent low scores would reflect a problem. Scores should be compared to patient outcomes, and studies should be conducted to determine whether a unit with high scores in areas such as discharge planning and patient teaching actually had fewer readmissions or complications. These studies are useful for comparing performance of these skills to patient outcome, as well as for monitoring the rating of these skills by management.

Each year a committee should be formulated to review the entire performance evaluation process. Management and staff personnel should review policies, procedures, average scores, information from quality assurance committees on patient care, and other information to determine the effectiveness of the system. Financial data should be compared to results of the performance evaluations to determine whether improving scores has decreased staffing needs, increased productivity, and decreased personnel costs.

An evaluation of management personnel, completed by employees,

Please complete the following and return it to the administrative secretary. Do not sign your name.

1. Do you think you are treated fairly and with respect by management, as an important part of this organization? Explain.

2. Are you provided with continual feedback concerning your strengths, weaknesses, and suggestions for improvement? Explain.

3. Do you think your efforts are reflected on your performance evaluation results? Explain.

4. Are you provided the support, guidance, and environment to perform at your best—to grow and develop? Explain.

5. Do you think that your hard work and achievements are rewarded? Explain.

6. Do you think that ineffective or unsatisfactory co-workers are allowed to remain in the organization and drain other employees? Or are they handled appropriately? Explain.

7. Do you feel you can talk to your immediate supervisor? Does he or she listen? Can you trust him or her? Explain.

8. Do you think that problems are handled appropriately on your unit? Are they corrected and worked on, or allowed to continue? Explain.

9. Do you feel you are involved in the decisions on your unit? Are you involved in planning changes, corrections, or improvements? Explain.

10. Do you enjoy working on your unit? Is there an atmosphere of friendliness and creativeness that makes working fun? Explain.

11. Do you feel that your immediate supervisor and management in general cares about you? Explain.

12. Additional comments:

Date ______________ Unit ______________

Figure 9–2. Management evaluation form completed by employees. *Note:* The nurse-administrator must approach this type of survey cautiously. When staff give negative feedback about a supervisor, they expect something to be done to change that person's behavior immediately. This is not always possible, and can create more problems than it solves. This must be kept in mind when eliciting this sort of information. Measures should be taken to explain the intent of the survey and what the staff can expect in the way of corrective action.

could be helpful in the overall evaluation. Maintaining complete confidentiality, employees can be allowed to evaluate their superiors. This evaluation could help determine employees' faith in the performance evaluation process and other aspects of the employer–employee relationship. As with any survey, the focus is on the *average* response and consistent input, not isolated incidents. Figure 9–2 provides an example of a management evaluation form.

If employees are provided an opportunity to evaluate management, it must be done so that results are used to reward or improve management performance. Administration must collect a unit's evaluations and have a neutral secretary tally results, so that the particular manager is not able to identify individual handwriting. Confidentiality is essential. In addition, the nurse-executive must review the results for each unit, and ensure follow-up. Managers must not be allowed to resent employee input, but must use it for growth and development. Managers must be accountable for their behavior, and this is one way to help monitor and correct problems. If the evaluation is used in conjunction with studies of patient outcomes, personnel data on turnover and absenteeism, and productivity reports, the nurse-executive can better evaluate the managers. The evaluation from employees can be useful for determining job satisfaction and other concerns or problems.

PERFORMANCE EVALUATIONS AND REWARD SYSTEMS

The performance evaluation must be linked to some sort of extrinsic reward system. Even the most self-motivated achiever will soon tire if effort does not result in some reward other than just self-satisfaction. People must feel that hard work will be worth the effort and will "get them somewhere." By linking reward to the performance evaluation, the evaluation can be used as one means to increase productivity and creativity. Some reward systems related to performance evaluation will be addressed in the following discussion. More will be explored in Chapter 11.

Monetary Reward Systems

Although money may not be the primary motivator for all employees, it helps. Salary increases to reward achievements, in combination with other retention efforts, can lead to increased productivity and job satisfaction. There are several ways to implement a monetary reward system. The most common is the merit raise system based upon the performance evaluation.

Merit Raise System. This is a system for providing a salary increase for exceeding job expectations. This is different from the yearly cost-of-living increase that is given to all employees. It is based completely on merit. The success of a merit raise system depends on the definition and means for evaluating merit. If a sound evaluation system that is trusted by employees is in effect, then a merit raise system can easily fall into place.

A merit raise policy must be developed that is understood and acceptable to employees. This policy must delineate the amount of the salary increase, as well as other details. Figure 9–3 provides an example.

Bonus System. In these difficult economic times, many organizations are reevaluating their annual cost-of-living raises. Some facilities may begin eliminating routine raises for all employees and basing salary increases *strictly* upon merit. They may raise the amount of the increase and institute additional bonus systems in order to promote excellence. This possibility falls in line with health care's transition into the business world. Many corporations and businesses reward outstanding employees with large bonuses. They believe that meeting minimum job requirements is no longer enough for success, so employees who make the greatest contributions receive the greatest rewards. Bonuses add up to thousands of dollars, but pay off the corporation in increased productivity and creative contributions.

How might a bonus system be incorporated into an organization's performance evaluation system? It could be done in several ways.

Annual Bonus. An organization may choose to maintain a minimum cost-of-living raise for *satisfactory* employees and award a lump sum of money to employees receiving *above average* or *excellent* ratings. This sum may change each year, depending upon the financial resources, but must be established and communicated for a 12-month period. By awarding a bonus rather than integrating the merit raise into the base pay, the organization reduces costs of other benefits based upon a percent of the employee's salary. In addition, the following year's salary increases are not calculated from the previous year's merit increase, but on a lower gross salary. A bonus is a one-time monetary reward, and does not accumulate and build upon itself as the traditional merit raise system can. But if the organization wants this to work, the bonus must be large enough to make the effort worthwhile. An $1000 bonus to an *excellent* employee may be equivalent to a 5-percent salary increase, but still save the organization money.

Merit Raise Plus Bonus System. An organization may abolish yearly salary increases and base raises strictly upon merit. In this case, the merit raise would be a monetary increase for *above average* and *excellent* ratings, similar to that of the example in Figure 9–2 (the exact percentage would vary depending upon the organization). Then bonuses would be awarded for additional achievements over and beyond the job description. Guidelines would be set by administration and concern areas such as research, leadership, creativity and innovation, education, or clinical contributions. Although guidelines would be fairly general, they would involve *achieving*

Definition: A merit raise is a raise in salary awarded to an employee for performance exceeding job expectations. Because *satisfactory* rating is considered to mean meeting job requirements, an *above average* or *excellent* rating is considered to mean that the employee is exceeding job expectations.

An employee who receives a *satisfactory* rating on performance evaluation will receive the across-the-board pay increase. All employees are eligible for the across-the-board raise unless they are on probation.

Employees on probation for any reason are not eligible for merit raises. Once removed from probation, they become eligible for a merit raise.

Employees are eligible for a merit raise at the time of their annual performance evaluation. The total scoring on the performance evaluation will determine if a raise is awarded:

Unsatisfactory	*Satisfactory*	*Above average*	*Excellent*
Does not meet job requirements	Meets job requirements	Exceeds job requirements	Outstanding performance
Probation	Across-the-board raise only	3 percent raise	5 percent raise

Performance evaluation scores are determined by the performance evaluation policy and scoring procedure.

Figure 9–3. Traditional merit raise policy.

organizational goals and *advancing the progress and success of the organization.* Each year an administrative board may outline organizational needs and receive applications from employees who wish to accept the challenge. Requirements may be that the employee has at least an *above average* rating and agrees to work toward the accomplishment on his or her own time. Employees may even form small groups to work together in a major research project or publication and share the bonus. Employees may also develop their own ideas for ways to progress organizational growth and request that the board allow their ideas to be entered into the bonus system. Again, the amount of the bonus must be worth the effort. When management studies and identifies relationships between creative contributions and financial gain, the amount of bonuses will rise. If improved image in the community through an educational project or increased professional status through a major publication can be related to future financial gain, the bonuses will rise. Creative organizations realize that these types of goals work to advance the organization and increase market shares in the long run.

Bonuses may be given in variations or combinations of the annual, or merit raise plus bonus systems already discussed. A bonus may serve to reward good performance and as a means to improve the financial standing of the organization by promoting creative contributions. A type of *gain sharing* may even be implemented, where units who show savings in personnel costs and reduce costs in patient care can receive a portion of the savings. Projects implemented by units to increase revenues through creative education or health promotion programs could result in a portion of the profits being shared among unit personnel. There are many mechanisms for providing financial rewards for performance. Of course, none should exist without the routine monitoring of quality of services and standards of practice.

And what of the *satisfactory* employee? In organizations where raises are only given to *above average* or *excellent* employees, the satisfactory employee is penalized. Such an employee may leave or improve. If the employee stays and chooses not to improve (or is unable to improve), he or she may develop an attitude problem. Management must provide counseling and guidance to ensure that this does not happen. All efforts are made to encourage and assist the employee to raise his or her rating. If attitude affects the employee's work, disciplinary measures must be taken. It is obvious that in this type of organizational setting, management is striving to retain only outstanding performers.

All organizations do not have the luxury of retaining only *above average* or *excellent* employees. The majority of their employees may only be at the *satisfactory* level. In this case, the organization must work to raise performance levels through bonus systems and merit raises (in conjunction with other personnel processes), but still provide salary increases for meeting job requirements. Employees may have difficulty adjusting to new incentive programs, and may demonstrate negative rather than positive responses. Remember, monetary reward systems are designed to enhance satisfaction and performance. The system must be appropriate for the needs of the organization.

Clinical Ladders

Many organizations are designing clinical ladder programs as a means for evaluating, promoting, and rewarding nurses in clinical practice. These programs vary, but usually consist of several clinical levels with specific job descriptions and criteria for evaluation. Criteria include clinical expertise and often leadership, educational, and research activities. Each level on the "ladder" represents an advancement in clinical practice. As nurses advance up the ladder, they are rewarded with a higher title, such as Clinical Nurse II, and a salary increase. Nurses often work with a preceptor or role model to gain the necessary skills, then are evaluated by a committee consisting of peers and management personnel.

Performance evaluation is an integral part of the clinical ladder. Each clinical level requires a specific performance evaluation tool, which could be compared to the sample criteria for performance evaluation in Appendix 9–3. *Satisfactory* criteria may be equivalent to requirements for a new graduate or first-year nurse. *Above average* criteria may be the requirement for Clinical Nurse II, and *excellent* criteria could be seen as the requirements for Clinical Nurse III. In order to advance, each nurse must have goals and objectives, complete selected training, then show evidence to a committee of achievement of the criteria. This comparison of the rating system to the clinical ladder is not to imply that the two systems are the same, but to facilitate understanding. The clinical ladder usually has more specific criteria for each level, and offers recognition by title change as well as salary increase. There is usually more peer involvement in the performance evaluation and advancement decision.

Clinical ladders require extensive policy and procedure development, and can be extremely time-consuming. If one is developed and presently working well, then by all means leave it in place. But if the aim is to improve clinical performance and provide recognition and reward for this performance, an effective evaluation system may serve this purpose. Implementing an effective performance evaluation process in conjunction with extrinsic reward and other personnel processes can accomplish similar results.

Career Ladders

Career ladder systems usually involve programs to counsel and guide nurses in advancing in their careers. They are mentioned here because it involves performance evaluation, and often is confused with the clinical ladder. Many programs integrate a clinical ladder advancement program with various other tracks, such as administrative ladders and research and educational advancement ladders. The career program assists the nurse in planning direction for the future and obtaining needed expertise to apply for advancement in his or her chosen area. The career ladder program helps the nurse to achieve the required clinical, administrative, or other competencies, then move up the appropriate track. Career ladder programs also can involve upward movement along the traditional administrative hierarchy, or even into job categories outside the organization. Clinical ladders are one component of the career ladder.

Promotions and Transfers

Performance evaluation is an integral part of internal recruitment and selection processes. From achievement on performance evaluations, managers can recommend employees for promotions. During the performance evaluation interview, the manager also receives input regarding future advancement goals. The personnel data form shown in Figure 6–2, is completed during the interview. Recommendations by managers go to administration and are recorded on the form shown in Figure 6–1, as well as on the individual evaluation form. Then when vacancies occur, or planning indicates a change in staffing or the need for new positions, this information can be retrieved. Human resource inventories assist in centralizing this information, which can then be channeled to nurse-recruiters and into selection processes.

Policies should be developed that set requirements for internal selection. These requirements should include the performance evaluations. As discussed in Chapter 6, "recruitment" job posting and other internal efforts call for a minimum of *satisfactory* on the performance evaluation. Some specific jobs may require *above average* or *excellent* ratings, and this may be a requirement for selection delineated on the "specific information concerning the job" (Appendix 6–2). Selection rating scales for internal selection should include management and peer recommendations and rating on the performance evaluation.

Effective performance evaluation builds on recruitment and selection processes by helping to retain satisfied employees, and develop and recommend employees to match existing and future openings. While employees can certainly take their own initiative to apply for an opening, they must know that their selection will be dependent upon their past and present performance in the organization.

CONCLUSION

Performance evaluation links to every aspect of human resource management. It is a key to effective recruitment and selection processes, as well as orientation. It is inherent in counseling and coaching, guides staff development, and is critical to maintaining good labor relations. It aims to retain productive and satisfied employees.

This chapter has outlined some guidelines for implementing an effective performance evaluation process. The appendices will provide some help in formulating tools and procedures. The chapter to follow on counseling and coaching will discuss procedures and considerations in managing the employee who has been performing below job expectations. As discussed earlier, the focus of performance evaluation is on employee growth, development, and well-being. But a mechanism must be provided for dismissing *unsatisfactory* employees following all efforts to assist in their development to *satisfactory* levels. Counseling and coaching explores these measures to improve unsatisfactory performance and guide behaviors, as well as presenting a progressive discipline procedure. This process is continuous with performance evaluation and closely integrated into the success of the other personnel processes.

SUGGESTED READING

Aroian, J., Grant, K. J., & Gilbert, J. P. Contracting for growth. *AJN,* 1984, *84*(8), 1042–1044.

Bell, M. L. Management by objectives. *JONA,* 1980, *10*(5), 19–26.

Brief, A. P. Developing a useable performance appraisal system. *JONA,* 1979, *9*(10), 7–10.

Calkin, J. D. Staff evaluation: An assessment of approaches. *Health Care Supervisor,* 1984, *2*(4), 68–78.

Darling, L. W., & McGrath, L. G. The cause and cost of promotion trauma. *JONA,* 1983, *13*(4), 29–33.

Davis, D. S. Evaluating advance practice nursing. *Nursing Management,* 1984, 15(3), 44–47.

DeVries, D. L. *Performance appraisal on the line.* New York: Wiley, 1981.

Fay, M. S. The grievance arbitration process—the experience of one nurse administrator. *JONA,* 1985, *15*(6), 11–16.

Freyd, M. *An appraisal of relative merits of types of rating scales and their use.* New York: American Management Association, 1967.

Golightly, C. MBO and performance appraisal. *JONA,* 1979, *9*(9), 11–20.

Goodykoontz, L. Performance evaluation of staff nurses. *Supervisor Nurse,* 1984, *12*(8), 39–43.

Greenfeld, E. F. *Performance appraisal: Promise and peril.* Ithaca, N.Y.: New York State School of Industrial and Labor Relations, Cornell University, 1981.

Henderson, R. I. *Performance appraisal: Theory to practice.* Reston, Va.: Reston, 1980.

Johnson, J., & Luciano, K. Managing by behaviors and results: Linking supervisory accountability to effective organizational control. *JONA,* 1983, *13*(2), 19–28.

Johnson, R. G. *The appraisal interview guide.* New York: Amacom, 1979.

Keil, E. C. *Performance appraisal and the manager.* New York: Lebham Freidman Books, 1977.

Kellogg, M. S. *What to do about performance appraisal.* New York: American Management Association, 1965.

Khan, M. K. Staff performance: A three-part appraisal. *Dimensions in Health Service,* 1983, *60*(1), 14–15, 22.

Koontz, H. *Appraising managers as managers.* New York: McGraw-Hill, 1971.

Lefton, R. E. *Effective motivation through performance appraisal: Dimensional appraisal strategies.* New York: Wiley, 1977.

Levenstein, A. Where nurses differ. *Nursing Management,* 1984, *15*(3), 64–65.

Levenstein, A. Back to feedback. *Nursing Management,* 1984, *15*(10), 60–61.

McIntyre, E. Clinical evaluation of a new critical care nurse. *Focus AACN,* 1982, *9*(5), 3–6.

Megel, M. A. Establishing a criterion-based performance appraisal for a department of nursing. *Nursing Clinics of North America,* 1983, *18*(3), 449–456.

Miller, M. Staff performance evaluation: What? Why? How? *JEN,* 1984, *10*(2), 74–84.

Morrissey, G. L. *Appraisal and development through objectives and results.* Reading, Mass.: Addison-Wesley, 1972.

Mullins, A. C., Colavecchio, R. E., & Tescher, B. Peer review: A model for professional accountability. *JONA,* 1979, *9*(12), 25–30.

Murphy, E. C. Module 6: Performance evaluation and the self-fulfilling prophecy. *Nursing Management* 1983, *14*(11), 59–61.

Newman, J. E., & Hinrichs, J. R. *Performance evaluation for professional personnel.* Scarsdale, N.Y.: Work in America Institute, 1980.

Odom, J. V. *Performance appraisal: Legal aspects.* Greensboro, N.C.: Center for Creative Leadership, 1979.

Pavett, C. M. Evaluation of the impact of feedback on performance and motivation. *Human Relations,* 1983, *36*(7), 641–654.

Pincus, J. Staff appraisal and development. *Nursing Mirror,* November 24, 1982, pp. 47–49.

Pucilo, N. P. How formal appraisal systems work. *Respiratory Therapy,* 1984, *14*(2), 37–43.

Richardson, K. Motivating critical care nurses through peer evaluation. *Critical Care Nurse,* 1982, *2*(4), 54–57.

Riley, M. Employee performance reviews that work. *JONA,* 1983, *12*(10), 32–33.

Siler, E. Performance standards using behavioral anchored rating scales. *American Journal of Infectious Control,* 1983, *11*(3), 31A–33A.

Sloma, R. S. *How to measure managerial performance.* New York: Macmillan, 1980.

Smith, H. P. *Performance appraisal and human development: A practical guide to effective managing.* Reading, Mass.: Addison-Wesley, 1977.

Snook, I. D. Management tools for the modern day health administrator. *Hospital Topics,* 1984, *62*(1), 11–12.

Spencer-Legler, M. A. Peer review in nursing: Specifics for implementation. *Ohio Nurses Review,* 1983, *58*(7), 8–10.

Umiker, W. O. Pay raises: Merit or seniority? *MLO,* 1983, *15*(9), 63–64.

APPENDIX 9–1

Standards of Medical–Surgical Nursing Practice*

Standard I. Assessment is the identification and gathering of data concerning the health status of the patient. This process is complete, continuous, and systematic, as evidenced by:

I. A comprehensive patient history and physical
  A. Patient interview
    Chief complaint
    History of present illness
    Allergies
    Medications
    Past medical history
    Cultural, environmental, and socioeconomic conditions
    Activities of daily living
    Personal habits
    Food and fluid preferences
    Appetite changes and weight changes
    Available and accessible human, community, and material resources
  B. Psychological assessment
    Emotional status
    Patterns of coping
    Concerns during hospitalization
  C. Physical assessment
    Personal hygiene and grooming
    Nutritional status
    Mental status
    Physical status
  D. Perception of illness
    Understanding of disease process or illness
    Understanding of reasons for hospitalization
    Desired outcome from hospitalization
II. The collection of data from available sources
    Patient, family, significant other
    Health care providers
    Individuals and/or agencies in the community
III. The collection of data by scientific methodology
    Interview
    Observation

---

*Reprinted with permission from Jernigan, D. K., & Young, A.P. *Standards, Job Descriptions, and Performance Evaluations for Nursing Practice.* E. Norwalk, Conn.: Appleton-Century-Crofts, 1983, pp. 72–74.

Inspection
Auscultation
Palpation
Reports and records

IV. The organization of data in a systematic arrangement. The arrangement provides:
Accurate collection
Complete collection
Accessibility
Confidentiality

V. The communication of data in an orderly fashion
Data are recorded by each shift daily
Data are updated by each shift daily
Data are revised and recorded as appropriate
Data are communicated verbally among health team daily

Standard II. Nursing care planning consists of determining patient problems and desired outcomes. Planning involves preparing the patient for home care. This is evidenced by:

I. The identification of present or potential patient problems from the patient assessment
Data are grouped into meaningful arrangements based upon scientific knowledge
Patient's health status is determined
Patient's health status is compared to the norms
Present and potential problems are identified
Problems are given priority according to impact upon the patient's health status

II. The formulation of desired outcomes
Patient (family, significant other) and nurse mutually agree upon the patient's present or potential health problems
Patient and nurse mutually agree upon desired outcomes
Desired outcomes are congruent with the patient problems and established norms
Desired outcomes are specific
Desired outcomes are measurable within a certain timeframe
Desired outcomes are consistent with other health providers' expectations
Desired outcomes are established to restore patient's optimal functioning capabilities

III. The incorporation of home health care into desired outcomes involves teaching
Disease process and complications
Medication

Diet
Exercise and activity
Self-care techniques and materials
Available support systems and resources

Standard III. The plan of care is implemented in order to achieve the desired outcome. This is evidenced by:

I. The formulation of nursing prescriptions that delineate actions to be taken. Prescribed actions:
 Are specific to identified patient problems and desired outcomes
 Are based on current scientific knowledge
 Incorporate principles of patient teaching
 Incorporate principles of psychosocial interactions
 Incorporate environmental factors influencing the patient's health
 Include human, material, and community resources
 Include keeping patient knowledgeable of health status and total health care plan

II. The implementation of actions delineated in the nursing prescriptions. Actions implemented:
 Actively involve the patient and family
 Are consistent with nursing prescriptions
 Are based upon current scientific knowledge
 Are flexible and individualized for each patient
 Include principles of safety
 Include principles of infection control

Standard IV. Outcomes of nursing actions are evaluated for further assessment and planning. This is evidenced by:

I. Evaluating the achievement of desired outcomes
 Data are collected concerning the patient's health status
 Data are compared to the specified desired outcomes
 The patient and nurse evaluate the achievement of desired outcomes

II. Reassessment of the nursing care plan
 Outcome of nursing actions direct the reassessment of identified patient problems
 Outcome of nursing actions direct reassessment of desired outcomes (assess the desired outcome to determine if appropriate, realistic, and in correct priority)
 Outcome of nursing actions direct reassessment of nursing prescriptions (assess the nursing prescriptions to determine if appropriate, realistic, and stated accurately)
 Nursing actions are assessed for effectiveness in achieving desired outcomes

III. Further planning as directed by the reassessment

Reassessment determines new patient present or potential problems

New patient problems direct the formulation and revision of desired outcomes

Revised desired outcomes direct new actions to be implemented toward desired outcomes

Desired outcomes are continually evaluated for achievement

The plan of care is continually evaluated and revised according to changes in the patient's health status

APPENDIX 9–2

Medical–Surgical Nurse: Performance Evaluation*

Note: The evaluator is expected to comment on all items rated "U" or "E".

Name ______________________ Employment date ______________
Rating period ________________ to ______________________
Department _________________ Job title ___________________

Instructions: Using the following rating scale, indicate the quality of performance by placing the appropriate letter on the line to the left of the item.

- U—Unsatisfactory (does not meet job requirements)
- S—Satisfactory (meets job requirements)
- A—Above average (exceeds job requirements)
- E—Excellent performance

I. Assessment

_____ 1. Assesses the number and level of personnel needed to provide quality patient care on the unit and collaborates with the head nurse or supervisor in adjusting staffing and assignments.

____

____

_____ 2. Assesses the delivery of nursing care on the unit and identifies problems and any need for improvements and changes.

____

____

_____ 3. Assesses the health status of assigned patients on the unit as outlined in the nursing standards.

____

____

3.1 Completes a comprehensive patient history and physical, including patient interview, psychological and physical assessment, as well as patient's perception of illness.

____

____

3.2 Collects data from the patient, family and significant others, health care providers, individuals, and/or agencies in the community.

____

____

*Adapted with permission from Jernigan, D. K. and Young, A. P. *Standards, Job Descriptions, and Performance Evaluations for Nursing Practice.* E. Norwalk, Conn.: Appleton-Century-Crofts, 1983, pp. 92–99.

3.3 Collects data by interview, observation, inspection, auscultation, palpation, and reports and records.

____

____

3.4 Organizes assessment data so that they are accurate, complete, and accessible, and remain confidential.

____

____

3.5 Communicates assessment data in an orderly fashion by recording, updating, and communicating among the health team daily and by revising as appropriate.

____

____

II. Planning

_____ 1. Serves on hospital committees and helps to review and revise policies and procedures, as directed by head nurse or supervisor.

____

____

_____ 2. Plans and develops self-objectives.

____

____

_____ 3. Plans ways to solve problems creatively and make innovative changes and improvements on the unit, in collaboration with supervisory personnel.

____

____

_____ 4. Completes a written care plan for assigned patients on the unit. Plans the care for individual patients as well as directs and supervises others in the planning of patients' care.

____

____

4.1 Identifies the patient's present or potential problems from the patient assessment.

____

a. Patient's health status is determined.

____

____

b. Health status is compared to the norms.

____

____

c. Problems are given priority according to impact upon the patient's health status.

____

____

4.2 Formulates desired outcomes, specific to patient problems and established norms.

____

____

4.3 Ensures that desired outcomes are mutually agreed upon by the patient and nurse, and are (a) specific, (b) measurable within a certain timeframe, and (c) consistent with other health providers' expectations.

____

____

4.4 Incorporates home health care into the patient's desired outcomes. This includes but is not limited to teaching about the disease process and complications, medications, diet, exercise and activities, self-care techniques and materials, and available support systems and resources.

____

____

III. Implementation

_____ 1. Implements activities necessary to meeting self-objectives.

____

____

_____ 2. Participates in implementing planned, creative changes and activities to improve nursing service.

____

____

_____ 3. Holds self accountable for the delivery of quality nursing care.

____

____

_____ 4. Promotes harmonious relationships and favorable attitudes among the health care team.

____

____

_____ 5. Supports and adheres to administrative and nursing service policies and procedures.

____

____

_____ 6. Assists with orientation of new employees.

____

____

_____ 7. Acts rapidly and effectively; manages self, patients, and other employees during any emergency situation.

____

____

_____ 8. Attends required in-service education programs.

_____ 9. Formulates nursing prescriptions that delineate actions to be taken. Prescribed actions:

9.1 Are specific to the patient's problems and the desired outcomes.

9.2 Are based on scientific knowledge.

9.3 Are based on principles of patient teaching.

9.4 Are based on principles of psychosocial interactions.

9.5 Are based on environmental factors influencing the patient's health.

9.6 Include human, material, and community resources.

9.7 Include keeping patient knowledgeable of health status and total health care plan.

_____10. Implements the actions delineated in the nursing prescriptions. Actions implemented:

10.1 Actively involve the patient and family.

10.2 Are based on current scientific knowledge.

10.3 Are flexible and individualized for each patient.

10.4 Include principles of safety.

10.5 Include principles of infection control.

_____11. Conforms to hospital dress code.

_____12. Is rarely sick or absent from work due to health.

_____13. Is prompt and attends report.

IV. Evaluation

_____ 1. Evaluates self-objectives; revises and formulates new objectives.

_____ 2. Evaluates the effectiveness of problem-solving techniques and the activities implemented to improve nursing service.

_____ 3. Contributes to the performance evaluation of nursing service personnel on the unit.

_____ 4. Participates in evaluation of R.N. orientation policies and procedures and recommends revisions to supervisor or head nurse.

_____ 5. Participates in the evaluation of in-service education programs.

_____ 6. Evaluates achievement or lack of achievement of desired outcomes.

6.1 Data are collected concerning the patient's health status.

6.2 Compares data to the specific desired outcomes.

6.3 Includes the patient's evaluation of the achievement of desired outcomes.

6.4 Reassesses nursing actions for effectiveness in achieving desired outcomes.

_____ 7. From evaluation of achievement or lack of achievement of desired outcomes, reassesses and revises the nursing care plan.

From evaluation:

7.1 Reassesses the patient problems.

7.2 Reassesses desired outcomes to determine if appropriate, realistic, and in correct priority.

7.3 Reassesses nursing prescriptions to determine if appropriate, realistic, and stated accurately.

From the reassessment:

7.4 Determines new patient present or potential problems.

7.5 From new patient problems, formulates and revises desired outcomes.

7.6 Revises nursing prescriptions.

7.7 Implements new actions in order to carry out revised prescription.

7.8 Continually evaluates desired outcomes for achievement or lack of achievement.

7.9 Continually evaluates and revises the nursing care plan according to changes in the patient's health status.

Medical–Surgical Registered Nurse: Scoring Procedure

Instructions: Total the number of each item and multiply times the appropriate number. Add these totals to make the score.

U ________ ×0 = ________
S ________ ×1 = ________
A ________ ×2 = ________
E ________ ×3 = ________ Total Score ________

Compare total score to the following scale to determine rank:

U	S	A	E
0 to 23	24 to 42	43 to 64	65 to 81

Overall performance review rank ________

ALL ITEMS IN THE FOLLOWING SECTION MUST BE COMPLETED.

A. Interviewer's comments on overall review. ____
____
____

B. Additional suggestions for overall work improvement and goals for next evaluation. ____
____
____

C. Self–objectives. ____
____
____
____
____
____
____

Date ________ Employee's signature ________________________
Date ________ Interviewer's signature ________________________
Date ________ Nurse-administrator ________________________

APPENDIX 9–3

Medical–Surgical Registered Nurse: Criteria for Performance Evaluation*

The following is a tool for completing the Registered Nurse Performance Evaluation Form. This is not intended as a comprehensive guide, but to provide examples by which to refer when completing the performance evaluation (see Medical–Surgical R.N. Performance Evaluation, Appendix 9–2).

I. Assessment

1. *Assesses the number and level of personnel needed to provide quality patient care on the unit and collaborates with the head nurse or supervisor in adjusting staffing and assignments.*

Explanation. Following report, the registered nurse assesses the number and expertise of the personnel and compares this with the patient classification to ensure that quality care can be delivered according to patients' needs. She assesses the assignments to see that they are fair, based on the patients' needs and the personnel's qualifications. According to her assessment, the R.N. makes adjustments in assignments, requests more help, or collaborates with the supervisor or head nurse on schedule changes for the next shift (or next day). This assessment is also a basis for deciding whether personnel can be sent to another hall or unit.

Evaluation Guide

U Considers only the number of patients, not the classification. "Never has enough help." Uncooperative in making changes in assignments or staffing. Rarely adjusts assignments, even with changes in census or patient acuity. Cannot give rationale to substantiate the need when requesting additional staff.

S Is aware of patient classification and needs, staff expertise, and ability to care for the patients. Substantiates reasons for requesting more help. Adjusts assignments based on the above rationale. Can determine whether number and level of personnel available are equivalent to the patient care required. Can determine whether assignments are appropriate. Is cooperative in accepting changes in staffing, or assignments, when requested by the supervisor or head nurse—based on patient classification and sound rationale.

A Performs all behaviors described in **S.** Continually assesses changes in

*Adapted with permission from Jernigan, D. K., & Young, A. P., *Standards, Job Descriptions, and Performance Evaluations for Nursing Practice.* E. Norwalk, Conn.: Appleton-Century-Crofts, 1983, pp. 42–53.

census and patient acuity and adjusts assignments and delegation of duties accordingly throughout the shift.

E Performs all behaviors in **A.** Assesses the staffing needs of the oncoming shift, collaborates with head nurse or supervisor, and can provide rationale for changes needed, according to this assessment. Considers the needs of the other units as well as his or her own unit, and includes this concern in decisions for staffing and assignment changes. Includes assessment rationale in suggesting changes or adjustments in the next day's staffing assignments.

2. *Assesses the delivery of nursing care on the unit and identifies problems and any need for improvement and changes.*

Explanation. The R.N. constantly observes the delivery of nursing care and the performance of the personnel under his or her direction. The R.N. makes rounds and assesses patients to see that appropriate care is being delivered to meet their needs. From this assessment, the R.N. identifies any problems that may be occurring on the unit, among personnel, etc. The R.N. identifies areas needing improvement or changes, or problems in the management of personnel concerning skills, knowledge, needed materials, or resources.

Evaluation Guide

U Never or rarely identifies needs on the unit. Goes without equipment or forms needed without verbalizing the deficiency. May verbalize problems and needs, but rarely has rationale on which to base the problems.

S When asked, will identify needs and problems on the unit. Gives rationale for these problems, from assessment.

A Is self-motivated to communicate assessment and identification of needs and problems to supervisory personnel. Identifies needs concerning additional knowledge and skills that would improve the delivery of care, based on sound rationale.

E Performs all behaviors described in **A.** Identifies potential needs and problems and communicates these to supervisory personnel.

3. *Assesses the health status of assigned patients on the unit as outlined in the nursing standards.*

   3.1 *Completes a comprehensive patient history and physical, including patient interview, psychological and physical assessment, as well as patient's perception of illness.*

3.2 *Collects data initially and on a continual basis from the patient, family, and significant others, health care providers, individuals, and/or agencies in the community.*

3.3 *Collects data by interview, observation, inspection, auscultation, palpation, and reports and records.*

3.4 *Organizes assessment data so that they are accurate, complete, accessible, and remain confidential.*

3.5 *Communicates assessment data in an orderly fashion by recording, updating, and communicating among the health team daily and revising as appropriate.*

Evaluation Guide

U Fails to meet criteria listed under assessment (3.1–3.5).

S Satisfies all criteria (3.1–3.5) and completes initial assessment note within 30 minutes.

A Performs all behaviors described in **S.** Completes assessment forms from previous shifts and adds pertinent information from the assessment. Seeks out additional information from all possible sources for the patient assessment. Communicates the patients' problems and care plan to the oncoming shift.

E Performs all behaviors described in **A.** Assesses slight alterations in the patients' health status and documents these changes.

II. Planning

1. *Serves on hospital committees and helps to review and revise policies and procedures, as directed by the head nurse or supervisor.*

Explanation. The R.N., as a professional, participates in nursing service committees (such as Quality Assurance or Policy and Procedure Committees).

Evaluation Guide

U Never or rarely serves on committees, even when requested.

S Serves on committees when requested.

A Volunteers to serve on committees, contributes, and actively participates.

E Volunteers to serve on committees, contributes, and actively participates. Demonstrates evidence of committee work on the unit. Includes information obtained from committee work in documentation, interactions, and direct patient care.

2. *Plans and develops self-objectives.*

Explanation. The R.N. assesses his or her own skills, knowledge, and interactions and identifies personal objectives. These objectives are goals to work toward and are intended to improve overall performance, as well as enhance professional growth, knowledge, and development.

Evaluation Guide

U Does not identify self-objectives from the performance evaluation.

S Plans and develops self-objectives and documents this on the annual evaluation and six-month interview session. Sets target dates for completion.

A Develops self-objectives from not only the performance evaluation, but from personal experiences and assessments as well. When developing objectives, sets priorities and identifies resources needed and areas of delegation. Documents this on the performance evaluation form and six-month interview session.

E Performs all behaviors described in **A.** Maintains an ongoing list of self-objectives, and from self-assessment, adds new objectives every three to six months. Plans self-objectives that foster creative innovations and achievement of organizational goals.

3. *Plans ways to solve problems creatively and make innovative changes and improvements on the unit, in collaboration with supervisory personnel.*

Explanation. From assessment of the delivery of nursing care, the R.N. plans ways to solve identified problems or to prevent potential problems. The R.N. should participate in planning ways to improve the care given on the unit. For example, if patients who are NPO are repeatedly being fed in the mornings, the R.N. identifies this as a problem. The R.N. further assesses reasons and causes for these occurrences. If the problem is identified as the personnel not checking the NPO list or trays before serving them, or that the NPO signs are not being read on the patients' doors before serving the tray, the R.N. would try to resolve this problem. One approach is to participate in the unit meeting and discuss the correct procedure with personnel. The R.N. may participate in planning the unit meeting and developing a better procedure for checking the trays.

Evaluation Guide

U Never particpates in planning ways to improve the activities on the unit.

S When asked will participate in planning ways to solve problems and make improvements on the unit. Attends 90 percent of unit and staff meetings to discuss needs and problems relating to patient care.

A Is self-motivated to communicate ideas and actively suggests solutions for problems and ways to improve activities on the unit. Attends 90 percent of unit and staff meetings.

E From assessment, identifies potential problems and plans creative ways to prevent future problems. Considers long-range improvements in the delivery of nursing care. Communicates creative approaches and innovative changes that will contribute to the evolution and progress of the organization. Attends 90 percent of unit and staff meetings.

4. *Completes a written care plan for assigned patients on the unit.*

   4.1 *Identifies the patient's present or potential problems from the patient assessment: (a) patient's health status is determined; (b) health status is compared to the norms; and (c) problems are given priority according to impact upon the patient's health status.*

   4.2 *Formulates desired outcomes, specific to the patient problems and established norms.*

   4.3 *Ensures that desired outcomes are mutually agreed upon by the patient and nurse, and are (a) specific; (b) measurable within a certain timeframe; and (c) consistent with other health providers' expectations.*

   4.4 *Incorporates home health care into the patient's desired outcomes. This includes but is not limited to teaching about the disease process and complications, medications, diet, exercise or activity, self-care techniques, and materials and available support systems and resources.*

Explanation. Plans the care for assigned patients, as outlined by the criteria, and directs others in the planning of patients' care.

Evaluation Guide

U Fails to meet the criteria outlined under "Care Planning."

S Satisfies all criteria listed under "Care Planning" and documents them within a 24-hour period.

A Following the initial assessment, formulates and documents the identified patient problems and desired outcomes on all new admissions during the 8-hour shift.

E Performs all behaviors described in **A.** From continual assessment, updates the problem list and desired outcomes for previous shifts on all assigned patients each day.

III. Implementation

1. *Implements activities necessary to meeting self-objectives.*

Explanation. The R.N. implements activities necessary to achieve the self-objectives developed and documented.

Evaluation Guide

U Does not implement activities to achieve self-objectives.

S With assistance from the head nurse, implements activities necessary to achieve self-objectives.

A Is self-motivated to initiate actions to achieve self-objectives. If unsuccessful, implements other planned actions.

E Performs all behaviors described in **A.** Is creative and utilizes resources and input from personnel in implementing activities necessary to achieve self-objectives.

2. *Participates in implementing planned, creative changes and activities to improve nursing service.*

Explanation. The R.N. participates in planned changes, such as initiating new forms or implementing new policies and procedures. The R.N. is supportive of changes and understands the rationale for changes.

Evaluation Guide

U Is uncooperative in implementing planned change.

S With encouragement from supervisory personnel, will participate in activities to improve nursing service.

A Volunteers and is enthusiastic about implementing planned change and activities to improve nursing service. Actively participates.

E Performs all behaviors described in **A.** Encourages others to participate in activities to improve nursing service. Is dedicated to making it work.

3. *Holds self accountable for the delivery of quality nursing care.*

Explanation. The R.N. can justify and explain his or her actions. Holds self answerable for all activities related to care of assigned patients.

Evaluation Guide

U Never or rarely takes responsibility for the care given to assigned patients. Always offers excuses or reasons for not being aware of activities relating to patient care.

S Can explain all nursing actions and is aware of the effect of actions on patient care.

A Can explain and takes responsibility for care given by self and personnel under authority, such as L.P.N.s, aides, and orderlies.

E Values self-accountability highly. Directs others' actions and requests information pertinent to patient care. Considers self as being integral to the patient's care and when on duty feels responsible for any activities concerning assigned patients, including procedures performed in other departments.

4. *Promotes harmonious relationships and favorable attitudes among the health care team.*

Explanation. The R.N. cooperates with other members of the health care team and does not allow personal differences to interfere with patient care. The R.N. sets an example for other employees by demonstrating a positive attitude about everyone "working together" for the betterment of the patient. The R.N. minimizes interpersonal conflicts and attempts to cooperate with others.

Evaluation Guide

U Exaggerates personal differences; is uncooperative about working with certain persons; displays a negative attitude when presented with changes.

S With encouragement from supervisory personnel, accepts changes and forgets personal differences, and attempts to "get along" with all members of the health care team.

A Is self-motivated to improve and maintain a good attitude and harmonious relations among other personnel and members of the health care team.

E Promotes positive relations and attitudes among personnel and acts as a role model by displaying enthusiasm and motivation for harmony among health care team.

5. *Supports and adheres to administrative and nursing service policies and procedures.*

Explanation. Is knowledgeable of and complies with policies and procedures.

Evaluation Guide

U Rarely is knowledgeable of policies or procedures affecting the registered nurse's practice and often does not comply with policies and procedures.

S Is knowledgeable of and complies with policies and procedures affecting nursing. When requested, assists with review and revision of policies and procedures.

A Performs all behaviors described in **S.** Refers to policy and procedure book to verify actions or answer questions by other staff members. Reviews the books periodically to maintain familiarity with policies and procedures.

E Performs all behaviors described in **A.** Always complies with policies and procedures. If does not, communicates the rationale for noncompliance to the supervisor and/or recommends revision in the policy or procedure.

6. *Assists with the orientation of new employees.*

Explanation. The R.N. works as a preceptor with a new R.N. on a day-to-day basis, according to the orientation procedure. The R.N. assists with the orientation of L.P.N.s, aides, orderlies, and unit secretary.

Evaluation Guide

U Refuses or is uncooperative in assisting with the orientation of new employees. If agrees to help, will not work closely or in supportive manner with the new employee.

S When asked, assists new employees in their orientation and role transition. Follows orientation procedures and provides explanations, demonstrations, and support to new employees.

A Performs all behaviors described in **S.** Requests to serve as preceptor. Is enthusiastic about helping new employees and works closely with head nurse and staff development to provide an effective orientation period.

E Performs all behaviors described in **A.** Makes new employees feel at home. Reviews and explains policies and procedures with which the employee is unfamiliar. Seeks out learning experiences that would be beneficial to the employee and is well aware of learning needs. Is open and responsive to forming mentoring relationships.

7. *Acts rapidly and effectively and manages self, patients, and other employees during any emergency situation.*

Explanation. The R.N. is knowledgeable of policies, procedures, and equipment needed during emergencies, remains calm and effectively manages self and all people involved in the emergency.

Evaluation Guide

U Is not familiar with emergency procedures or equipment and tends to lose control during emergencies.

S Follows policies and procedures during emergencies. Remains calm and maintains control. Is familiar with emergency equipment.

A Performs all behaviors described in **S.** Manages and directs L.P.N., aides, orderlies, patients, and families during emergencies.

E Performs all behaviors described in **A.** Provides a calming effect for other personnel. Provides emotional support for families and patients when appropriate. Takes charge until the appropriate persons arrive on the scene.

8. *Attends required in-service education programs.*

Evaluation Guide

U Does not attend all required in-service education programs according to policies.

S Attends all required in-service education programs according to policies.

A Performs all behaviors described in **S.** Attends 90 percent of all in-service programs offered for R.N.s.

E Performs all behaviors described in **A.** When requested, actively participates in the planning and implementation of in-service programs.

Recommends needed in-service programs. Actively participates with questions, comments, and suggestions during the programs.

9. *Formulates nursing prescriptions that delineate actions to be taken. Prescribed actions:*

   9.1 *Are specific to the patient's problem and the desired outcomes.*

   9.2 *Are based on scientific knowledge.*

   9.3 *Are based on principles of patient teaching.*

   9.4 *Are based on principles of psychosocial interactions.*

   9.5 *Are based on environmental factors influencing the patient's health.*

   9.6 *Include human, material, and community resources.*

   9.7 *Include keeping patient knowledgeable of health status and total health care plan.*

Explanation. After identifying patient problems and desired outcomes, the R.N. prescribes actions to be taken in order to achieve desired outcomes. These actions are documented on the nursing care plan. The prescriptions include the seven criteria outlined above.

Evaluation Guide

U Fails to meet the criteria outlined (9.1–9.7).

S Satisfies all criteria outlined above and documents this within a 24-hour period.

A Performs all behaviors described in **S.** Formulates and documents nursing prescriptions that delineate actions to be taken on all new admissions during that 8-hour shift.

E Performs all behaviors described in **A.** From continual assessment and planning, adds to nursing prescriptions written from previous shifts on all assigned patients, each day.

10. *Implements the actions delineated in the nursing prescriptions. Actions implemented:*

    10.1 *Actively involve the patient and family.*

    10.2 *Are based on current scientific knowledge.*

    10.3 *Are flexible and individualized for each patient.*

    10.4 *Include principles of safety.*

    10.5 *Include principles of infection control.*

Explanation. After formulating nursing prescriptions, the R.N. implements the nursing actions delineated. All actions implemented are documented in the nurses' notes and reflect the total nursing care plan.

Evaluation Guide

U Fails to meet the criteria outlined (10.1–10.5).

S Satisfies all criteria outlined above and documents actions taken each shift.

A Performs all behaviors described in **S.** Collaborates with physician and other members of the health care team in implementing actions.

E Performs all behaviors described in **A.** Utilizes creative and innovative techniques in implementing actions. Involves staff in actions and teaches the rationale and scientific basis for the actions.

11. *Conforms to hospital dress code (according to policy).*

Evaluation Guide

U Seldom conforms to dress code policy.

S Usually conforms (90 percent of the time) to dress code policy.

A Always conforms to dress code policy.

E Is always immaculately dressed and groomed. Appears spotlessly clean, fresh, with shined shoes at all times.

12. *Is rarely sick or absent from work due to health.*

Explanation. Absenteeism is defined according to number of occurrences. An occurrence can be one day or more days, related to a particular illness. For example, one "call-in" with the flu with two days of illness would be one occurrence. The head nurse counsels employees approaching six occurrences.

Evaluation Guide

U Six occurrences.

S Five occurrences. Always calls in advance according to policy.

A Two to four occurrences per year.

E One or no occurrences per year.

13. *Is prompt and attends report (20 minutes prior to shift).*

Evaluation Guide

U Tardy six times per year. Often runs 15–20 minutes late.

S Tardy five times (within 5–10 minutes). Always calls when running late.

A Tardy three to four times per year (within 5 minutes).

E Tardy only two times per year or less.

IV. Evaluation

1. *Evaluates self-objectives; revises and formulates new objectives.*

Explanation. The R.N. evaluates his or her self-objectives to determine if the objectives have been achieved, and to determine progress. The R.N. reassesses objectives to determine if they are realistic. From the evaluation, new or revised self-objectives and strategies are developed.

Evaluation Guide

U Does not evaluate and revise self-objectives. Allows same objectives to continue month after month, with no improvement or change.

S Evaluates achievement of self-objectives documented on evaluation form at the annual and six-month evaluation. Makes revisions and sets new objectives at that time.

A Obtains input from peers and supervisory personnel when evaluating self-objectives. Provides rationale and pertinent facts to substantiate the evaluation results. Documents the results.

E Performs all behaviors described in **A.** Evaluates, revises, and sets self-objectives every three months and maintains documentation. Implements new, creative strategies to alter plans and achieve objectives.

2. *Evaluates the effectiveness of problem-solving techniques and the activities implemented to improve nursing service.*

Explanation. After participating in planning methods to solve problems and implementing the plan, the R.N. evaluates the outcomes to determine if the problem has been solved. If the problem has not been solved, the R.N. reassesses the problem and actions taken and participates in determining new techniques to solve the problem. Other problems may also be identified by this evaluation.

Evaluation Guide

U Never or rarely evaluates effectiveness of change or of problem-solving activities. Never notices improvement or effects of activities to improve nursing service.

S When requested, will provide an evaluation of activities and problem-solving techniques. Can base evaluation on sound rationale with evidence of improvement.

A Is self-motivated to evaluate nursing service activities. Communicates evidence substantiating evaluation of nursing service activities to supervisory personnel. Provides appropriate amount of time for planned change to occur before evaluating effectiveness of the change.

E Performs all behaviors described in **A.** From evaluation, identifies new problems and new areas in need of work. Revises plan of action accordingly, and includes creative strategies in this revision. Communicates evaluation and revision to supervisory personnel.

3. *Contributes to the performance evaluations of nursing service personnel on the unit.*

Explanation. The R.N. provides input to the head nurse and supervisor concerning the performance of peers, the L.P.N.s, aides, orderlies, and unit secretaries on the unit, in regard to patient and unit outcomes. The R.N. provides input concerning their contribution to progress on the unit. Also completes self-evaluation as described in performance evaluation policy.

Evaluation Guide

U When asked, does not provide pertinent or substantial input to the supervisor concerning the performance of other employees under his or her direction.

S When asked, can provide pertinent and substantial input concerning the employees' performance under direction. Closely evaluates the performance of new employees under direction and provides input for improvement.

A Performs all behaviors described in **S.** Gives specific information concerning an employee's teamwork, creativeness, concientiousness, and the outcome of the employee's patient care. Participates in appeal committee concerning performance evaluation decisions.

E Performs behaviors described in **A.** Participates in peer review committee, studies patient outcomes on the unit, and continually supports those attempting to improve their performance. Serves as a teacher and role model.

4. *Participates in the evaluation of in-service education programs.*

Explanation. The R.N. provides input to the staff development and supervisory personnel concerning appropriateness, content, and delivery of inservice education programs. The R.N. communicates learning needs and whether these needs were met to nurse-educators following the program. The R.N. identifies staff development needs and provides feedback concerning the utilization of learning on the unit. The R.N. communicates ideas for improving the in-service programs.

Evaluation Guide

U Never or rarely provides feedback concerning the need for inservice programs or the utilization of information obtained from the programs. Rarely evaluates the educational offerings.

S When asked will communicate an evaluation of the in-service program attended.

A Is self-motivated to evaluate in-service programs and to communicate this evaluation. Bases evaluation on sound rationale. Identifies strengths and weaknesses of in-service programs and ways to use the knowledge gained on the unit.

E Performs all behaviors described in **A.** Actively utilizes knowledge gained from in-services on the unit and evaluates the effectiveness of new techniques and knowledge. Recommends revisions in program content from this evaluation. Requests clarification and explanations from staff development or supervisory personnel concerning content of programs and communicates ways to improve educational offerings.

5. *Evaluates achievement or lack of achievement of desired outcomes.*

   5.1 *Data are collected concerning the patient's health status.*

   5.2 *Data are compared to the specific desired outcomes.*

   5.3 *The patient and nurse evaluate the achievement of desired outcomes.*

Evaluation Guide

U Fails to meet criteria (5.1–5.3).

S Satisfies criteria listed above and documents achievement or lack of achievement of desired outcomes in nurses' notes.

A Performs all behaviors described in **S.** Collaborates with the patient, health care team, and other personnel in evaluating achievement of desired outcomes. Discusses achievement or lack of achievement at shift report.

E Performs all behaviors described in **A.** Includes assessment of slight alterations in the patient's health status and in the evaluation of achievement of desired outcomes.

6. *From evaluation of achievement or lack of achievement of desired outcomes, reassesses and revises the nursing care plan.*

   6.1 *Reassesses the patient problems.*

   6.2 *Reassesses desired outcomes to determine if appropriate, realistic, and in correct priority.*

   6.3 *Reassesses nursing prescriptions to determine if appropriate, realistic, and stated accurately.*

   6.4 *Reassesses nursing actions for effectiveness in achieving desired outcomes.*

   From the reassessment:

   6.5 *Determines new patient present or potential problems.*

   6.6 *From new patient problems, formulates and revises desired outcomes.*

   6.7 *Revises nursing prescriptions.*

   6.8 *Implements new actions in order to carry out revised prescriptions.*

   6.9 *Continually evaluates desired outcomes for achievement or lack of achievement.*

   6.10 *Continually evaluates and revises the nursing care plan according to changes in the patient's health status.*

Evaluation Guide

U Fails to meet criteria (6.1–6.10) and to document revisions in the plan of care.

S Satisfies criteria listed above and documents revisions in the plan of care.

A Gathers data from all possible sources and collaborates with all members of the health care team (as appropriate) in reassessing and revising the nursing care plan.

E Reassesses and revises (as appropriate) the nursing care plan on all assigned patients each day and documents this on the nurses' notes and care plan each day.

APPENDIX 9–4

Performance Evaluation Scoring Procedure*

In the following procedure, a *satisfactory* ranking means that at least 90 percent of the items on the performance evaluation are rated as *satisfactory* (if not, the overall score would not reflect satisfactory achievement of the nursing standards); *above average* ranking means that at least 80 percent of all items are rated as *above average;* and *excellent* ranking means that at least 80 percent of all items on the performance evaluation are rated as *excellent.* Refer to the scoring procedure form at the end of the performance evaluation on page 239.

1. Add up the number of "U", "S", "A," and "E" ratings. Write these totals in the blanks on the scoring sheet at the end of the evaluation form.
2. Multiply each total by the designated number. A "U" gets zero points, an "S" gets one point, an "A" receives two points, and an "E" receives three points.
3. The products of this multiplication are totaled, and their sum equals the total score.
4. Compare this total score to the numbers comprising each rank. Wherever this number falls is the rank of that particular employee. For example, if "A" is 43–64, an employee who scored a total of 51 points would receive an *above average* rating.

The following is an example of how to develop the four ranking categories:

A particular performance evaluation has a total of 49 items. Multiply *49* in this manner:

0 × 49 = 0 (U)
1 × 49 = 49 (S)
2 × 49 = 98 (A)
3 × 49 = 147 (E)

U	S	A	E
0 to 43	44 to 77	78 to 117	118 to 147

Then take the "S" number (49). Multiply it by 90 percent to receive 44.1. Because 0.1 is less than 0.5, it can be dropped. Write this number in the spot indicated above. This is the minimum score that can be made to receive an *S* ranking. Then take the "A" score (98), and multiply it by 80 percent to receive 78.4. Again, 0.4 is less than 0.5 and can be dropped. Write this number in the *A* spot as shown above. This becomes the mini-

*Adapted with permission from Jernigan, D. K., & Young, A. P., *Standards, Job Descriptions, and Performance Evaluations for Nursing Practice.* E. Norwalk, Conn.: Appleton-Century-Crofts, 1983, pp. 56–57.

mum score that can be made to receive an *above average* ranking. Anything less (77) becomes the top score for the *satisfactory* ranking. Take the "E" total (147) and multiply it by 80 percent to receive 117.6. Because 0.6 is greater than 0.5, it raises the number to 118.

This becomes the minimum score that can be made to receive an *excellent* ranking. It is written in the first blank under *E* as shown above. One number less (117) becomes the top score for the *A* ranking as shown. The top *E* score would indicate all items had received an *excellent* rating, or three points. This is derived by multiplying 3 times 49 items to equal 147. The *U* ranks from 0 to one point below the *satisfactory* ranking (43).

Each performance evaluation must be tabulated in the above manner, as each one (R.N., L.P.N., aide, etc.) has a different number of items. The scores are typed on the back of each form, made available to the staff, and used when evaluating the performance ranking.

APPENDIX 9–5

Sample Six-month Interview and Evaluation Form*

Six months following the annual evaluation, a formal interview and evaluation period is provided for each employee. The head nurse and employee set a time to meet and discuss performance and progress towards goals. The employee receives input concerning areas in need of improvement and suggestions for change, as well as strengths and excellent performance. Any *unsatisfactory* performance is communicated and documented and *must be improved to satisfactory* prior to the annual evaluation period. The interview period allows evaluation of self-objectives and validation of self-evaluation. The growth and development needs of the employee are discussed. The following form provides a guideline for discussion and documentation:

Date ____________ Name ____________ Unit ____________

1. Self-evaluation of performance over past six months:

2. Progress towards self-objectives, revisions, and new self-objectives developed during last six months:

3. Strengths in performance (include *excellent* performance):

4. Weaknesses in performance (include *unsatisfactory* performance):

5. Discussion of personal and career needs and goals:

6. Changes or new self-objectives for next six months:

7. Suggestions for specific knowledge, skills, or needed training over next six months. Guide for improvement of performance:

8. Additional discussion, recommendations, or comments:

Date ________________________ Employee Signature ____________
Date ________________________ Interviewer Signature ____________

*This form becomes part of the employee's personnel file and is used in the annual evaluation review.

APPENDIX 9–6

Employee Special Progress Report Form

Unusual occurrences, outstanding employee performance and activities, and critical incidents should be recorded and discussed with the employee. This form is a guide for documenting unusually *good* or *bad* occurrences. Outstanding performance should be recognized and documented, and forwarded to the vice-president for nursing. Critical incidents requiring warnings or discipline must be documented with corrective actions. This special form can be used to document any type of unusual activities, and becomes part of the employee's permanent personnel record.

Name ______________ Date ______________ Unit ______________

1. Describe the occurrence, including date, time, location, and outcome. State the facts and whether observed by you (the manager) or reported to you:

2. Describe the action taken by the supervisor:

3. Additional comments:

4. Employee comments:

I have read and understand the above:

Date ____________ Employee Signature______________

Date ____________ Supervisor Signature ______________

10 The Counseling and Coaching Process

Counseling and coaching are the two parts of a process that links a need or deficiency with results; it is intimately linked to the performance evaluation process and is part of growth and development. As employees are continually evaluated, they must be provided counsel, support, and direction in implementing their roles and responsibilities and developing with the organization. The counseling and coaching process can assist employees to perform up to their abilities and actualize their potentials.

The process of counseling and coaching is ongoing and occurs both formally and informally. It is used for the employee who is seeking job enrichment and growth or for the underachiever who is not performing up to potential. It is also used for borderline performers and those who are evaluated as unsatisfactory. Counseling and coaching are important parts of a nurse administrator's work and occur through all aspects of human resource management.

This chapter will focus on counseling and coaching as they relate to the marginal and unsatisfactory employee. Of course, it is equally important to counsel and coach better employees who are contributing to the organization. Managers must not become so totally sidetracked in working with the problem employees that little energy is left for those specially talented individuals who need extra guidance. But employees experiencing malcontent, maladjustment to change, or other types of disequilibrium pose a persistent problem for the nurse-administrator. They are an obstacle to efficient functioning and can disrupt the performance of other, better-adjusted employees. They must be guided in taking ownership of their problems or behaviors and in becoming self-directing and productive, and they must be assisted in achieving stability and satisfactory performance. When this assistance or these efforts fail, they must then be guided into other work more suitable to their needs, expectations, and abilities. While counseling and coaching are positive approaches to directing improvement and growth, their concern is as much for organizational harmony as for individual well-being. At the point where all efforts fail to assist the employee in maintaining standards, and the employee will not take responsibility for improving behaviors, the process shifts to progressive discipline and eventually outplacement. The stability, balance, and integrity of the work environment must be maintained for the workforce as a whole. Counseling involves exchanging ideas, talking things out, and providing advice and recommendations. Coaching involves teaching and directing another person's actions and behavior. Together, counseling and coaching can help employees correct deficiencies and meet or even exceed job expectations.

THE MARGINAL AND UNSATISFACTORY EMPLOYEE

An employee performing below or barely at expected levels is a concern to the nurse-administrator for a variety of reasons. In many cases, this employee is not meeting minimum standards of practice. Secondly, poor performance can drain morale on the unit. By chronic absences, complaining, promoting interpersonal conflicts, or through continued mistakes and omissions in patient care, such a person's conduct causes resentment and frustration for the other employees. Thirdly, this employee becomes a financial drain on the organization. Poor attitude or poor performance causes decreased productivity (the employee may put little effort into work), decreased efficiency (caused by accidents, errors, and communication breakdowns), and increased expense through overtime paid to other employees to cover his or her absences and tardiness. In addition, the decreased morale becomes costly in terms of increasing absenteeism, decreased productivity, and turnover on that unit; the frustrated and resentful employees tire of the dissatisfying working conditions. It becomes exceedingly difficult to recruit and retain high-quality employees on this unit. Then, with increased turnover come increased costs for recruitment, selection, and orientation. The cost in administrative time to handle an increased number of grievances and labor relations problems, or in conflict resolutions and solving interpersonal problems, begins to mount. Poor performers cause a vicious cycle of poor morale and increased costs to the organization.

The common response to the problem employee is for the manager to (a) get tough, (b) be extra nice, (c) call in a third party for help, or (d) make the employee *want* to quit. Managers also expect instant results. None of these tactics are successful in improving the situation, although calling in a third party may be indicated at some point during the counseling and coaching process.

Other typical management traps occur when dealing with a difficult employee. These are

1. Being afraid of the employee's response to a confrontation
2. Feeling sorry for the employee
3. Giving special treatment to an employee
4. Fearing confrontation of an employee in a minority group
5. Ignoring the problem
6. Leaving the employee alone because of seniority

Often, when the problem is allowed to continue, the manager will attempt to correct the situation by actually doing the employee's work and filling in for discrepancies. In many cases the employee is transferred rather than corrected. Often the problem grows until it is out of control, and the manager wants to get rid of the problem. Hence no attempts to improve and coach the employee are made, and, of course, nothing is documented.[1]

Solutions are not reached through these ineffective management practices. An organized and effective counseling and coaching process is vital to the well-being of the employee, as well as to the organization. The manager must keep in mind the basic aims and purposes of counseling and coaching, and integrate these into everyday practice. These can be summarized in the following statements.

1. The primary concerns in counseling and coaching are the welfare of the employee and the organization.
2. Counseling and coaching are based on a genuine respect for human beings and their importance to the organization.
3. Counseling and coaching aim to develop a satisfied and competent employee who will strive to improve.
4. Counseling and coaching provide employees a means for emotional support, ventilation of feelings, and assistance in developing the skills to solve or cope with personal problems.
5. Counseling and coaching provide employees with a means for developing self-awareness and perceptions that will assist in solving work-related problems.
6. Counseling and coaching integrate the employee's family, physical and mental health, and needs and values when assisting him or her to meet potential.
7. Counseling and coaching aim to develop and improve interpersonal relations and employee trust in the organization.
8. Counseling and coaching are a part of growth and development, and aim to improve and assist the employee in meeting his or her needs.

9. Counseling and coaching aim to guide the employee in assuming responsibility for his or her own behavior, and seeking self-improvement.
10. Counseling and coaching are means with which to communicate that the organization is concerned and responsive to employee needs and problems.

ORGANIZING THE COUNSELING AND COACHING PROCESS

The most effective means for implementing the counseling and coaching process is through the employee's immediate supervisor. This supervisor is responsible for evaluating the employee's performance, has observed this employee on a daily basis, and should be the most accessible support system. The supervisor is in the position to develop effective communication, trust, and mutual problem solving, which provides the environment for counseling and coaching. In addition, the supervisor's background of ongoing management development should prepare him or her for this important process.

An in-house employee counseling and employee assistance program can also be developed. With the increasing pressures and problems facing employees at home and at work, these types of programs are becoming widespread. They provide a wide range of services, from legal assistance to drug and alcohol assistance. They work toward providing a healthy work environment and decreasing absenteeism, accidents, and employee grievances. These programs assist with career planning, provide information on policies and procedures, and provide mental health services. The employee assistance program may be provided by in-house specialists or through contact with an outside clinic or counselor.[2]

An in-house counseling and coaching service could be headed by a psychologist, a psychiatrist, or a clinical nurse specialist in mental health. This person could be consulted via a referral from the first-line supervisor or be directly approached by the employee. Following assessment, other referrals could be made to various department heads, outside clinics, or even back to the head nurse for a meeting with the specialist and the employee to discuss problems. This mental health specialist serves to provide confidential, nonbiased counseling and coaching to help solve interpersonal work problems or to overcome other stress-producing situations.

In conjunction with counseling and coaching processes, peer support groups can be organized to allow nurses to manage work-related problems together. Groups may be formed to discuss health-related issues of concern, work environment frustrations and issues, and ways to overcome stress and burnout. Group discussions can be held by individual units or formed by counselors with interdisciplinary group members. The type of groups or peer counseling will depend on the nature of the problem and the purpose or desired outcome. But peer discussions and assistance can be very helpful as a support system and a means for overcoming problems affecting employees' work. Peer groups should be organized and implemented by an effective, health-oriented group leader.[3]

All employees require support and guidance at some point during their employment. Even outstanding nurses may encounter personal difficulties that can eventually affect their work. Counseling and coaching should be organized so that they are readily available to employees and can meet their needs. The first-line nurse-manager is critical to an effective process and for following up on in-house counseling programs. An organized, continuous approach must be taken by all management personnel.

STEPS IN COUNSELING AND COACHING

The counseling and coaching process is a means to define problems and analyze underlying causes, and also to devise strategies to improve or correct the problem or situation. An employee who performs below expectations is identified and assisted to improve performance. During this process, interpersonal, family, or other problems causing an unsatisfactory behavior are identified and discussed. Solutions may be worked out mutually by the manager and employee or call for other measures, such as peer assistance, an in-house mental health specialist, or referral to a legal or financial advisor. The process gets to the root of employee problems and provides assistance in solving them. It involves four basic steps:

1. Identification of the problem
2. Analysis of nonperformance or behavior problems
3. Development of strategies for improvement
4. Action, evaluation, and follow-up

The following text will discuss each of these steps.

Identification of the Problem

Managers should learn to identify problems and borderline behaviors early on, so that poor performance practices do not become a habit or develop into serious management problems. Identification of performance problems is part of the performance evaluation process, and would be reflected in the annual and six-month interview and evaluation period. But, as stated in Chapter 9, there should be no surprises. Borderline and unsatisfactory behaviors are identified through ongoing assessment, and employees are provided continual feedback on deficiencies and needs for improvement. Managers must initiate on-the-spot counseling and coaching when observing an unacceptable behavior. By the time the formal evaluation period arrives, evaluation of any areas as *U* will have been preceded by a counseling and coaching process. Because the behavior was not corrected, it would most likely dictate initiation of progressive discipline or some other action. Discipline is utilized only after the employee has failed to respond to other measures of assistance and support.

What constitutes a problem or unsatisfactory behavior? Common behavior problems and potential problems can be categorized into three main areas: technical, personal, and interpersonal deficiencies. The following provide examples of common problems in each of these three areas.

Technical Deficiencies

1. Fails to meet job expectations as defined in the criteria for performance evaluation
2. Fails to carry out policies and procedures, contractual agreements, or terms of employment
3. Is involved in frequent accidents
4. Commits numerous mistakes and omissions

Personal Deficiencies

1. Is chronically late or absent
2. Expresses dissatisfaction, hostility, pessimism, and a large number of grievances
3. Is often ill at work, complains of many physical and personal problems, and may leave early due to these problems
4. Lacks initiative, shows indifference, often is unavailable when needed, and may show lack of concern over patients and their families

Interpersonal Deficiencies

1. Is involved in ongoing personality conflicts with others
2. Often refuses or is unable to contribute to the unit's culture and practice its philosophy—may resist the team's planned projects and changes
3. Often is rude and unfriendly to students and new employees, causing an unpleasant work environment and affecting the orientation process

Some of these behaviors are common and can be seen in even the best employees from time to time. Normal complaining and arguing will occur in the day-to-day work routine, and can even serve to ventilate feelings and frustrations.[4] But when behaviors begin to recur and show disruption or interruption in the functioning of unit activities and patient care, or if they are leading to a decrease in morale, the nurse-administrator must intervene.[5] Some employees may exhibit the above problem behaviors in a borderline fashion. Their performance may be marginal, and improve only when under scrutiny by administration. These employees should be identified as *Unsatisfactory* and included in the counseling and coaching process.

In identification of the problem, the exact behavior must be specified, and not simply stated as "an attitude problem," etc. Not only must the unacceptable behavior be defined; specific examples of this behavior should be provided (exact dates and incidents are best). The deficient behavior should then be compared to job expectations, policies, and so on, to show deviation from standards and reason for the behavior being unacceptable. The nurse-administrator should do an initial investigation prior to the counseling session. This investigation should include an assessment of

The Severity of the Incident. Is the incident important enough to mention, or are other problems more serious and in need of attention? Care should be taken not to be unreasonable or expect perfection. A one-time incident may simply warrant watching—make a note of the date and occurrence, and quietly observe. Often employees are aware of problems and correct them themselves.

How Long the Behavior Has Existed. If this behavior has been exhibited previously, how was it managed? What documentation is available? Are several employees exhibiting this behavior? If so, one person cannot be singled out and corrected. If behaviors have been allowed to continue without management intervention, correction may involve group meetings with discussion, and communication of future enforcement of policies.

Whether Administration has Contributed to the Problem. Determine possible causes of the problem due to management practices such as poor communications, ineffective orientation and training, poor working conditions, ineffective selection, or a breakdown in other personnel processes. Always consider the possibility of lack of knowledge or poor management practices.

An Employee's Work History. Review length of service, contributions, previous performance evaluations, and general track record. This can give valuable clues to the nature of a problem and its progression.

Points to Keep in Mind. During this investigation, keep in mind the need for fairness and objectivity. A prior confrontation or negative feedback about this employee should not be allowed to interfere with the proper management of the situation. A clear, unbiased mind is important to effective decision making. If this is impossible, another nurse-administrator should be called upon to manage the problem. Remember that the focus is on both the optimum functioning of the organization, and an unhappy or troubled human being who needs help. The objective must be to find the cause of the problem and assist the employee to correct or improve. Most employees can be of value to the organization despite this deficient behavior. Also, recruitment, rehiring, and training of new employees is costly. When possible, attempt to salvage all employees.[6]

If a behavior or incident is severe enough to warrant suspension, immediate probation, or dismissal, prepare documentation, discussed later in this chapter. Provide the personnel policies that support this action. Ensure that employees are aware of policies and that they have been uniformly applied to everyone. Never act in haste or call a meeting when angry. Arrange the meeting shortly after the incident or problem has occurred, but after allowing time for the calming of emotions. It is not wise to schedule a meeting after an extremely difficult day or following the 11 P.M. to 7 A.M. shift. Employees may be overly tired and not in a mood for communicating.

Analysis of Nonperformance or Behavior Problems

Following the initial investigation, a meeting should be arranged to discuss the problem with the employee. This meeting should take place in a relaxed environment, without interruptions or the possibility of being overheard. The purpose of this first counseling session is to

1. Communicate the existence of a problem to the employee
2. Allow the employee to explain or express his or her opinions and thoughts on the subject
3. Collect information concerning the cause of the behavior or problem
4. Focus on the employee's strengths and importance in the organization, and communicate caring, concern, and emotional support
5. Begin to formulate ideas and strategies for problem solving

Each employee is different, and each situation must be managed differently. The problem should be explained, with its resulting effects, such as deviation from standards, policies, procedures, or drain on morale. It is best to approach the first session more as a concerned friend than as an authoritative manager. The employee must sense openmindedness and your desire to understand the situation more fully.

The counselor's emotions should be kept under control during the meeting, allowing the employee to relay his or her perception of the situation. An employee who becomes upset, defensive, or argumentative must be allowed to work through initial denial or anger with an objective listener.

Many employees are aware of discrepancies and have ready insights into causes and solutions. Others may not perceive the existence of a problem and require specific facts about dates, incidents, and repercussions from the incident. The employee should be asked whether he or she understands the problem, and be allowed to disagree with your perception. If the employee disagrees, acknowledge the difference of opinion, but reinforce the need to maintain standards and adhere to policies. The employee must understand that some solution must be reached for correcting the problem and that you will assist in remedying the situation.[7]

The management approach will depend on the employee's response during this meeting. If the employee remains defensive, hostile, or uncommunicative, schedule another meeting in a day or two, allowing time to think about what has been discussed. If the employee is open to suggestions and wants to improve, proceed with the next step—strategies for improvement. If he or she continues to be uncooperative, there are several options that can be taken, depending on the nature of the problem:

1. The employee can be referred to another manager who will be better able to communicate with him or her
2. The employee can be referred to a counselor within the organization, who might help in discussing the problem
3. Disciplinary measures may have to be initiated, especially if the behavior involves noncompliance with a policy or job expectation

It is important that this first meeting communicate a nonthreatening concern for the employee and a willingness to assist in overcoming any obstacles or reasons for certain behaviors. Through mutual discussion and exchange, the cause of the behavior should be identified and mutually analyzed. Is it work-related and under management's control? Is it work related but out of management's control? Is it personal? The problem must be defined, along with the underlying causes, and agreed upon by the employee.[1]

There are numerous reasons for noncompliant behavior or poor performance. By understanding common causes of poor performance, managers can learn to spot certain behaviors that indicate potential problems. The following are a few examples of common problems that result in performance deficiencies.

1. *Burnout.* Apathy, discouragement, and indifference due to continued, repetitive, unstimulating, or unusually difficult work schedules lead to burnout. Lack of feedback and rewards, lack of autonomy, inflexibility, and continual stressors and crises can also cause burnout.[8]
2. *Cop-Out.* Temporary boredom, dissatisfaction, and apathy due to bad fortune or rejection can result in cop-out. Being passed over for a promotion, a plateau in professional advancement, not being accepted by peers, or failing at some endeavor can result in cop-out by some employees. Behaviors such as laziness, lack of interest, and anger may also be seen. Cop-out should be distinguished from burnout prior to developing strategies for improvement.[8]

3. *Return to Nursing Due to Economic Pressures.* Many individuals have retired from nursing due to dissatisfaction with salaries, shift work, working conditions, or other aspects of the work. The need for two incomes, divorces, being laid off from other jobs, children in college, and a number of other reasons may have forced them back into nursing. This, along with undesirable shift work and scheduling, can cause much dissatisfaction and many behavioral problems.
4. *Personal Loss.* Marital difficulties resulting in divorce, death of a loved one, a troubled adolescent who rejects the family, financial crises, and other personal or family stressors can lead to a feeling of loss and depression. These employees may only temporarily exhibit performance problems, or may allow their personal lives to affect their work.[8]
5. *Drug or Alcohol Abuse.* Poor performance can result from dependence on drugs or alcohol. The substance abuser poses a special problem for management. Due to the nature of the work, these employees could seriously endanger the safety and lives of patients. Therefore, they cannot be allowed to provide care. Activities such as stealing patient's medications must also be investigated.
6. *Lack of Knowledge.* Unsatisfactory performance can be due to lack of knowledge. When communications are unclear or expectations are not defined, performance may be deficient due to simply not understanding. Lack of prior training in a skill or procedure could also result in poor performance.
7. *Inability to Learn or Perform Competently.* Occasionally an employee will be motivated to perform, but does not have the intellectual aptitude or the motor abilities. Also, an employee may not have the emotional maturity to handle stressful situations, or to deal with patients and families.
8. *Emotional Disturbance.* Certain employees may be overly sensitive, defensive, hostile, or unresponsive due to emotional problems. They may have poor self-images or distorted perceptions of reality. These people make working conditions very difficult for other employees, and often have unhappy patients.
9. *Failing Health.* Employees experiencing physical conditions that limit their ability to perform the job may experience unsatisfactory behaviors. Chronic illnesses or physical limitations can result in performance below expected standards.

Once the cause of a problem can be identified and analyzed, a plan can be devised for correcting the situation. This plan is developed mutually by the employee and the nurse-manager.

Development of Strategies for Improvement

The strategy for problem solving will depend upon the employee's needs and the nature of the problem. Possible approaches could include

1. Planning special training and staff development programs.
2. Referral to in-house specialists. A plan delineating the nature of the corrective action with needed time span would be forwarded to the nurse-manager under strict confidentiality. In some extremely personal cases, only the expected behaviors and time span are revealed. Employees must comply with the agreement or progressive disciplinary measures are instituted.
3. Peer assistance programs or groups. The employee and manager define expected behaviors and time span for improvement, then the employee works with a group to correct the problem.
4. Contract development. The employee and manager mutually outline expected behaviors, management assistance, and employee activities in a specific timeframe. This is a type of negotiation where both parties compromise.
5. Referral to physician, psychiatrist, or outside clinic. Depending on the problem, employees may need certain types of treatment and follow-up.
6. Correction of ineffective management practices contributing to the problem.
7. Transfer, shift change, or scheduling change. Sometimes the solution to a problem is relatively simple.
8. Job enrichment. Problems can occur due to job dissatisfaction or lack of advancement opportunities. Efforts should be taken to provide a challenging and rewarding work environment.
9. Advise and recommend. Management may simply recommend altering behaviors. Through the counseling and exchange period, the problem can sometimes be solved.
10. Change the job, change the work, resignation, early retirement, or dismissal. Depending on the severity of the problem, the previous attempts to correct it, the likelihood of success, and the time and investment needed for success, one of these strategies may be implemented. A job change may involve job sharing or changing the job description. A change of the work could involve redistributing responsibilities or the type of work performed. The needs of the employee are considered in this decision. Options such as resignation and early retirement may be offered. Dismissal decisions depend on the nature of the problem (as defined in policies) and the ability by the employee to improve in the agreed-upon timeframe.

Specific Strategies for Improvement. Specific strategies will relate to the specific problem and might include a combination of the above approaches. Some examples of strategies for improvement include:

For the "Burnout." Use peer assistance groups, transfer to less stressful unit, and provide improved working conditions.

For the "Cop-Out"

1. Provide training and opportunities to advance at any age or level in the organization
2. Involve the employee's family in discussion of career directions and work satisfaction
3. Challenge employees to maintain standards and continually improve through performance evaluations, reward systems, and recognizing creativity
4. Identify the source of the apathy and provide positive reinforcement for strengths and good performance[8]

Employees Who Have Been Forced to Return to Nursing. These employees must be identified and provided emotional support. Efforts to provide peer assistance and flexible, convenient scheduling should be made. Special benefits such as child care may also help these employees to manage their problems. Their concerns and grievances must be heard objectively. Good working conditions and involvement in decision making may improve their performance.

Employees Experiencing a Personal Loss. Management must set plans with employees to limit the problem's effect at work. These plans should identify a reasonable time span for coping and adjusting, minimum job expectations until the problem is solved, and support mechanisms such as clergy, professional counselors, and family therapy. Managers must provide support while maintaining unit functioning. Emphasis should be to let work help employees get through their problems. Sometimes a leave of absence or sick leave may become necessary.[8]

Drug or Alcohol Abusers. Each organization has its own methods for identifying and managing these employees. Nurses observed taking patient narcotics are often fired on the spot. The same often applies for employees who show signs and symptoms of consuming alcohol on the job. A manager who suspects drug or alcohol abuse should have the employee closely monitored to be sure. Often employees will deny a direct question and must be approached with the "evidence." Also, termination must be for just cause, as discussed later, so should be based on documented evidence versus hearsay. The state board of nursing should be notified of suspected substance abuse, and will assist in investigating the circumstances.

Some states and facilities are organizing peer assistance programs where abusers enter detoxification programs and work with a peer. Upon completion of the program they are allowed to resume their positions on a probationary basis. Support for the success of these programs in rehabilitating impaired nurses is mixed. The nurse-administrator should form a task force to discuss this issue and determine policies and procedures for managing these cases.

Lack of Knowledge. Job expectations must be reviewed prior to hiring and during orientation, and the terms of employment must be agreed upon and signed by both managers and employees. This serves as proof that employees were informed of job expectations. The self-assessment and competency-based education during the orientation program also ensure that minimum requirements for performance are obtained. Any changes, new policies, and new procedures must be communicated and documented by initialling of the policy by employees; proof of attendance at in-service must be maintained. Meetings must be scheduled often enough so all employees have the opportunity to attend, and their attendance should be part of the performance evaluation. Procedure books must be current and accessible, and any new equipment or procedure must be preceded by classes and training. If unsatisfactory performance is due to lack of knowledge, the reason should be investigated, and appropriate classes and training provided.

The Employee Who is Unable to Learn or Perform Competently. This employee must be provided guidance, assistance, and training to obtain the necessary skills within a reasonable period of time. But if after time, energy, and guidance, the employee continues to perform below competencies, he or she must be assisted in finding a suitable position. A transfer to a less stressful unit than emergency or intensive care, for example, may solve the problem. If efforts to find work that the employee can perform fail, he or she must be dismissed.

The Emotionally Disturbed Employee. These employees may require extensive psychotherapy and counseling. If there is an in-house counselor, they should be referred to this counselor. The organization must determine the employee's potential for improvement, and the reasonable length of time it can afford to offer. Sometimes, when concern and caring are demonstrated, these employees begin to make improvements.

Employees Suffering from Failing Health. In cases such as back problems, arthritic conditions, diabetes, and other illnesses that limit scheduling or assignments of an employee, all attempts should be made to accommodate the limitations. Job assignments and shift rotations should be individualized within reason; that is, not placing undue financial hardship on the facility or unfair workload on the other employees. If a physical condition is affecting job performance, this should be identified and necessary assistance provided. Lengthy and frequent absences should be handled according to policies covering the number of occurrences and length of time an employee can be off and still expect to resume the same position and schedule. These policies must be uniformly applied.

Planning Strategies for Improvement. This should be a mutual process. Managers assist employees to solve their own problems. Through support and counseling, the employee must gain insight into the behavior, and take ownership of his or her performance. If efforts to counsel and coach fail, employees must be confronted with the behavior problem and given a choice. They may be asked whether they can meet the job requirements and if they want to continue working in the organization. Given time to reflect and make a decision, they then must take responsibility for either complying or being terminated—the decision is placed in their hands.[7]

Many employees will respond to a caring manager who has a genuine interest in his or her well-being. Sometimes simply allowing ventilation of a frustration or issue will solve the problem. The counseling session can also be a management tool to explain the need for certain policies or practices, as well as establishing a trusting and rewarding relationship.

Counseling and coaching can also be a way to gain important insight into structural and organizational problems. When assessing behavior problems and developing strategies for improvement, the system should be examined for inefficiencies or breakdowns. Poor management practices must be corrected. Common management problems include[9]:

1. Lack of incentive, reward systems, or motivational environment
2. Incongruent values and philosophy between the staff and administration
3. Improper job assignment or selection processes
4. Promoting to management position without proper training and preparation
5. Poor supervision
6. Lack of job standards and expectations

Inequities in treatment, ineffective performance evaluation procedures, and lack of or ineffective grievance procedures also point to management ineffectiveness. Management must continually look for early signs of problems, such as a persisting issue or complaint by employees. These issues are important to them and can magnify if not identified and resolved. Communication must be kept open, and managers must keep in touch with the staff. A manager who first identifies a problem employee should do a self-evaluation, because problems may be due to management practices.[1] Poor management practices must not be tolerated by the vice-president for nursing, and they must be recognized early and corrected immediately. Nothing is more of a drain on morale, productivity, and operations than poor management practices.

Action, Evaluation, and Follow-up

Once problems are assessed and analyzed and strategies are planned for improvement, the plans must be put into action. Employees are assisted in implementing plans, and are evaluated according to the established criteria. A follow-up date must be set to ensure continued compliance. If strategies fail and no improvement is seen, progressive discipline may become necessary. There are many considerations in ensuring a fair and objective disciplinary process. The remainder of this text will deal with these issues and concerns.

PROGRESSIVE DISCIPLINE

Progressive discipline involves a series of steps to correct an employee problem. The steps involve progressive warnings or reprimands concerning the deviation from minimum standards. The usual procedure is the sequence from verbal warning to written warning and possibly to suspension and then dismissal. Each step should address only one behavior problem at a time. There need not be a set time period for proceeding from one step to another. If immediate improvement is expected, and this expectation is communicated to the employee, then the next step can be instituted shortly after the preceding step. Also, one step may be repeated rather than progressing to the next step if an employee has made a genuine effort to improve.[10] Each step should involve certain elements:

Verbal Warning

This may be an informal discussion on the unit, following an incident or observation by the manager. It may also be included in the counseling process, during the problem solving and analysis stage. Or the manager may call a meeting with an employee and verbally warn him or her of the consequences of a continued unsatisfactory behavior. A verbal warning should

1. Let the employee know he or she has deviated from an expected behavior
2. Allow the employee to discuss and explain his or her point of view
3. Communicate to the employee the exact behavior improvement expected
4. State the amount of time allowed for this improvement to occur
5. Include assistance, support, and coaching by management for employee improvement
6. Communicate the seriousness of the problem, if not corrected
7. Plan for a follow-up meeting, if appropriate

A verbal warning provides the employee a chance to improve without damage to his or her record, performance evaluation results, or ego. Although criticism is never enjoyable, many employees may unintentionally deviate from expected behaviors and appreciate being given an early opportunity to improve. If this improvement is upheld, there is no reason for management to document it on the performance evaluation as "unsatisfactory," or in the personnel record (though managers should make note of the incident as their own personal reminder). Employees must be rewarded for their efforts by maintaining a clean record. If the behavior persists, a written warning should be issued.

Written Warning

If the problem continues, the second step in progressive discipline is the written warning. A meeting is called by the manager, and the employee is told again of the problem. It is explained how he or she had been previously warned of the need to improve, but had failed to do so. The employee is given an ultimatum—comply with expected standards or find work elsewhere. "It is your decision." The employee is then given a copy of the written warning, which should include

1. A statement of the problem or deficient behavior
2. The prior verbal warning and need to improve
3. Any assistance given by management such as counseling, training, resources, and other support to help him or her improve
4. A description of the standard, contractual agreement, or job expectation that was violated
5. Further assistance to be provided by management
6. The exact expected outcome and the time span for improvement
7. The consequences of not improving
8. The follow-up date

The employee should be allowed a written response if desired, and should sign that he or she has read and understands the information. A refusal to sign should be noted on the form by the manager.

Suspension

Following verbal and written warnings, a suspension may be the next disciplinary action or step. Again, the explanation given above under "Written Warning" is provided, and a second written statement concerning lack of compliance and resulting suspension should be signed by the employee. Also included is immediate dismissal if the problem is not corrected following the suspension. A suspension communicates management's intent to correct the situation, and aims to impress the employee with the seriousness of the behavior problem. The time period for suspension (during which the employee is not paid) should be appropriate for the problem. Suspended employees are told to leave the facility immediately, and informed when to report back to work.

Some organizations do not use suspension in progressive discipline.

They provide a second written warning prior to dismissal. Other organizations use suspension only when further investigating a serious occurrence, until further actions are decided. Suspension without pay may also be instituted as a disciplinary action for certain critical incidents.

Critical Incidents

Certain behaviors are completely unacceptable to the organization and can be categorized as "critical incidents." These incidents should be defined in the personnel handbook, with a statement of the consequences, such as "one-week suspension without pay" or "immediate dismissal." The incidents will require immediate disciplinary action, and can justify bypassing the progressive discipline process. Examples of critical incidents include insubordination, theft, destruction of property, releasing confidential information, successive unauthorized absences, and many others.

Probation

It is common for many employees to temporarily improve following disciplinary measures, only to slip back into unsatisfactory behaviors after a few months. These employees should be closely observed and issued a final warning at the first sign of the deviant behavior. With continual marginal behaviors and short-lived improvements, they may be placed on probation for six months to a year. In the probationary report (which they must sign), they should be informed of specific behaviors that will result in immediate dismissal during this time period. In addition, unsatisfactory behaviors must be reflected on the performance evaluation. Failure to improve and *maintain* this improvement from the six-month to the annual performance evaluation would result in two consecutive *U* ratings in that performance area. And, as explained in Chapter 9, policy can require that employees are not allowed to score two *U* ratings in a row. One *unsatisfactory* rating can result in probationary status, and subsequent failure to improve can result in dismissal. Counseling and coaching, discipline, and performance evaluation systems must work as one. Management must develop policies that assist in ridding the system of unsatisfactory people who are unable or unwilling to improve, despite all assistance.

Dismissal

Following failure of all actions and interventions, dismissal may be the only solution. It follows in the sequence of the progressive discipline process. It should be noted, however, that the time span between the last written or final warning must be considered. An employee issued a verbal and written warning four to six months earlier may receive another written warning, rather than being dismissed. Depending on the seriousness of the problem, the employee must again be provided with a warning and a means to improve.

During the dismissal interview, management must retrace prior events leading up to the dismissal, and have the employee sign his or her understanding (signatures do not indicate agreement, only understanding of the content; all disciplinary forms should state this fact). A witness present during the interview is helpful, especially if the employee refuses to sign. This witness should be nonbiased toward management or the employee.

Management must have definite policies concerning progressive discipline, and they must be understood by all employees. The responsibility for counseling, coaching, and progressive discipline should be placed at the level closest to the employee, although supervisors and the vice-president for nursing may be consulted or may intervene when problems are not managed appropriately. Nurse-managers must be continually monitored to ensure that all policies are enforced appropriately, fairly, and uniformly.

Exit Interviews

Exit interviews are normally conducted following a voluntary resignation. The exit interview is a management tool to explore the real reasons for resigning, learn about employee attitudes, and gain insight and information about the actual goings-on in the organization. It is an important procedure to improve recruitment, selection, and retention processes. On occasion an exit interview may be conducted for an employee who has been dismissed. The supervisor or vice-president for nursing may want to smooth over feelings and show that the organization does care, even through things could not be worked out. An employee is allowed to ventilate anger and other feelings, and the supervisor listens. The interview thus serves as a sort of counseling session. After emotions are expressed, the supervisor focuses on the employee's strengths and talents and gears the conversation toward the future. Guidance and recommendations are made regarding future employment. The employee is given hints about behaviors, appearance, and attitudes that may help in finding another job.

The exit interview is also used to answer questions concerning severance pay or benefits that may be granted for a period of time. Most organizations have policies that dictate losing accrued vacation, holidays, and other benefits if discharged. Some organizations may want to work out other arrangements with the employee. If the employee has been chronically borderline or causing a drain on morale and productivity, he or she may be asked to resign. Willingness to leave could be accompanied by a severance package of continued salary and benefits for an agreed-upon period of time. Sometimes a lump sum of money is offered. The announced reason for resignation is mutually agreed upon, and the whole process is kept confidential. Agreements of this sort usually occur with middle managers and above, but could conceivably occur with a staff nurse. Management thus saves the time, energy, and financial drain of progressive disciplinary procedures, training programs, appeals proceedings, and sometimes legal battles. A mutual agreement allows the employee to "save face" and maintain benefits while looking for another job. The agreement usually includes a release by the employee for any future legal charges or suits against the employer.

Outplacement Service (OPS)

Outplacement is an organized service for employees who have been dismissed or forced to resign from an organization. It is a means for supporting these employees and helping them get through the initial trauma, as well as to begin providing coaching that will assist them in finding a new job. It is usually a service for higher-paid employees, because it is believed that lower-salaried workers have less difficulty finding a comparable job. Outplacement counselors can work for the organization, or be outside consultants who contract for this service. They usually charge the organization 15 percent of an employee's salary.[11]

Outplacement service is a support for employees, and is considered part of their severance agreement. It smooths the termination process, decreases lawsuits, improves personnel relations, increases the morale of other employees, and decreases the cost of termination. The OPS counselor is ready and waiting during the dismissal interview (often in the next room), and takes over after the employee is told of termination. The counselor begins focusing on reemployment and provides guidance in assessing strengths, marketing skills, development of resumes, skill in interviewing, and other strategies to find work. The counselor also supports the employee during the search, and provides office space and assistance for phone calls and writing letters. The purpose of OPS is to neutralize the trauma, rebuild confidence, plan job searches, and support the employee throughout this process.[11]

Kangery[12] states that due to economic conditions, mergers, and corporate restructuring, many nurse-executives are being fired or forced to resign. A new administration often forms a new executive team, or a new nurse-administrator forms his or her own management team. This means more outplacement of nurse-managers. Outplacement counselors are used to assess alternative possibilities other than termination, such as job restructuring, transfer, and coaching. The counselor provides guidance to the vice-president for nursing in planning the termination interview. Following the dismissal, the counselor explains severance pay and benefits, and begins relocating the individual. Outplacement counseling helps the employee cope with job loss, and smooths the transition from the organization to a new area of employment.[12] This is another means to show concern and respect for every employee, and confirms administration's commitment to its human resources. Despite the fact that this employee has been dismissed, other employees can see that the process was executed with as much compassion, dignity, and support as possible.

DUE PROCESS AND TERMINATION FOR JUST CAUSE

If an organization is unionized, it will be required to dismiss employees only for just cause, and to provide them "due process" during the entire disciplinary process. But nonunionized organizations also have an obligation to be equitable and ensure these same conditions for employees. Not only will this help to deter unionization and decrease grievances and legal battles; it will also communicate a commitment to and concern for its human resources. The following text discusses employer responsibilities and considerations to ensure fair personnel practices throughout the progressive discipline process.

Nurse-administrators may have to prove that an employee was disciplined or dismissed for just cause and was provided due process throughout proceedings. *Just cause* involves

1. Proving an employee violated a rule or committed an offense
2. Justifying the punishment of the offense
3. Proving the appropriateness of the punishment to the offense[13]

Disciplinary actions must be taken for good reason. They must be justified and follow progressive discipline procedures. As mentioned earlier, critical incidents such as falsifying reports, forging signatures, willful violation of hospital rules, and committing several offenses in a short timespan may justify dismissal without progressive discipline. Nurse-administrators, however, must be prepared to provide evidence of their actions.[13]

Due process must also be provided to all employees. This would include ensuring that

1. All personnel have knowledge of policies and procedures and information in the personnel handbook. They must be informed of deficiencies or problems, and the problem must be related to their work in the organization, and be reasonable. Expectations must be fully communicated with suggestions provided for improvement.
2. Prior warnings must be given concerning problems, along with the consequences if the problem is not corrected. Employees must know expected behavior, know of impending disciplinary measures, and be given assistance and a reasonable time period to correct deficiencies.
3. An objective assessment must be made by administration concerning the deficiency and circumstances. An investigation must be fair and comprehensive, and include hearing the employee's side and explanation.
4. All discipline must be progressive, allowing adequate warning and chances to improve (excluding behaviors that are critical and call for severe and immediate discipline).

5. Documentation of the problem must be maintained, with facts concerning the investigation, assistance, training, and the action taken. All such documentation must be brought to the employee's attention prior to placement in the permanent record.
6. Corrective action must be consistent with the seriousness of the problem, and it must be reasonable.
7. All policies, procedures, and corrective or disciplinary actions must be applied uniformly and consistently, and past performance considered.[14]

Administrators have a responsibility to ensure just cause and due process, and provide fair personnel practices. Bolden[14] summarizes some key points to include in policies and procedures for employee evaluation and discipline.

1. All managers responsible for evaluating employees must be knowledgeable of policies, procedures, and the performance evaluation process prior to assessing performance.
2. Persons preparing the performance evaluation must discuss it with the employee, who can sign an agreement or make a written response, which becomes part of the personnel record.
3. Unsatisfactory behavior is communicated in writing, along with recommendations and assistance for correcting deficiencies. A specific time period must be given for correcting unsatisfactory behavior.
4. Policies should be developed explaining any behaviors that can cause immediate dismissal, i.e., incompetency, gross insubordination, willful neglect of duty, or misconduct while on duty.
5. Any *unsatisfactory* ratings on the performance evaluation must be preceded by due process, progressive discipline, and failure of the employee to correct unsatisfactory behavior.
6. Any disciplinary action or dismissal must be for just cause, and will be overruled through grievance proceedings if management fails to follow established policies and procedures.
7. Employees can appeal disciplinary decisions. Decisions may be overruled and provide employees with additional training and assistance to correct deficiencies. Appeals hearing must be held within two weeks of a written notice.[14]

Progressive discipline procedures can lead to employee dismissal from the organization. The nurse-administrator must understand the importance of ensuring employees' rights and protecting employees from wrongful discharge. The following text will discuss the concept of "termination at will" and measures to prevent wrongful discharge and frequent financial losses resulting from lengthy litigation.

TERMINATION AT WILL

Kingsley[11] states that the concept of termination at will was established through the courts in 1884. This legalized the employer's right to fire an employee for any reason or without a reason, and for an employee to comply or quit. The Wagner Act of 1935 limited termination at will by barring employers from firing personnel due to membership in unions or participating in union activities; dismissal must be for just cause. Protection from termination at will increased with the passage of other legislation. The Civil Rights Act of 1964 barred discimination in employment practices (including discipline and dismissal) based upon sex, age, national origin, race, or religion. The Rehabilitation Act of 1973 protects nonunionized handicapped or disabled employees from discrimination.

Employees in the above classes may file suit against employers, stating they were terminated for discriminatory purposes. Employers must maintain documentation of just cause and progressive discipline, and show evidence of due process.[11]

Joiner[15] discusses the erosion of the termination-at-will doctrine, and states that more and more employees are filing suits for wrongful discharge. There is an increasing concern for worker job protection and right to a fair process. The right to terminate at will is restricted in many states by state laws and court decisions. Although these restrictions vary from state to state, the following are some examples:

1. Protection of employees from discharge due to filing for workers' compensation claims, refusing to commit perjury, serving jury duty, and reporting harmful or unethical employer practices (whistle-blowing).
2. Protection of employees from discharge due to an oral promise of good faith, or an implied contract. A personnel policy stating "discharge for just cause" or an oral promise of job security made by a supervisor or recruiter serves as a binding contract and would require just cause for termination. Even a continued length of service can be justification to have just cause prior to termination.
3. Protection of employees against termination for reasons contrary to public policies. This includes engaging in activities discussed in (1) above, and refusing to engage in sexual acts, refusing to engage in price-fixing, and serving in the military.

Joiner further states that the consequences to employers from suits involve large monetary penalties, bad publicity, and even difficulty in recruiting and selecting new employees. The following identifies some ways to protect employees as well as to prevent litigation.

1. Ensure that all interviewers and management personnel are aware of the binding effect of oral promises regarding job security

2. Be aware of all personnel policies, and apply them uniformly
3. Provide progressive discipline and in-house grievance procedures
4. Ensure current and thorough job descriptions and fair and accurate performance evaluations[15]
5. Establish specific policies describing the consequences of violating job descriptions and work rules. Have employees sign these policies
6. Ensure that employment applications, personnel manuals, and posted notices and communications spell out what you want them to say and are practiced
7. When disciplining, always deal with the worst "offenders" first
8. Have the employee present his or her "side" in front of a witness and in writing, and investigate the employee's story prior to action
9. Be consistent with all discipline
10. Pretend you are an impartial jury when examining the case[16]
11. Consider having all terminations reviewed by a person or committee, offering severance pay for a release from future claims; provide exit interviews and outplacement counseling. A committee can be formed to review all facts and evidence prior to disciplinary proceedings or discharge. This committee can include legal advisors and other consultants to review the fairness, just cause, and due process of the proceedings. It could also act as a "jury" to ensure appropriate documentation and justification of terminations

There is no absolute defense against suits, and employers should accept current trends and plan ways to improve employee relations. Sound personnel practices, increased job security, and participation by personnel will help to reduce negative attitudes and improve productivity.[15]

GRIEVANCE PROCEDURES

Many organizations are implementing grievance procedures to improve employee satisfaction, productivity, and help in deterring unionization. As termination at will is being eroded, and employees' knowledge and expectations concerning their protection, equal opportunities, and rights are greater, organizations must take steps to change with the times.[17]

O'Brien and Drost[18] state that most employees join unions due to job dissatisfaction. The first-line manager has the greatest effect on this dissatisfaction. Many employees cannot find other work and need to keep working, so stay in their positions but exhibit poor attitudes and performance. They think nothing will help and have little interaction with members of the administrative team other than their first-line manager. Due to this isolation, they think they will receive the same treatment if they approach managers higher up on the hierarchy. A formal or established means for communicating and working out grievances will serve as one means to overcome this problem.

According to Balfour,[17] there are five types of grievance procedures that can be implemented, each with various pros and cons. By implementing one or a variation of the procedures, an avenue for communicating dissatisfaction is created, along with a system of "justice" for the employee. The following presents a summary of each type of grievance procedure described by Balfour.

Open Door Policy

This exists when an employee is able to approach the supervisor with a complaint at any time. The employee has the freedom to walk into the supervisor's office and discuss a problem or voice dissatisfaction. This can be quite effective if the supervisor will listen objectively and follow through. It will be ineffective if the manager thinks he or she is being fair but, in reality, views the employee's complaints as unjustified and fails to listen or take action. This is not good management. It also is ineffective for the employee who has difficulty expressing himself or herself, and cannot exert influence.

Ombudsman

This is the use of a mediator who can listen to employee disputes and complaints and act as an advocate. This person must be highly respected, an expert in the field, and possess excellent communication and interpersonal skills. Employees can go to the mediator, who will be interested, concerned, and assist in finding a remedy for legitimate grievances. The mediator often negotiates a settlement resulting in a "win–win" situation.[17]

Step Procedures

This is a series of steps to resolve conflict where a complaint is heard at the next higher step if it is not resolved. There are several ways to implement a step procedure. The grievance procedure described in Chapter 9 concerning performance evaluation disputes is one example of the traditional step procedure (see section on the appeals process). If top management cannot resolve the problem to the employee's satisfaction, a grievance committee may hear the case and make a decision. This committee could consist of peers and managers and serve as a jury, determining the verdict either by majority vote or unanimity. (Also see Chapter 9, section on appeal or grievance board.) Grievance committee members are usually impartial, objective, and attempt to be open minded. But Balfour[17] recommends that labor relations decisions be made by experts in personnel administration.

In some cases, the employee may take a grievance to another final authority, as spelled out in their procedures. The final authority could be an outside arbitrator, in-house hearing office, or objective expert. This decision would be final.

Hearing Officers

A hearing officer can be an employee who is paid by the organization to mediate between management and employees on a full-time basis. This person must be perceived as honest, fair, and an expert in labor relations. The hearing officer is presented with the grievance and makes the final decision. The employee is not assisted in presenting his or her case. Unfortunately, the loser in the decision (management or employee) often resents this system as well as the officer.

Outside Arbitration

This is where the employer and employees both pay an arbitrator's fee, who, as an outsider, determines a decision. In unionized organizations the cost is spread among all members. In nonunionized settings the cost is set for each individual case, and can be too expensive for some employees.

Balfour[17] states that for the nonunionized setting, the ombudsman procedure seems to be the most effective system, in that employees and management must be involved in working out their differences. The mediator assists in the negotiations. A step procedure can create a win–lose decision versus a mutual decision or compromise between parties. The employee may also need an advocate's assistance through the proceedings and in presenting his or her case. In order to be effective, a step procedure must resolve the problem at the lowest possible level, where those most involved and concerned with the issues work on the resolution.

Whichever procedure is chosen, it must be communicated and accepted by all, and be applied consistently. It must be easy to use and protect against retaliation. It must also be a speedy process that results in decisions based upon merit. Employees must believe that the system will result in fair and accurate outcomes.

CONCLUSION

Counseling and coaching is a process that helps employees to understand their problems and improve performance. It provides a humanistic means to resolve work-related issues while being sensitive to employee well-being. It can improve productivity and job satisfaction. Through mutual exchange, sharing, advice, and guidance, an employee can be assisted in fulfilling potential and performing up to his or her abilities.

For the marginal or unsatisfactory performer, the process is a means for "ownership" of the behaviors—taking responsibility and improving behavior. Employees are given a choice and all the help and guidance they need to improve. If they refuse help and will not take responsibility for their actions, progressive discipline is instituted. Although the intent continues to be for improvement and assistance by management, the steps are in place to dismiss the employee who is unwilling to be a part of the organization. Counseling and coaching is carried through to dismissal, where employees are helped through the termination process and coached in finding new employment. When all efforts at maintaining employment have been exhausted, the employee is counseled and coached in future career decisions and alternatives.

The human resource is the most important element in the success of the organization. But one unhappy and dissatisfied human being can affect all others. Therefore, management must take steps to counsel and coach dissatisfied employees, and correct problems and frustrations. But an unsatisfactory or unfit employee cannot be allowed to remain in the organization, or all personnel processes will be affected and the good, productive employees will suffer. Mechanisms must be established to correct unsatisfactory behavior. Counseling and coaching is one such mechanism.

The nurse-administrator is concerned about correcting problem behaviors and managing the underachiever, but also wants to improve the total performance of the nursing staff. In addition to counseling and coaching, other steps can be taken to improve this performance and productivity. Morale, job satisfaction, reward systems, and a number of other factors are related to employee performance and behaviors. These factors can be assessed, organized, and implemented through the process of retention and productivity to enhance and maximize employee performance. Performance evaluation and counseling and coaching are continuous with the process of retention and productivity. This process is another step toward effective human resource management, and is the subject of our next chapter.

REFERENCES

1. Roseman, E. *Managing the problem employee.* New York: AMACOM, American Management Association, 1982, pp. 12–40.
2. Holoviak, S. J., & Holoviak, S. B. The benefits of in-house counseling. *Personnel,* 1984, *61*(4), 53–58.
3. Scully, R. Staff support groups: Helping nurses to help themselves. *JONA,* 1981, *11*(3), 48–51.
4. Arndt, C., & Huckaby, L. D. *Nursing administration: Theory for practice with a systems approach* (2nd ed.). St. Louis: Mosby, 1980, pp. 197–201.
5. Kepler, T. L. Mastering the people skills. *JONA,* 1980, *10*(11), 15–20.
6. Hatfield, B. P. Re-positioning the mal-adjusted employee. *Hospital Topics,* July/August 1981, p. 19.

7. Murphy, E. C. Discipline: Who owns the responsibility? *Nursing Management*, 1983, *14*(7), 59.
8. Glicken, M. D., & Janka, K. Beyond burnout: The cop-out syndrome. *Personnel*, 1984, *61*(6), 65–70.
9. Lachman, V. D. Increasing productivity through performance evaluation. *JONA*, 1984, *14*(12), 7–13.
10. Jobes, M. Maryvale Samaritan Hospital's personnel policy manual. Phoenix, Ariz: Maryvale Samaritan Hospital, 1984.
11. Kingsley, D. T. *How to fire an employee*. New York: Facts on File Publications, 1984, pp. 90, 106, 120–130.
12. Kangery, R. Outplacement service for the nurse executive. *JONA*, 1984, *14*(7&8), 11–15.
13. Kjervik, D. K. Progressive discipline in nursing: Arbitrator's decisions. *JONA*, 1984, *14*(4), 34–37.
14. Bolden, J. H. *Legal aspects of employee evaluation in Florida school districts. Instructional Module I.* Tallahassee, Florida: Department of Educational Leadership, F.S.U., 1983, pp. 1–16.
15. Joiner, E. A. Erosion of the employment-at-will doctrine. *Personnel*, 1984, *61*(5), 12–18.
16. Panken, P. M. How to keep a firing from backfiring. *Nation's Business*, June 1983, pp. 74, 75.
17. Balfour, A. Five types of non-union grievance systems. *Personnel*, 1984, *61*(2), 67–75.
18. O'Brien, F. P., & Drost, D. A. Non-union grievance procedures: Not just an anti-union strategy. *Personnel*, 1984, *61*(5), 61–62, 66.

SUGGESTED READING

Baer, W. E. *Discipline and discharge under the labor agreement*. New York: American Management Association, 1972.

Barnes, G. Wrongful dismissal: An expensive mistake. *Dimensions in Health Service*, 1982, *59*(9), 10–15.

Bray, K. A. Effective disciplinary action . . . essential to the success of any nurse manager. *Critical Care Nurse*, 1982, *2*(6), 10.

Carone, P. A., Kieffer, S. N., Krinsky, L. W., & Yolles, S. F. (Eds.). *Misfits in industry*. New York: SP Medical and Scientific Books, 1978.

Carr, A. Labour relations and discipline . . . what makes a good manager. *Nursing Mirror*, 1982, *155*(22), 39–40.

Combe, J. D. Peer review: The emerging successful application. *Employee Relations Law Journal*, 1984, *7*(4), 659–671.

D'Aprix, R. Organizational communication. *Hospital Forum*, 1983, *26*(3), 24–33.

Deegan, A. X. *Coaching: A management skill for improving individual performance*. Reading, Mass: Addison-Wesley, 1979.

Felin, A. G. The risks of blowing the whistle. *AJN*, 1983, *83*(10), 1387–1390.

Finkle, A. L. Can a manager discipline a public employee? *Review of Public Personnel Administration*, 1984, *4*(3), 83–87.

Fischer, F. H., & Rapport, S. Discharge for contractual "just cause." In *Employee termination handbook: Legal and psychological guidelines for employees.* Englewood Cliffs, New Jersey: Executive Enterprises, Prentice-Hall, 1981.

Fournies, F. *Coaching for improved work performance.* New York: Van Nostrand, 1978.

Fox, A. C. Progressive discipline: Policy and process. In *Employee termination handbook: legal and psychological guidelines for employees.* Englewood Cliffs, New Jersey: Executive Enterprises, Prentice-Hall, 1981, p. 157.

Frayne, C. A., & Hunsaker, P. L. Strategies for successful interpersonal negotiating. *Personnel,* 1984, *61*(3), 70–76.

Garcia, L. A. A guide to progressive disciplinary measures. *Medical Laboratory Observer,* 1983, *15*(9), 93–96.

Gordon, M. E., & Miller, S. J. Grievances: A review of research and practice. *Personnel Psychology,* 1984, *37*(1), pp. 117–140.

Harney, E. L. Discipline without punishment. *AORN J,* 1983, *37*(5), 914–920.

Heshizer, B. An MBO approach to discipline. *Supervisory Management,* 1984, *29*(3), 2–8.

Horty, J. F. Truth's a strong weapon in firing workers. *Modern Health Care,* 1983, *13*(1), 136.

Kabb, G. M. Chemical dependency: Helping your staff. *JONA,* 1984, *14*(11), 18–23.

Kruchko, J. G., & Dube, L. E. A new right for non-union workers. *Personnel,* 1983, *60*(6), 59–64.

Kuzmits, F. E. Is your organization ready for no-fault absenteeism? *Personnel Administration,* 1984, *29*(12), 119–127.

Levenstein, A. Maintaining discipline. *Nursing Management,* 1982, *13*(12), 35–37.

LoBosco, M. Nonunion grievance procedures. *Personnel,* 1985, *62*(1), 61–64.

Mager, R., & Pipe, P. *Analyzing performance problems.* Belmont, Calif.: Pitman Learning, 1970.

Marriner, A. Discipline of personnel. *Supervisor Nurse,* 1976, *7*(11), 15–17.

Metzger, N. The supervisor's role in the disciplinary and grievance procedure. *Health Care Supervisor,* 1983, *2*(1), 77–86.

Meyer, A. L. A framework for assessing performance problems. *JONA,* 1984, *14*(5), 40–43.

Moore, J. F. A supervisory challenge: The difficult employee. *Health Care Supervisor,* 1983, *1*(3), 12–16.

Morin, W. J., & Yorks, L. *Outplacement techniques: A positive approach to terminating employees.* New York: AMACOM, 1982.

Murphy, E. C. The bookends of management: Hiring and firing. *Nursing Management,* 1983, *14*(12), 21–24.

Pulich, M. A. Train first-line supervisors to handle discipline. *Personnel Journal,* 1983, *62*(12), 980.

Regan Report on Nursing Law, Nursing misconduct: Illegal drug possession . . . The position that a board of nursing or hospital should take. 1983, *24*(2), 2.

Regan Report on Nursing Law. Termination of employment: Employer's rights: Maus vs. National Living Centers. 1982, *23*(7), 2.

Steinmetz, L. L. *Managing the marginal and unsatisfactory performer.* Reading, Mass.: Addison-Wesley, 1969.

Stevens, B. Performance appraisal: What the nurse executive expects from it. *JONA,* 1976, *6*(10), 26–31.

Stillman, S. M., & Strasser, B. L. Helping critical care nurses with work-related stress. *JONA*, 1980, *10*(1), 28–31.

Tidwell, G. L. Employment at will: Limitations in the public sector. *Public Personnel Management Journal*, 1984, *13*(3), 293–303.

U.S. Department of Labor. *A working woman's guide to her job rights.* Washington, D.C.: U.S. Government Printing Office, Superintendent of Documents, 1984.

Wahn, E. V. Off-duty employee misconduct: How should it be handled. *Dimensions in Health Services*, 1983, *60*(1), 31–32.

Walton, F. Employment law . . . appeal hearing saved the day. *Health and Social Service Journal*, 1983, *93*(4845), 541–542.

Walton, F. Employment law . . . getting the contract right. *Health and Social Service Journal*, 1983, *93*(4829), 534.

Walton, F. Employment law . . . termination of employment. *Health and Social Service Journal*, 1982, *92*(4811), 1028–1029.

Whitis, R., & Whitis, G. The exit interview: A nursing management tool. *JONA*, 1983, *13*(10), 13–16.

11 The Process of Retention and Productivity

Everyone is well aware of the need for a productive work force in these times of economic constraint. The focus is on *retaining productive people;* that is, to retain employees who will achieve organizational goals in the most efficient means possible. *Retention* means maintaining the steady work force, or decreasing turnover. *Productivity* means obtaining the desired results, with no waste of time, energy, or resources, at the lowest possible costs. Because turnover increases costs and decreases efficiency, it can greatly reduce productivity. Retention is the best recruitment tool, and reduces costs of orientation, exit interviews, and other administrative costs involved with turnover. Certainly these cost savings contribute to a more productive nursing service—no waste of time, energy, or resources at the lowest possible cost. But retention alone is not enough. The staff must be productive. While retaining personnel does save money and energy, these people must be *motivated to do the work.* They must have motivations congruent with organizational goals and purposes. They must obtain the desired results.

Retention and productivity are *mutually dependent.* One cannot be approached without considering the other, and the effectiveness of one depends upon the effectiveness of the other. Productivity cannot be obtained without first reducing turnover and retaining employees. If there is continual turnover, not only are costs high to prepare these new employees for their roles, but there is a low degree of commitment to organizational goals. It takes time to socialize individuals into a new culture and create a sense of belonging. Once these feelings are nurtured, individuals can begin developing commitment and striving to achieve organizational goals. In the proper environment, they can develop personal gratification along with the desire to be part of a team. This process is slow, and cannot possibly take place in a setting of constant turnover. In such a setting, cultures cannot take root and motivations cannot become congruent. Turnover must be held in check before efforts to build a productive work force can be successful.

Conversely, a productive work force can reduce turnover. A work force that is applying its efforts efficiently and accomplishing goals is more likely to retain its employees. When employees feel useful, successful in their work, and part of a team, they are more apt to remain in the organization. Many of the conditions necessary for building productivity also satisfy human needs and perceptions affecting the desire to stay with the organization. Productivity enhances teamwork and commitment, and plays an important role in retaining employees.

This chapter will explore the various components and factors affecting the process of retention and productivity. A model for effective retention and productivity will demonstrate the interactions and integration of components involved in successful outcomes. It should be noted that the content in this chapter is based on and applies many theories of motivation, but does not provide an exploratory review of these theories. It is important for the reader to review theories on human behavior, motivation, productivity, and organizational behaviors in conjunction with this content. The Suggested Reading listing at the end of the chapter provides a guide for further study. Also, this chapter focuses on the *human side of productivity*. Analysis of productivity through work flow studies, nursing costs per patient, efficiency studies, staffing reports, and other statistical means are critical to evaluate and improve productivity in the organization. The "numbers" are necessary to simplify, coordinate, evaluate, and quantify, and should be studied, explored, and applied in conjunction with the material in this chapter. It would require several volumes to cover all aspects of retention and productivity. Because it is the people who do the work, this chapter will examine the human side of productivity. Attention should be given to cost reductions and quantifying efficiency and effectiveness, but emphasis should be on improvement of the human resources. A competent, committed, and energetic team is the best mechanism for achieving retention and productivity. Factors such as morale, job satisfaction, and motivation will in the long run determine the results.

A MODEL FOR RETENTION AND PRODUCTIVITY

The essential interaction for achieving retention and productivity can be shown as

$$\text{Job satisfaction} \; \underset{\leftarrow}{\overset{\rightarrow}{+}} \; \begin{matrix}\text{Motivation} \\ \text{congruence}\end{matrix} = \text{Retention and productivity}$$

Job satisfaction alone cannot result in productivity. The appropriate amount of tension or stimulus must exist to elicit a productive outlay of energy. This outlay of energy must be *congruent* for personal as well as organizational purposes (that is, "motivation congruence"). All employees are motivated in some manner, so the existence of motivation alone is not enough. Motivations must be to fulfill individual, group, and organizational needs, and to achieve a unified goal. Although separated for clarification and discussion, many of the components of job satisfaction also affect motivation congruence, and vice versa.

JOB SATISFACTION

Satisfaction is the state of having needs fulfilled, being free of uncertainty, being content, and receiving what is due. Job satisfaction is the state of having needs fulfilled, being secure and content, and receiving what is due from one's work. It concerns the individual's feelings, perceptions, and attitude about the quality of work life.

Job satisfaction does not ensure productivity, but it is one of the determinants of productivity. First, it is directly related to retention. Dissatisfaction with work is a key factor in absenteeism and turnover. A satisfied worker is more likely to remain in the organization. If job satisfaction is directly related to retention, and retention and productivity are mutually dependent, then job satisfaction is also related to productivity. Second, job satisfaction is a prerequisite condition to productivity. An employee cannot maintain a high level of energy output and seek high-level achievement without first having certain needs met. As in Maslow's hierarchy of needs, job satisfaction—security, perception of equity and receiving one's due, and feelings of trust, belonging, and competency—must be obtained *before* one can become productive and maintain that productiveness. Meeting these needs for job satisfaction will not in itself ensure productivity, but is the essential first step. Because a dissatisfied worker will use energies to seek satisfaction concerning fair pay, congenial work groups, and equitable treatment, etc., the need for job satisfaction must be met before motivation congruence can be attained.

The following text describes the components of job satisfaction. These include: environmental change, personal needs and expectations, the work environment, perceptions, groups, and competency. It must be noted that there is a close interrelationship between the components of motivation congruence and the components of job satisfaction. For many individuals, feeling satisfied with one's work also includes possessing shared values, receiving significant rewards, and maintaining open communications and a feeling of control. For our purposes, job satisfaction will include the main conditions and elements affecting satisfaction and setting the stage for motivation congruence.

Environmental Change

Job satisfaction is directly affected by environmental change. Environmental change must be assessed and predicted in order to set the stage for job satisfaction; therefore, it is listed as a separate component. Some of the changes affecting workers, the work, and the work environment will be mentioned here.

Various changes affect the worker. Nurses, who are predominantly female, have more career options; are staying in the work force longer, delaying marriage and family; are more aware of their rights; and are more politically active. As a whole they have become more assertive and seek job satisfaction, professional respect, and control over their practice. Change has also affected work in many ways, especially in terms of decreasing length of stay and costs. With the aging population, increased acuity, and high technology, nurses' work is more demanding and complex. Discharge planning, prevention of complications, outpatient care, and group educational classes have become more important, as have self-care units and family participation. Knowledge of geriatrics, computers, and time management is now essential in many work areas. Organizations must provide the right structures, support, and resources for the changing work, and the workers must obtain needed skills and knowledge to reach competency and achieve job satisfaction. In addition, the worker must adapt attitudes, values, and expectations concerning the changing nature of work in order to be secure and satisfied with this work.

Change affects the work environment in additional ways. The heavy emphasis on cost control versus human needs and development can lead to dissatisfaction, poor morale, and lower productivity. Turnover of top administrative teams creates uncertainty and insecurity in employees. Animosity among physicians over increased competition and erosion of control can lead to adverse physician–nurse relationships and a nonproductive work environment. Lack of communication, secrecy, and an increased workload for nurses can lead to job dissatisfaction. Management must be constantly attuned to the effects of change on workers, the work, and the work environment, and take steps to foster and maintain job satisfaction. This will require an ongoing and changing effort.

Personal Needs and Expectations

Understanding the needs, values, drives, attitudes, and expectations of employees is necessary for satisfying those needs. What does a new employee expect from the organization? This should be determined during recruitment and selection to ensure that expectations are realistic and can be met. What are the needs that drive and motivate employees? Similarities and patterns can be identified through surveys, exit interviews, one-to-one communication, and during performance evaluation interviews. Nurses of similar backgrounds and upbringing, educational preparation, age group, and geographic location often have some common expectations. Values, attitudes, and motivations of employees often become more similar through close working interaction over a period of time. This evolving "culture" communicates its needs and attitudes by its response to change, concern with certain issues and problems, and behavior with patients, physicians, and administration. Careful listening will pick up their interests, concerns, and needs. Because people often cannot identify what it is they really want, observation and listening is important. Understanding inner needs, values, and expectations is not always easy, so management must develop an intuition toward its workforce along with an understanding of human nature. This, along with listening, observing, *and* the use of interviews and surveys, will reveal the needs and expectations that must be satisfied. This assessment must be ongoing.

There is a certain order and consistency to human behavior, and management must always keep this in mind. The need for dignity and respect, trust, and a sense of belonging remain consistent. The need to control or have influence over decisions affecting work, a feeling of value about one's work, and the need for a supportive, congenial atmosphere continue to exist over time. The need for fair treatment, two-way communications, job security, just wages, and benefits (in comparison to other facilities and comparable work in other fields) appears to remain consistent. By staying closely in touch with employees and showing concern, caring, and respect, management can not only identify employee needs and concerns, but also find the means to satisfy these needs. Close interaction and communication can set the stage so that management and employees can find solutions together. This, in itself, is a satisfying experience.

Work Environment

When needs, values, drives, and expectations are identified, the appropriate work environment to foster job satisfaction must be provided. It is obvious that management cannot meet every need of every employee. But *conditions* can be provided in the work environment to allow freedom to pursue individual goals and creative needs. Support and counseling can be provided for employees with problems or unrealistic expectations. And the organization must respond to issues of concern to employees by clarifying or perhaps changing the work environment or management practices. The work environment must be one that responds as needed to enhance job satisfaction. Here are listed some examples of what is included in the work environment:

1. Organizational structure—centralized, participative, autonomous
2. Job design

3. Physician–nurse relations
4. Workload and staffing
5. Scheduling system
6. Support services
7. Interdepartmental relations
8. Job content
9. Job assignment methodology
10. Job roles and responsibilities
11. Available consultants, specialists, and resources
12. Interpersonal relations and employee relations with management
13. Support and training for adjusting to new roles and responsibilities
14. Involvement, influence, and control over own work and unit activities
15. Valuing of employees' worth and role in organizational success (evidenced by seeking their opinions, suggestions, and inclusion in decision making, as well as using their ideas)
16. Types of communication, such as open, two-way, and informal versus downward and formal
17. Mutual trust and respect between employees and management
18. Assistance to employees for problem solving and conflict resolution
19. Adequate supplies and equipment

While there are certainly other factors included in the work environment, those listed here can be instrumental in affecting job satisfaction. The type of work environment, such as self-scheduling, participative management, collaborative practice, and primary versus functional or team nursing would depend on the needs, values, and expectations of employees *and* the organizational goals and values. Most often the organizational goals can be met by meeting many employee needs. An organization can still accomplish quality patient care (according to its standards) and improve its image in the community by meeting the employee need for involvement and more control of a unit's activities. If these personal and organizational goals are merged, employees are more satisfied and more likely to be productive.

Perceptions

How an individual sees and comprehends the environment affects that individual's satisfaction with that environment. And how the individual takes in what is seen and heard affects his or her feelings, attitudes, and expectations. An employee's perceptions are determined by self-image, past experiences, assumptions about others, ability to understand, and willingness to see the truth.

Employees' self-image, or mental picture of themselves, can affect their needs and values. It can also affect how they interpret and understand their experiences. A person with a poor self-image and little self-confidence may perceive a busy manager as "being unfriendly" or "being upset or angry." Because of low self-image, this person may interpret events and others' behaviors in ways that will verify his or her self-image. Performance may also be poor, in keeping with the poor self-image. Due to lack of self-confidence, insecurities, and feelings of failure, an employee's highest need may be to feel accepted and liked by peers, or by management. This need to be accepted could be the person's chief motivator.

The confident employee with a positive self-image would also tend to interpret events to verify perception of self. A supervisor who "didn't speak to me" was simply busy and was thinking of other things. This employee's performance would be geared to reinforce the positive self-image. The employee may have high achievement needs or, if affiliation is needed, may be the group leader.

Managers must work not only to assess employees' self-image, but to improve this image. If the manager communicates trust and confidence in an employee's ability, the employee will begin to trust and have self-confidence. By feeling important, needed, trusted, and competent, an employee will work to live up to these feelings, or the positive self-image. The employee will begin to perceive the world in a more positive way, and respond according to these perceptions. Understanding and developing positive self-images is an important step in building a satisfied and confident nursing staff.

Perceptions are also affected by a person's past experience, assumptions about others, and the ability *and* willingness to see reality. Experiences in life can affect how one views the present and future. Dissatisfying experiences such as poor relationships, lack of achievement of career goals, unhappy family life, and others can cause a negative outlook and attitude. *Life dissatisfaction* or *satisfaction* greatly affects the ability to attain job satisfaction. If one perceives life with pessimism due to past experiences, then negative expectations will be attached to all experiences, including work. If a person expects poor interpersonal relationships, lack of appropriate rewards and recognition, etc., that person will perceive all interactions in that light and never be satisfied. Management must understand the relationship of life experience to job satisfaction. Working to build positive self-images will help, but counseling may be necessary. A person who is unable or unwilling to be satisfied can drain morale and cause dissatisfaction for other employees. Causes for dissatisfaction must be determined and steps taken to alleviate dissatisfiers. Occasionally individuals may have to be assisted in finding other work, due to their negative effect on other employees.

What one assumes about the self and others is a by-product of self-image and experiences. An employee may assume that a supervisor is "out to get me" and perceive the supervisor's remarks on the performance evaluation as overly critical and punitive. Employees' assumptions are often based upon what they are willing or want to believe and their ability to understand their surroundings. Due to negative feelings and expectations, they may unconsciously interpret events negatively, and assume the worst; they may receive unclear messages from administration, and so be unable to perceive these messages accurately. Therefore, they will assume reality to be different, due to misunderstanding.

Communication is a critical tool for correcting assumptions. Management must continually explain actions and provide rationale with all requests or delegation. Employees must not be allowed to *assume* the reasons behind actions; they must be given clear explanations. Managers must stay close to employees to understand their assumptions and clear up misunderstandings. They must use words that are clear and appropriate for employees' educational levels, and see that they understand. Having employees restate instructions or explain rationale will verify that they understand. An environment of open communication, where employees can ask questions and freely discuss feelings and beliefs, will help correct faulty assumptions.

In addition, how management behaves affects assumptions. Stating that all employees are free to ask questions and voice concerns, but always being too busy to listen, communicates a different message. Stating that management cares about employee concerns while listening with arms folded tightly around chest and with a tense, unfriendly expression does not communicate the spoken message. Management's body language and actions affect employees' assumptions and perceptions. Positive verbal and nonverbal communications that consistently show respect, caring, trust, *and* willingness to listen and discuss concerns will help to correct faulty assumptions. Management must continually assess assumptions and seek to verify or correct them. Correcting faulty assumptions is probably one of the most time-consuming, but most critical, parts of a manager's work. Accurate assumptions about the organization can affect the degree of job satisfaction. Group meetings, open forums, one-on-one discussions, and open communication are essential to assess and correct assumptions.

An employee's perceptions of the organization and management will affect behavior at work. How the employee interprets the work environment determines how he or she views rewards, interactions, causes for performance problems, fairness of treatment, and work conditions. Perception of these conditions can determine satisfaction or dissatisfaction. Providing the proper environment is not enough; management must ensure that employees *perceive* this environment to be satisfying and rewarding.

Groups

A group is a collection of people for a common purpose. There are formal groups, which are a structure of the formal organization (such as a task force or quality circle), and informal groups. This section will concern the effect of informal groups on job satisfaction.

Informal groups are a key to job satisfaction. The influence and actions of these groups, like aspects of the work environment, greatly affect the quality of work life for individuals, as well as shaping behaviors and attitudes of the group members.

What are informal groups, and why are they formed? An informal group is a collection of people who have something in common. They are not officially recognized by the administration; that is, they are not on the organizational chart or part of formal plans. But over a period of time these group members gain strength through mutual support and sharing, and influence the work environment of the organization. Informal group members interact with one another, form relationships, and share common goals.

Why are groups formed? It is a natural phenomenon for people to form groups. Family structures, a collection of friends, neighborhood gatherings, church meetings, social clubs—all involve group activities. People tend to flock to others with similar interests, attitudes, or values.

Informal groups are also formed when people interact over a period of time. This interaction tends to result in sharing of experiences, interdependence, and similar interests. Informal groups are commonly found within departments and shifts, due to close proximity and interactions.

People join groups for various purposes. Due to their personal needs and self-image, they may have a strong need to belong. Others with strong needs for achievement and recognition may join groups to gain status and informal power. With growing uncertainty and economic pressures in organizations, employees will turn to their informal groups for the security and sense of belonging they cannot find in the formal system. This feeling of safety in numbers, sharing of troubles and concerns, can make work easier to tolerate. Participating in informal groups can also provide a feeling of control that may be eroding in the formal structure. Informal groups can offer friendship, support, and belonging. When human relations are poor and communication is closed, informal groups can become a source of strength to employees, and grow to be a powerful force in the organization.

Even under optimum manager–employee relations, informal groups exist and exert control over the organization. This control is due to the numbers of people with shared concerns, and the influence the group has over its members. Over time, groups form their own culture, with values, attitudes, and expectations. They behave in ways to fulfill these needs and expectations. They develop unwritten rules of behavior for group members. They even develop a self-image, assumptions, and perceptions about work and the organization.

For example, many nurse-administrators are familiar with the informal group of "old-timers." This group of nurses usually began working with the organization many years ago and have strong ties with one another, as well as with certain department heads and perhaps physicians. They have lunch and breaks together, and often have a "following" of group members who are impressed with their power, inside knowledge, or status. An informal group leader usually emerges. Although this informal group can be supportive and helpful to management, members may also try to preserve the "good old days" by resisting change and maintaining a negative attitude toward the "new" administration. They may exert pressure on group members to conform by positive or negative reinforcement. A member who verbally approves of an administrative plan or action may be ridiculed, ignored, or even ostracized from the group. A member who openly opposes management may be congratulated and given some special "inside" information. In some cases this group perceives all management personnel as untrustworthy and "out to get them." They assume that seniority does not matter, nor does loyalty, and so work to undermine those in authority.

Such a group obviously works against the organization. Its members may risk management's disapproval to remain in the group. The degree of conformity will depend on the need for acceptance and approval by group members, as well as fear of group retaliation. Retaliation can vary from rejection from the group, gossiping about the ex-member, and withholding information and assistance during work, to open hostility.

Not all groups are detrimental to the organization. Some serve more of a social purpose—to make work more fun. Others are motivated for clinical competency and work together to solve patient problems and improve group members' skills. But the groups do become cohesive, and tend to perceive the organization according to *how it affects their group.* A group strives to continue existing. Group behavior toward the organization is greatly affected by management's attitude toward the group and the work environment. Informal groups tend to work with the organization when

1. The groups are recognized as contributing to the organization and are consulted on work-related matters
2. The groups are allowed to interact and work together, with no attempts to "break them up"
3. The groups are involved in planning and implementing change, and when allowed to participate, take a personal interest in the outcome
4. The groups are asked to assist in clearing up misunderstandings or problems and to provide input regarding employee concerns and needs
5. The management practices consistently show caring, concern, respect, and trust

Informal groups can greatly affect job satisfaction. By influencing conformity, they shape individual perceptions and behaviors, altering the requirements for need fulfillment and the conditions under which they can be satisfied. Control over attitudes and values affects members' ability and willingness to be satisfied with their work.

Group behaviors and interactions with other groups or with management also affect the work environment. Disharmony, conflicts, and hostility create an unhappy environment and dissatisfying work life. In addition, the treatment of an individual by a group can affect job satisfaction. A person may experience conflict between role and group conformity, feel frustrated when not accepted into a group, or be ostracized if group rules of conduct are broken. This treatment can cause job dissatisfaction.

Conversely, groups can create a happy, congenial, and friendly work environment. They can provide strong interpersonal relationships and support and promote positive self-images and attitudes. This type of environment promotes retention and job satisfaction.

Management must identify informal groups and their leaders, and assess their needs, values, expectations, and perceptions. New employees can be assigned to work areas with "appropriate" group members who can contribute to their socialization into the organization. By understanding group characteristics, management can predict the effect of certain actions on the group, and strive to integrate group needs with organizational needs. Steps can be taken to use the creative talents and skills of groups, and allow them some control over their work. When informal groups see that they are not threatened and that management values their contribution to quality service, a more satisfying and cooperative environment begins to develop.

Competency

Job satisfaction is directly affected by an individual's *perceived and actual competency.* The sense of being competent in one's work is essential to being satisfied with that work. The actual ability to skillfully implement a role and responsibility creates a satisfying work environment for others as well as successful results from effort by the individual.

Competency is the state of being appropriately qualified, able, and fit, as well as having the capacity to achieve a goal. Human beings must *feel* competent in their work or they will experience role stress, feelings of inadequacy, insecurity, frustration, and dissatisfaction. In addition, environmental change creates new tensions and the need to continually adapt to retain, improve or alter competencies. A perception of competence is necessary for a positive self-image and perceptions of self and the organization, and to satisfy basic human needs for belonging, security, and self-respect. An individual must feel competent before responding to higher expectations and incentives in the environment.

Actual competency must be achieved in order to meet minimum job expectations and properly implement that job. Without this, an atmosphere of errors, inadequacies, ineffectiveness, and inefficiencies will develop. Competent and satisfied workers will become frustrated and overburdened, draining morale and decreasing productivity. In addition, an incompetent worker will fail to achieve expectations, goals, or results from efforts. Inability to "succeed" leads to dissatisfaction.

The individual with a perception of competence is more satisfied and therefore contributes to a satisfying work environment for others. An individual who is qualified and able to function in his or her role contributes to an effective and satisfying work environment for all employees.

Achievement of appropriate qualifications, skills, and knowledge for a role is a requirement for properly implementing that role. As minimum-level competency is achieved, new skills, knowledge, and goals can be achieved. Individuals will continually strive to achieve a higher level of competency, given the proper support, environment, and incentives. However in order to obtain higher level expectations and skills, the minimum expectations must first be achieved. Perceived and actual competency for role implementation is a prerequisite for successful growth and development.

Achieving perceived and actual competency is an ongoing process. Management must communicate attitudes and expectations of competency to the workforce. The attitude and belief that employees are competent will be transmitted over time, until employees internalize these attitudes and perceive themselves as competent. But, of course, this is not enough. They must be given the support, guidance, and resources to become competent and maintain competency. From recruitment, jobs must be analyzed along with cultural expectations, in order to match people with the appropriate work. Candidates must be recruited who have the skills and potential for meeting expectations. The best candidate for the job must be selected. Orientation processes must provide support and guidance for adjusting to new roles and the opportunity to learn needed skills and knowledge. The socialization into the organization should result in a cultural fit, interpersonal competence, and sense of mastery of required skills. The outcome of orientation should be minimum-level competency and the beginning of the ongoing growth and development process. The performance evaluation and coaching and counseling serve to maintain competency and guide continued growth and development. Staff development is ingrained in all growth and development processes, from orientation to counseling. Achievement and maintenance of competency is part of all personnel processes, is essential for a satisfying work environment, and is necessary for continued growth and development and achievement of motivation congruence.

Conclusion

Being secure and feeling that one is receiving what is due from one's work is job satisfaction. It is a very personal experience, and one that continually changes as attitudes, needs, perceptions, and the environment change. Achievement of job satisfaction depends upon personal needs and expectations, perceptions, the work environment, informal group activity and behavior, the effects of environmental change, and achieving competency. Each of these components of job satisfaction have been briefly explored.

Each of these components act together and affects attainment of job satisfaction. Properly balanced and managed, these components can be used to create a satisfied work force. This is an essential step to achieving motivation congruence, and eventually, retention and productivity.

MOTIVATION CONGRUENCE

Motivation congruence is the process of channeling individual and group motivations to achieve personal and organizational goals. This is dependent upon job satisfaction. Part of the manager's job in providing a satisfying work environment is to assess individual and group needs and expectations. By an understanding of these, employees' motivations can be understood. Employees' goals and motivations for need fulfillment are the basis for applying appropriate strategies and components for motivation congruence. So not only is job satisfaction necessary in order to attain motivation congruence, but understanding its components is required for using appropriate motivational strategies. In addition, the components for motivation congruence are interdependent. Psychic rewards must be used in combination with external incentives, opportunities to succeed, etc., in order to be effective. Each component interacts for overall success, and each component continually changes in response to employee and organizational change. The following section will discuss each component affecting motivation congruence. These include perception of control, peer pressure, opportunities to succeed, open communication, growth and development, psychic rewards, external incentives, and control of operations.

Perception of Control

While people's needs and expectations continually change, there seems to be a consistent, underlying need for "control" that remains steady. This need may vary in intensity and among individuals, but its existence continues. The need for control is qualified with the word "perception." This is because whether or not total control actually exists, it is the employee's own sense or feeling of control that matters. People need to feel that they can affect their environment in some way and can influence the outcome of success or failure. A feeling of control over one's own destiny is not only important for job satisfaction, but necessary for an innovative and productive organization. As a person gains confidence in his or her ability to affect decisions and operations concerning her work, that person will become more a part of those operations, and motivated to achieve their success. As individuals have more control over planning and implementing change, they begin to "own" the activities and become committed to achieving the goal. A growing perception of control over what happens on one's unit results in a perpetual cycle of productivity—more control, more ownership, more commitment, and more motivation to its success. As success is attained, with the proper rewards and incentives, improved self-image and self-confidence result in increased self-determination and continued motivation to achieve.

When a person feels that he or she can control what happens in the future, that person will take more of an interest in work activities. The person who understands that he or she is responsible for the outcome will be more motivated to achieve results. The appropriate amount of freedom, with support and guidance, provides the stimulus or "tension" to enhance motivation toward goals. A person who feels he or she has no control over what happens, or events never change despite continued efforts, will quit trying.

Management can provide freedom and allow control by staff over unit activities while still guiding the course of actions. For instance, organizational goals can be communicated and clarified; then the staff can be allowed freedom in attaining objectives that help meet organization goals. Management may approve a unit's objectives, but allow the staff to implement plans as they see fit. While a watchful eye over activities may exist, staff members are allowed to experiment and test activities and to make mistakes. In the long run, personal satisfaction and group goals will be met, along with organizational purposes.

The need for control varies among personnel and within facilities. Many employees may need only to control the outcome of their own actions and to feel they have some influence over their status in the organization (such as outcome of performance evaluation ratings, raises, promotions, or recognition). Others may have a great need to control unit activities and decisions. Whatever the priority or degree of need for control, employees must be taught that what they do *counts* and affects the overall success of the organization. They must be given appropriate amounts of control—depending on their past experiences, degree of self-confidence, and their abilities—until they begin to take ownership over their activities. Then, in time, the perpetual cycle is begun. They become self-determining and motivated toward success. As they gain small successes, improve their self-images, and control their work activities, they become more committed to the organization.

Employee control can vary from self-governance to self-scheduling. It can simply involve employee participation on planning committees or employee task forces for problem solving, recruitment, or selection of new employees. Quality circles can be implemented to allow employee participation and control over unit problems and improvement. Primary nursing may offer the type of control needed over clinical practice. The development of a career development program, with employee participation, can provide the direction and control for future progression in the organization.

There are many ways to provide employee freedom and control. The effectiveness of each will depend on the culture, experiences, and needs of the staff. Whatever strategy is employed, certain points should be kept in mind to enhance the perception of control.

1. Some degree of decentralization is necessary for employees to be motivated to the outcomes of their unit, and to begin to attain ownership over the results from their efforts.
2. Employees must understand the values, goals, and purpose of the organization so that they can attain an identity in the organization. When they understand what they are working toward, they can take some interest in the outcome.
3. Employees must be involved in setting standards, planning goals and objectives, and determining changes and activities that affect them. This involvement will facilitate their acceptance and motivation toward the success of these activities.
4. Employees must be given the information and support necessary for implementing control. When given the freedom to plan and implement an activity, or to control a unit's functioning, employees will fail unless prepared and supported for this new control. Background information, financial data, adequate time for meetings, space and material resources, and staff development for group dynamic, problem solving or communication skills, etc., may be required. Employees must be able to adapt to this new control and be equipped to handle it. They must be provided with the skills and knowledge they need to be able to succeed.
5. The boundaries of control must be clear and understood by all. Expectations and responsibilities must be communicated along with the degree of freedom in implementing those responsibilities. If nurses understand that they are free to "do what works" without interference, they can proceed with certainty. If management approval is required prior to employee actions, disapproval must be justified and accompanied by sound rationale. If employees are told they have control but not given the administrative support needed to implement ideas, they will perceive a lack of real control and fail to own their actions. The boundaries of actual control are understood by management's support of and response to employee effort. This becomes evident through verbal and nonverbal administrative behavior.

Peer Pressure

Peters and Waterman write that peer pressure is the greatest motivator of employees.[1] The pressure exerted within groups, from internal competition teams or from peer evaluation, can have a key effect on motivation congruence and productivity.

The influence of groups on their members was discussed earlier. Group leaders and members expect one another to conform to their norms and expectations, and often go to great lengths to ensure this conformity. Just as the informal group can affect the quality of work life and job satisfaction, it plays a role in productivity and motivation. When a group's motivations and values are consistent with organizational goals and values, productivity is greatly enhanced. Group members are influenced to conform to these values and are pressured to achieve organizational goals.

The congruence of group motivations with organizational goals is a difficult task to achieve and requires ongoing vigilance by administration. But when informal groups have something to gain, whether it be status, increased autonomy, or recognition, they will be more motivated to work with the organization. The use of strategies discussed in the earlier section on groups along with psychic rewards and external incentives for *group* behaviors and activities can result in motivation congruence. The manager must view groups as a whole and apply principles and strategies similar to those used with an individual. Groups require job satisfaction based on their needs, the work environment, changes, their perceptions, and a sense of competency, just as the individual requires job satisfaction to be productive. Groups respond to a perception of control, pressure, and competition from other groups, and all the other components required for motivation congruence. When working for retention and productivity, managers must apply strategies for both individuals *and* groups in order to achieve maximum success.

Internal competition is a powerful force for both individuals and groups. Competition for ideas, cost reductions, completion of projects, or decrease in absenteeism result in peer pressure to win. People want to be the best and, if given the opportunity, will exert pressure on group members to achieve goals. Dressler[2] states that the best way to motivate employees for organizational goals and to improve productivity is to use internal competition. He states that identifying the desired behavior, developing a graph displaying results on each unit, and verbally praising good performance will result in increased productivity. Employees on each unit can visualize their performance as compared to that of other shifts or units, and will be motivated to increase productivity so as to improve their position on the graph.

Internal competition is not effective for all endeavors or purposes, but can improve the cohesiveness of groups and increase the production of ideas and results. As groups tend to segregate themselves from the rest of the organization, combining groups and departments in competition is helpful for overcoming barriers. Although competition may be intense, communications are opened, interests are aroused, and pressure is applied to reach results. And everyone is working toward organizational purposes, creating a sense of purpose or mission for the total whole.

Pressure exerted through peer approval and evaluation is also a great motivator. When staff are involved in peer review of standards and patient outcomes, peer evaluation of formal group projects and activities, the results can be impressive. Individuals want the approval of their colleagues and will be motivated to attain this approval. Involvement of employees in assurance of quality and evaluation of objectives and planned change will enhance productivity. Just as group participation enhances motivation through the perception of control, it also contributes to motivation congruence by the effects of peer pressures.

Peer pressure often influences the nonproductive or unmotivated employee to improve performance. People compare their performance to that of those around them, so often will improve performance in order to keep up. A competent, motivated, and enthusiastic work force tends to create a type of internal competition for excellence. As mentioned earlier, success breeds success. In addition, groups will assist the slow or nonproductive employee to gain skills and knowledge needed for improvement—especially when competing with other groups. The unmotivated underachiever will usually be coerced by group tactics to conform. Peer pressure is a great motivator.

In addition, groups can be used as a motivational strategy. Forming quality circles or small task forces results in increased productivity. Group members share a common goal, work closely together to achieve that goal, and take ownership of the outcome. This creates enthusiasm, a sense of belonging, sharing, and participation. It also results in increased knowledge and understanding of the organization and others' roles and responsibilities. Using formal groups for specific activities enhances job satisfaction, motivation congruence, and retention and productivity.

Opportunities to Succeed

One of the essential elements in motivation congruence is the opportunity to succeed. Providing opportunities for success includes creating situations where employees can attain a sense of accomplishment, and providing the tools, guidance, and support for success.

Situations and structures can be developed that provide employees many avenues for success. A clinical ladder program should have clear criteria and expectations that must be met in order to advance. This is an explicit mechanism for accomplishing goals and attaining success in clinical areas. Criteria for achieving above average or outstanding ratings on performance evaluations provide opportunities to succeed. By clearly meeting the defined expectations and criteria, an employee can achieve an outstanding rating. Assisting employees in developing realistic self-objectives provides an opportunity to succeed. As discussed in Chapter 9, the manager guides these self-objectives in conjunction with organizational objectives, and ensures that they are attainable and realistic. Once employees have written directions for improvement, they can work toward that improvement and attain success. The accomplishment of self-objectives works to achieve organizational goals and a personal sense of accomplishment.

Bonus systems for ideas and innovative contributions set up avenues for success. If employees have good ideas, they are given a way to implement these ideas through these special systems. Bonus systems, as discussed in Chapter 9, provide an opportunity for reward, recognition, and involvement, while working for organizational goals. The development of projects and challenges to meet an organizational need creates an opportunity for success.

Team contests, interdepartmental competition, and task forces for problem solving also set up numerous avenues for attaining success. It is essential that administration offer a variety of situations where employees can have a chance to shine. Then rewards such as recognition, trophies, parties, awards, pictures in the lobby, free lunches, bonuses, paid days off, etc., should be developed to reinforce their efforts.

When opportunities for success are provided, they must be attainable, and the staff must have a chance of meeting the challenge. Unrealistic expectations are as good as no expectations, because the staff will perceive them as impossible to achieve. Standards should be high, but within reach and the staff must be provided staff development, resources, and coaching to enable them to achieve these standards. They must perceive that they can do it, and be helped along the way before they will exert energy towards a goal. By communicating confidence in their abilities, and providing counseling on ways to improve, management can help them to succeed. Support groups, special training programs, work with clinical specialists and preceptors, one-to-one counseling and coaching, all involve showing staff how they can attain their goals. Employees must obtain the skills, knowledge, and ability to accomplish goals before they can succeed. Then they must *see* the results of their efforts.

Everyone wants to feel good about themselves and their accomplishments. When they sense they are not only competent, but excel in some way, they are more motivated to continue the behaviors that brought them success. And success improves self-confidence and the desire to continue succeeding. Realistic opportunities for small successes must be available on an ongoing basis so that the feeling of accomplishment is ongoing. This contributes to retention and productivity.

Open Communication

The importance of open communication has been stressed throughout this book. Its role in motivation and productivity cannot be overemphasized. A communicative environment is necessary for job satisfaction, and essential for motivation congruence. An open, informal, and easy means for self-expression goes hand in hand with a healthy, enthusiastic workforce. An atmosphere of secrecy and "formal chain of command" creates an attitude of distrust. When administrators are visible, accessible, and easy to talk to, a close, working relationship can be developed between management and the staff.

An atmosphere of informality, with open-door policies, first-name basis, and relaxed and impromptu problem-solving meetings tends to improve communication. Staff need to know they can express their thoughts and opinions without being judged or punished. They need to know that they will be heard. Active listening is one of the essential parts of a manager's job. Fostering the freedom to speak *and* be heard demonstrates management's respect and valuing of employees' ideas and opinions. Providing open forums to discuss issues, holding regular unit meetings, and interacting informally on a daily basis all provide a means for communication.

Communication also includes informing employees about happenings in the organization, future plans, and any events that affect their work. Employees should not read about a new organizational project in the community's newspaper. They should be told *first*, and included in the planning of projects. If employees are included in planning and current news and information, they will feel a part of the organization and more committed to its goals.

Lastly, communication involves nonverbal expressions and follow-up actions. If managers avoid eye contact, constantly glance at their watches, leave in the middle of a discussion or allow constant phone calls and interruptions, they are not opening communication. If they become angry, impatient, or judgmental when listening to ideas or suggestions, they are not opening communication. If they always listen agreeably but never follow through or act upon suggestions, they are shutting off communication; the staff will realize that it is useless to express an idea or concern, because nothing will ever be done to remedy the situation or follow through. All problems cannot be solved, but management must take steps to use suggestions and implement ideas. They must show the concern to solve problems and work with the staff to overcome obstacles and clear up misconceptions. Active listening is often the solution to a problem, but reaching a decision and implementing the actions is also essential to continue communication. When employees know they will be heard and their ideas used, they will be motivated to continue contributing suggestions. They will feel they play a part in the organization's success, so will work to achieve its goals.

Growth and Development

The sense of continually renewing, learning, growing, and improving plays an important part in retention and productivity. The feeling of mastery of new skills, developing creative talents, fulfilling potentials, and actualizing new knowledge results in a sense of well-being and inner gratification. The feeling of mastery and inner gratification contributes to a positive self-image, self-confidence, and the motivation to seek continued improvement. Remaining stagnant in one's knowledge and skills only contributes to complacency, boredom, and lack of interest in work. Management must provide ongoing guidance and encouragement for continued growth and development. Beginning with orientation and through performance evaluation, coaching and counseling, and staff development, support and guidance must be provided for ways to improve. The organization must be committed to lifelong learning and provide opportunities, resources, and support for continued growth and development of its employees.

Growth and development play a big part in meeting personal needs for achievement, sense of competency, recognition, and self-respect. Employees who are stimulated to learn and improve will contribute to developing a progressive and innovative organization. As people gain new competencies and develop talents, they are more satisfied, motivated to achieve new goals, and contribute more to organizational success. Through role modeling and maintaining high expectations, management must make learning, growth, and development a part of everyday organizational life.

Psychic Rewards

All motivational strategies must be linked to incentives and rewards for continued motivation congruence. A person does not usually maintain high energies to achieve goals *only* for inner satisfaction. Although this plays a large part in motivation, it is not enough. By offering rewards that are significant to a person's needs and values, the appropriate amount of tension is created. This tension stimulates the motivation to meet needs—it serves as an incentive.

Psychic rewards are one type of incentive. Many of the components previously discussed do result in a sense of gratification, satisfaction, and achievement, and are psychic income. But when they are supplemented by the manager's praise and recognition, or *psychic reward,* motivation congruence is greatly enhanced.

Psychic income is feeling special, needed, successful, and knowing when a job was done well. It involves a sense of worth and gratification and is intensified when combined with psychic reward, or attention and recognition from others for good performance. Management can provide psychic rewards "free of charge." By praising good performance, giving attention and recognition to successful activities, and providing feedback, employees are motivated to continue the behaviors that have brought reward.

Managers often neglect psychic rewards because they appear too obvious and simple. But motivational strategies and incentive programs cannot be effective without also meeting the basic needs for approval, recognition, and knowing one is doing well. When employees receive psychic rewards from managers (and peers), they will feel successful and be motivated to continue this success. Psychic rewards also result in a good feeling by employees toward management and the organization.

One simple method for providing psychic rewards is through positive reinforcement. When good behavior or performance is observed, praise is given. Of course, employees cannot be praised every time they meet expectations or perform well, so the reinforcement should be random and intermittent. Employees will not know exactly when their reward will come, and so will continue good performance. New behaviors should be reinforced consistently at first, and always shortly after they are observed. Then, in order to maintain good performance, reinforcement provides rewards occasionally and irregularly, though continuously.[3]

Psychic income results from celebrating an employee's achievements, awarding team efforts, and other means for recognition. Management can also reward employees by talking with them, showing interest in them as people, consulting them for ideas and opinions, and praising good suggestions. Employees should be allowed to present ideas to management, *and receive credit*. Psychic rewards also include respect, concern, and caring for each individual by management.

Part of motivation, retention, and productivity depends upon appropriate and adequate psychic rewards. Successful workers who are highly compensated for their performance are often starved for "a pat on the back." It is so easy to give, and yet so often neglected. Managers must learn that the intangibles can be the key to success. Receiving psychic rewards can make the difference.

External Incentives

External incentives are another major determiner of motivation congruence. They are based on the fact that effort must result in improved or desired performance, and this in turn must result in significant rewards. The reward must be valued as important to the individual—it must meet an unfulfilled need, and it must be worth the effort. The amount of effort required, and the goal or desired performance, must be realistic. All the discussion of previous components concerning opportunities to succeed, ability to achieve goals, and confidence to try apply to this component.

Psychic rewards are one way to provide incentives. But there are other types of incentives that combine with psychic reward to result in optimum motivation congruence. Merit raises, cash bonuses, profit sharing, and incentive programs are examples of external incentives. Career development and clinical ladder programs offer salary increases and raises in status. Paid time off and awards of merchandise ranging from a turkey to a television are types of external incentives. The reward must be seen as needed or important to the individual, and offer psychic income, too.

Merit raises and bonus systems were addressed in Chapter 9 on performance evaluation. These were fairly traditional approaches to external incentives. Many organizations are developing innovative mechanisms for rewarding employees for contributing to organizational improvement. For instance, the "idea bank" is an incentive program to generate cost-saving ideas. Employees put ideas for ways to save money in a light-bulb-shaped bank. An employee committee evaluates the cost-saving merits of each idea, and the good ideas are implemented. Employees are rewarded by receiving a check for 10 percent of the first-year savings to the organization. Employees earn anywhere from $500 to $800 in bonuses, and hospitals have reported savings of $25,000 a year from this program.[4]

Certain points should be considered when implementing incentive programs. They must be implemented in conjunction with other motivational components, and be applied to a *satisfied* workforce. In the absence of the proper environment and conditions, external incentives will not be enough. In addition:

1. Rewards must be based on good performance
2. Incentives must be in combination with nonmonetary, psychic income
3. Rewards must be frequent enough to be meaningful, but not given so often that they become expected and routine
4. Rewards must be fairly and uniformly applied, based on measurable results or behaviors
5. Incentives must be in conjunction with close management of performance. Reward systems are not enough to ensure quality performance
6. Incentive plans must be simple, understood by all, and accepted by the staff as worthwhile

External rewards and incentives must be continually provided and based on the assessed needs and values of the work force. In combination with the other components of motivation congruence, they can directly affect retention and productivity.

Control of Operations

Although the application of these various components of job satisfaction and motivation will result in retention and productivity, there is an additional element that must be present. This is the management practice of controlling operations. Retention and productivity do not come *strictly* from "humanistic" management. Proper work flow, facility design, job analysis and simplification, staffing based on patient acuity and expertise, and financial management and control of operations are required for success. The systems and work must be analyzed, refined, and made efficient. Resources must be available. Communications and functions must be *coordinated*. The work and total organization must be evaluated for efficiency and effectiveness, and improvements secured.

As stated in the introduction to this chapter, this discussion has centered on the human side of productivity. But it must be emphasized that *all* of the components must be present, effective, and work together in order to achieve and maintain retention and productivity. The coordination, evaluation, and control of operations for maximum efficiency and quality is essential. Part of retaining a productive workforce depends on sound management practices for coordinating and control. This, in combination with the components for job satisfaction and motivation congruence, will ensure success.

Shared Values

Lastly, the need for shared values must be emphasized. Rewards and systems must be developed that result in employee need fulfillment while attaining organizational goals. Guidance, coaching, positive reinforcement, and incentives serve to achieve this goal. Mutual need fulfillment, however, does not necessarily create the sharing of values. Employees must believe in the importance of *some* aspects of the organization, and value the worth of the work.

It has been stated that perception of control and increased participation promote involvement, understanding, and "ownership" of the activity. These are necessary strategies to facilitate shared values. Effective recruitment and selection processes ensure appropriate attitudes and values to fit the job, and orientation assists with further development for the transition into new roles. But fostering shared values depends on more than this; it depends on a clear understanding of one's work and how that work contributes to the whole. It depends on a perception of the mission or purpose of the organization, and a belief that this is good; it depends on identifying with this mission, and developing a commitment to its achievement.

How might this commitment be obtained? By practicing and using all the components of job satisfaction and motivation congruence; by openly discussing and explaining organizational long-range and short-range plans; most importantly, by continually reminding employees of the reason they are there and their role in the organization's success.

Peters and Waterman[1] write that organizational values are the beliefs and common cause that guide all actions. They are what make the organization different or better. If a hospital believes it can provide the friendliest, warmest, and most personalized service in the community, this belief should continually be communicated to employees. This goal should be integrated into all activities, posted on bulletin boards, and never be forgotten. By continually seeing, hearing, and being involved in achieving this goal, employees will take ownership of it and begin sharing its value.

Reducing costs or increasing productivity is not a value that can be internalized and shared for long. Employees do not become emotionally involved in "numbers," but they can begin to share values concerning quality, personalized service, or being "the best." Administrators must identify how their organization can be the best at something, and become committed to this goal. Then employees can identify personally with these goals, contribute to the outcome, and be part of a "winning team." They can understand the total picture, why they are there, and how they can play a part in the outcome. They can have identity in the organization, and know where it is headed. By understanding and identifying with its mission, they can become committed to it.

Conclusion

Motivation congruence entails applying conditions and strategies to stimulate motivations towards personal *and* organizational purposes. It involves setting the appropriate challenge and "tension" that will result in a productive outlay of energy toward satisfaction of the whole—individual, group, and organization. Each of the components presented is necessary to and affects the achievement of motivation congruence. Each is dependent on the others for success, and all contribute to maximizing mutual need fulfillment.

Retention and productivity are dependent upon job satisfaction and motivation congruence. There is a continual interaction and interdependence between the components of each. Closed communications, limited opportunities to succeed, and lack of control over work all can and do affect job satisfaction. The lack of motivation toward organizational goals results in these motivations being channeled in other directions, often in nonproductive directions. This eventually affects personal needs and expectations, group interactions, and the work environment, and can cause job dissatisfaction. People are all motivated in some way, so when lacking direction and purpose, will choose the purpose that best suits their personal needs. But when given appropriate conditions, incentives, and rewards, they will channel their motivations in a more unified direction.

In addition to noncongruent motivations affecting job satisfaction, simply the *lack* of stimulation and interest results in diminished job satisfaction. People become bored, complacent, and lack the psychic income that follows achievement. They become dissatisfied and often do not understand the reason. An environment that lacks challenge and stimulation (and reward) or has noncongruent motivations will eventually result in job dissatisfaction.

Motivation congruence cannot be maintained without first achieving *and* maintaining job satisfaction. There must be basic need fulfillment before the individual can focus on other goals and purposes. Competency must be achieved before mastery over new skills and advancement in growth and development can occur. Job satisfaction sets the foundation for motivation congruence, but as with all aspects of management, requires on-going vigilance. The conditions in each component continually change and strategies must be adjusted appropriately.

Retention and productivity are the result of many components and interactions, not just one strategy or intervention. Managers must understand that a career ladder or merit raise system is not the answer. By using an understanding of human nature and change, along with the components of job satisfaction and motivation congruence, the stage may be set for success.

RETENTION AND PRODUCTIVITY AND THE PERSONNEL PROCESSES

This whole book is about retention and productivity. Throughout each chapter, strategies, principles, and concepts have been explored that facilitate the morale, growth and development, and self-gratification of the human resource. Each personnel process serves not only to maintain and develop competent people, but to tap and develop their talents and potential for personal *and* organizational success. Retention and productivity are integrated in and dependent upon each personnel process. The components for job satisfaction and motivation congruence must be a part of the planning and implementation of each process.

The next chapter concerns the personnel process of staff development, and its role in tapping and maximizing human talents and potentials. Because achieving competencies, growth and development, and expertise for obtaining goals is essential to retention and productivity, the need for effective staff development is evident. Effective staff development serves to facilitate and foster retention and productivity.

REFERENCES

1. Peters, T. J., & Waterman, R. H. *In search of excellence: Lessons from America's best-run companies.* New York: Warner Books, 1982, pp. 51–52, 279.
2. Dressler, G. *Improving productivity at work: Motivating today's employees.* New York: Harper & Row, 1984, p. 7.
3. Rosenbaum, B. L. *How to motivate today's workers.* New York: McGraw-Hill, 1982, p. 66.
4. Alabama Hospital Association. *Hospital Profiles.* Montgomery, Ala.: Alabama Hospital Association, 1985, *15*(2), p. 3.

SUGGESTED READING

Abdel-Halim, A. A. Social support and managerial affective responses to job stress. *Journal of Occupational Behavior,* 1982, *3*(4), 281–295.

Alson, J. P. Awarding bonuses the Japanese way. *Business Horizons,* 1982, *25*(3) 46–50.

American Academy of Nursing Task Force on Nursing Practice in Hospitals. *Magnet hospitals—Attraction and retention of professional nurses.* Kansas City, Mo.: ANA, 1983.

Argyris, C. *Integrating the individual and the organization.* New York: Wiley, 1964.

Berns, J. S. The application of job satisfaction theory to the nursing profession. *Nursing Leadership,* 1982, *5*(1), 27–33.

Best, F. Short-time compensation in North America: Trends and prospects. *Personnel,* 1985, *62*(1), 34–41.

Bobbe, R., & Schaffer, R. Want productivity improvement? Manage it! *Administrative Management,* 1982, *43,* 22–25.

Calabrese, R. Interaction skills for nurse managers. *Nursing Management*, 1982, *13*(5), 29–30.

Case, B. B. Moving your staff toward excellent performance. *Nursing Management*, 1983, *14*(12), 45–48.

Champagne, P. J. Using labor management committees to improve productivity. *Human Resource Management*, 1982, *21*(2), 67–73.

Cleverley, W. O., & Mullen, R. P. Management incentive systems and economic performance in health care organizations. *Health Care Management Review*, 1982, *7*(1), 7–20.

Crickmer, B. Lessons of leadership: The ins of management by an outsider. *Nation's Business*, 1981, *69*, 56–60.

D'Aprix, R. *Communicating for productivity*. New York: Harper & Row, 1982.

Davis, K. *Human behavior at work: Human relations and organizational behavior* (4th ed.). New York: McGraw-Hill, 1972.

Davidson, J. P. Remarks—Managing cycles of productivity. *Personnel Journal*, 1982, *61*(470), 420–422.

Dowling, W. F., & Sayles, L. R. *How managers motivate: The imperatives of supervision*. New York: McGraw-Hill, 1971.

Dwortzan, B. The ABCs of incentive programs. *Personnel Journal*, 1982, *61*(470), 436–442.

Eddy, W. B., & Burke, W. W. (Eds.). *Behavioral science and the manager's role*. San Diego: University Associates, Inc., 1980.

Fiedler, F. E. *A theory of leadership effectiveness*. New York: McGraw-Hill, 1967.

Foengen, J. H. Let's personalize the workplace. *Personnel Journal*, 1982, *61*, 642–643.

Frederick, S. Why John and Mary won't work. *Inc*, 1981, *3*, 70–71.

Friese, P., & Stefura, E. Job sharing, a solution to the personal energy crisis. *The Canadian Nurse*, 1983, *79*(1), 20–23.

Friss, L. An expanded conceptualization of job satisfaction and career style. *Nursing Leadership*, 1981, *4*(4), 13–21.

Froebe, D., Deets, C., & Knox, S. What motivates nurses to join and remain with an organization? *Nursing Leadership*, 1983, *6*(1), 22–33.

Gellerman, S. W. *Motivation and productivity*. New York: Macmillan, 1963.

Giblin, E. J. The challenge facing human resources. *Personnel*, 1984, *61*(4), 4–10.

Gilbert, T. F. A question of performance. Part I: The PROBE model. *Training and Development Journal*, 1982, *36*, 21–30.

Gilbert, T. F. A question of performance. Part II: Applying the PROBE model. *Training and Development Journal*, 1982, *36*, 85–89.

Ginsburg, S. G. Diagnosing and treating managerial malaise. *Personnel*, 1984, *61*(4), 34–40.

Goble, F. G. *Productivity: Getting employees to care*. New York: AMACOM, 1980.

Gorman, T. What ails the health professions? *American Teacher*, 1981, *65*(8), 10–11.

Grady, S. Employee-owned companies. *Working Woman*, 1981, *6*, 44.

Gryner, F. M. *Quality circles: A team approach to problem solving*. New York: AMACOM, 1981.

Guest, D. What's new in motivation. *Personnel Management*, 1984.

Harvey, F. W. A working model of behavior. *Supervisory Management*, 1982, *27*, 16–20.

Henderson, R. I. Designing a reward system for today's employee. *Business Magazine*, 1982, *32*(3), 2–12.

Herzberg, F., Mauser, B., & Synderman, B. B. *The motivation to work* (2nd ed.). New York: Wiley.

Higgins, J. Sharing out profits. *Personnel Management,* 1984.

Homans, G. C. *The human group.* New York: Harcourt, Brace & World, 1950.

Joselow, F. Exploring the office landscape. *Working Woman,* 1981, *6,* 55–59.

Kamy, E. M. Office productivity. *Industrial Management,* 1982, *24*(3), 29–31.

Kaminski-da Roza, V. A. Workshop that optimizes the older worker's productivity. *Personnel,* 1984, *61*(2), 47–56.

Knowles, H., & Knowles, M. *Introduction to group dynamics.* New York: Association Press, 1959.

Lachman, V. D. Increasing productivity through performance evaluation. *JONA,* 1984, *14*(12), 7–13.

Lancaster, J. Creating a climate for excellence. *JONA,* 1985, *15*(1), 16–19.

Lavandero, R. Nurse burnout: What can we learn? *JONA,* Nov/Dec 1981, 17–22.

Lee, J. A. *The gold and the garbage in management theories and prescriptions.* Athens, Ohio: Ohio University Press, 1980.

Levenstein, A. Toward creative self-management. *Nursing Management,* 1983, *14*(1), 22–23.

Lewin, K. *Field theory in social science.* New York: Harper & Row, 1951.

Likert, R. *New patterns of management.* New York: McGraw-Hill, 1961.

Lippit, G. L. *Organizational renewal: Achieving viability in a changing world.* New York: Appleton-Century-Crofts, 1969.

List, C. E. How to make quality circles work for your organization. *Personnel Journal,* 1982, *61,* 652.

Marriner, A. Development of management thought. *JONA,* Sept. 1979, pp. 21–31.

Maslow, A. *Motivation and personality.* New York: Harper & Row, 1954.

McClelland, D. C. Achievement motivation can be developed. *Harvard Business Review,* 1965, *43*(6), pp. 6–25.

McClure, M. Managing the professional nurse. Part I. The organizational theories. *JONA,* 1984, *14*(2), 15–21.

McClure, M. Managing the professional nurse. Part II. Applying management theory to the challenges. *JONA,* 1984, *14*(3), 11–17.

McElroy, M. W. The productivity myth. *Info Systems,* 1982, *29,* 140–141.

McGregor, D. *The human side of enterprise.* New York: McGraw-Hill, 1960.

Mills, T. M. *The sociology of small groups.* Englewood Cliffs, N.J.: Prentice-Hall, 1967.

Morath, J. Putting leaders, consultant and teachers on the line. *Nursing Management,* 1983, *14*(1), 50–52.

Pryor, M. G. The dissatisfaction profile: The key obstacle to motivation. *Industrial Management* (US), 1982, *24*(3), 7–11.

Sayles, L. R., & Strauss, G. *Human behavior in organizations.* Englewood Cliffs, N.J.: Prentice-Hall, 1966.

Schein, D. *Organizational psychology.* Englewood Cliffs, N.J.: Prentice-Hall, 1974.

Smith, I. Matching the incentive to the performer. *Personnel Management,* 1984.

Snyder, C. A., & Luthaus, F. Using OB MOD to increase hospital productivity. *Personnel Administration,* 1982, *27,* 67–68.

Solomon, G., & Bouloutian, A. Build a performance system—Not a training system. *Training and Development Journal,* 1982, *36,* 32–34.

12 The Process of Staff Development

An organization is only as good as the people in it. Stimulated, vital, progressive people make for a vital, progressive, and self-renewing organization. As stated in the preface and throughout this entire text, the success of any organization depends on developing and maximizing its human resources. Although each personnel process is an essential link to this "developing and maximizing," staff development serves to unify all growth and development to achieve wholeness—merging personal fulfillment with organizational purposes for overall organizational development. The purpose of this chapter is to explore systems, principles, and strategies that lead to an effective staff development process—one that will achieve ongoing organizational development. It will explore staff development in a general sense and in its relation to human resource management. It will then discuss organizing staff development and examine each of its four components. Finally, a model for unit-level staff development programs will be presented. This model will outline a guide for planning and implementing a learning experience, from the assessment phase through evaluation.

WHAT EXACTLY IS STAFF DEVELOPMENT?

Traditionally, staff development has consisted of in-service education, continuing education, and orientation. In-service education involves specific training for skills related to the job or a performance deficiency, or information pertaining to new developments in the organization. Continuing education is broader in scope, and involves planned learning experiences to enhance nursing practice, administration, research, or education.[1] Orientation involves preparing new employees for required competencies and fostering their socialization into the organizational culture. But staff development involves more than this. It also involves enhancing individual fulfillment of potentials and organizational development. It must consist of a variety of functions, from informal, spontaneous teaching and competency-based education to culture development and community health education. Staff development involves learning, in all dimensions and aspects of the organization. It involves facilitating the growth, development, and renewal of individuals and the organization as a whole. It is integrated into all areas of organizational life, and greatly determines the quality of this life.

Staff development is an ongoing process. This process can be seen as consisting of four major components: organizational development, operations, community relations, and research. Together these components interact and exchange as a process to promote human resource development and the achievement of organizational goals. Each of these components will be explored later in the chapter.

The process of staff development is usually implemented through a department entitled "in-service education," "continuing education," "human resource development," or "education." The director of this particular department is responsible for the outcome of these processes. For simplicity, the term "staff development" will be used to represent all such departments responsible for these educational processes and components. The department head will be called "the director of staff development." Note throughout the following text that traditional in-service, orientation, and continuing education functions are maintained within the four components for staff development. But widened functions related to fostering individual fulfillment, creativity, and organizational growth and vitality are also intact.

Before exploring the specifics in the staff development process, staff development as a whole must be clearly understood.

STAFF DEVELOPMENT AND HUMAN RESOURCE MANAGEMENT

Staff development is intimately connected to all areas of human resource management. Effective staff development depends upon recruitment of quality candidates who will grow with the organization, selection of the right person for the right job, and effective adjustments and socialization into the workplace. The conditions must be right so that the individual is ready to learn, and has satisfied basic needs of survival, security, and acceptance. Only qualified employees will be able to effectively and efficiently reach the desired level of competence necessary for proper function of the organization. Only when an employee is properly matched to the environment can he or she focus on actualizing potentials and continued growth and development.

Similarly, performance evaluation and coaching and counseling processes affect staff development. Continued learning and improvement is rewarded and reinforced through performance evaluation, just as learning needs are identified along with objectives for correcting and improving performance. A valid, reliable, objective, and trusted performance evaluation system will serve to relate performance to learning and help measure behavioral changes resulting from staff development experiences. Coaching and counseling further separate management and attitudinal needs from educational needs, correct unsatisfactory performance that interferes with the functioning and well-being of the organization, and ensure that individual attention is given to employees in need of help. Barriers and obstacles must be removed before learning can take place. This is all part of creating an environment for continual learning.

Retention and productivity, and labor relations also greatly determine the effectiveness of staff development. Employees must be satisfied in the workplace and motivated to seek growth and improvement in order for learning to occur and be transferred to the practice area. It is not enough to be exposed to new information. Employees must be motivated to change behaviors and use their new knowledge. The principles and processes of retention and productivity lead to this motivation, and are necessary for the success of staff development activities. The same holds true for employer–employee relations. An environment of mutual respect, trust, and cooperation based on shared values and unified purposes creates a climate for growth and development. Openness to ideas, communication, and concern for individual welfare all contribute to the conditions necessary for continued organizational development. Each of the personnel processes is critical in establishing this climate.

Just as staff development depends on effective personnel processes, it in turn is a crucial part of these processes and necessary to their effectiveness.

Recruitment

The changing work force is now seeking self-actualization in the workplace. This work force desires a means for career growth and advancement, self-development, and continued education. The process of staff development plays a big role in satisfying these needs and attracting qualified applicants. It also is closely related to internal recruitment and long-range planning for human resources. As future positions are anticipated along with the need for advanced or new skills, staff development educators will assist in preparing employees for these new roles. Individual development programs involving home study, courses in nearby schools, self-learning modules, and special clinical training will be developed and coordinated through staff development activities. Group training for future managers or new units will take place through staff development—all for the purpose of internal recruitment.

Selection

Staff development activities during the internal recruitment stage will greatly determine the qualifications of an applicant for selection. Candidates must demonstrate competency or show evidence of needed behaviors prior to being selected. Effective staff development will assist in attaining these competencies and in selecting the right person for the right job. In addition, managers will be trained in interviewing techniques and selection processes through the staff development department.

Orientation

The entire orientation process is conducted through the staff development department. While closely coordinated with administration, socialization, identification of goals and learning needs, and development of needed competencies occur through staff development.

Performance Evaluation

The entire performance evaluation process focuses on growth and development and requires management expertise in staff development activities. The staff development department works with nurse-managers to assist them in gaining the skills necessary for effective performance evaluation. Employees' self-evaluation and self-objectives completed during the evaluation process serve as growth and development goals and provide direction for learning. Staff development consultants assist employees in meeting their goals and guide their learning and self-development. Performance evaluations provide standards by which employees can determine needs and seek development activities to meet those needs. Staff development is necessary to assist employees to maintain and improve performance.

Counseling and Coaching

Effective counseling and coaching are dependent upon staff development processes. Special educational assistance must be provided to individuals with learning difficulties or performance problems due to inadequate skills or preparation. Staff development personnel are consulted to assist in the counseling and coaching process, and often contract with these employees for special skills development.

Retention and Productivity

Staff development plays a big role in retaining productive employees. Their job satisfaction will be influenced by their ability to adapt to change and maintain needed competencies. Staff development provides resources, activities, and assistance in this adaptation. Retention and productivity also depend on a satisfying work environment, opportunities to master new skills and competencies, and a climate that stimulates and rewards continual learning and improvement. Staff development processes focus on developing this type of climate and work closely with administration to ensure management's commitment to and reinforcement of staff development. Staff involvement in needs analysis, strategies to foster and allow expression of creative talents, and learning activities that promote positive self-images and an understanding of one's role in the whole organization are all staff development activities that affect retention and productivity.

Labor Relations

Staff development provides opportunities to satisfy personal achievement and competency needs and communicates concern and caring for the individual employee. This plays a big role in maintaining effective employee–employer relations. Staff development strategies such as allowing independence through self-directed learning and self-evaluation; involvement of employees in needs analysis and program development; offering guidance and assistance for testing new ideas and gaining new skills—all communicate trust, respect, and interest in the employee as an individual. Staff development greatly influences the employer–employee relationship.

ORGANIZING FOR THE STAFF DEVELOPMENT PROCESS

Staff development must be integrated into all aspects of organizational life, and greatly determines the quality of this life. In order to achieve these goals, the staff development department must be appropriately placed in the organizational structure and hierarchy. This organization must promote optimum communication, coordination, control, and use of educational resources. Most of all, it must promote effective outcomes. The exact organizational design will depend on a facility's unique situation, philosophy, and needs. This design often falls between a centralized and decentralized approach, and may be hospital-wide or directly under the nursing department.

A centralized staff development department may possess more clout in some institutions, and so be able to obtain larger budgetary allowances, proportionally speaking, than a decentralized department. A centralized hospital-wide department, if effective, can integrate all services and em-

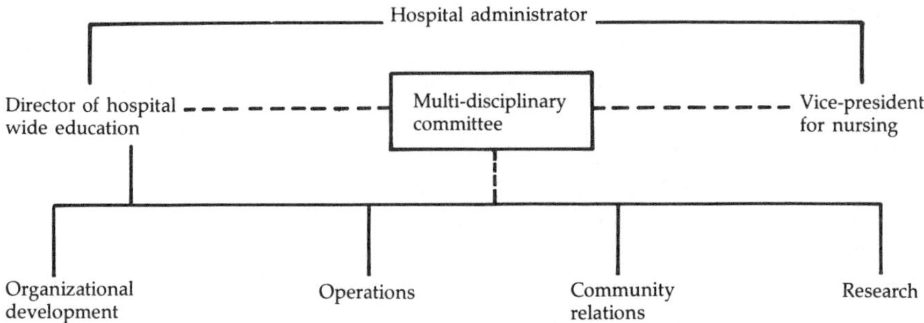

Figure 12–1. Hospital-wide staff development model.

ployees, standardize procedures, and prevent duplication or waste of materials and equipment. All the pros of efficiency, coordinated planning, and integration that come with centralization can be seen in a hospital-wide approach. On the negative side, centralization can cause educational processes to become detached from unit-level needs, and can lack flexibility and creativity. In decentralization, specific learning needs can be identified, and individualized programs can be offered to meet those needs. Decentralization allows flexibility, creativity, ongoing staff interaction and involvement, and facilitates a close working relationship between educators and the staff. Conversely, with decentralization, services may be duplicated and efficiency in resource use may be decreased. There is often no centralized, uniform plan to coordinate and control long-range development. Each unit "does its own thing." Despite the pros and cons, either organizational design can be *and is* effective, given the proper setting, conditions, and leadership.

Some facilities function under a centralized department and department head, but maintain many decentralized staff development activities on the unit level. This is a centralized–decentralized approach. Although

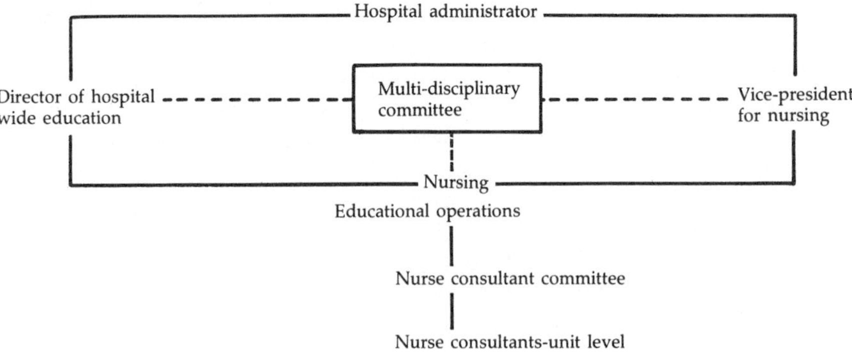

Figure 12–2. Relationship of hospital-wide education to nursing service.

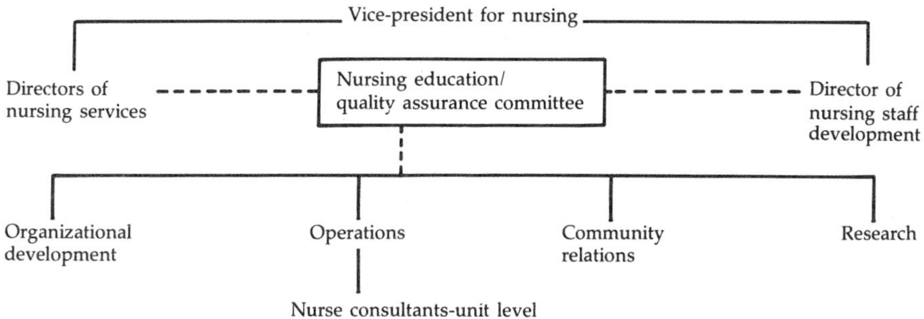

Figure 12–3. Nursing staff development model.

educational activities are organized in a centralized area, the staff development operations for each specific department or unit are decentralized. Staff development programs are provided for overall organizational needs and goals, but individualized according to specific unit needs and requirements. This approach provides the needed decentralization that prevents the detachment from unit needs, lack of flexibility, or lack of creativity that can accompany centralization. It allows the centralization needed for standardization and efficiency, along with individualized, interactive decentralization. The following text will examine this centralized–decentralized approach for a hospital-wide and a nursing staff development department. Obviously, there are a multitude of other variations and arrangements. These two were chosen simply as examples, and as a means to explore the four components in the staff development process.

Figures 12–1 and 12–3 show examples of hospital-wide versus nursing staff development departments. Each of the four components of staff development can be seen in both arrangements. Figure 12–2 relates hospital-wide education to the nursing operations component.

In a hospital-wide staff development department, the director of hospital-wide education can be answerable directly to the hospital administrator, and equal to the vice-president for nursing (in some cases the director of education answers to the vice-president for nursing or to some other administrator). Although the vice-president may have no authority over this person, there must be a cooperative and communicating working relationship.

The director of hospital-wide education directs the assessment, planning, implementation, and evaluation for each of the components of staff development, and ensures the integration of these components into total organizational life. To facilitate this process, a multidisciplinary committee may be formed in an advisory capacity. This committee can help integrate various departments with staff development. It can work to coordinate the four components of staff development to long-range plans and hospital-wide strategies. Additional activities involving needs, assessment, contingency planning, program development, and other processes may be facilitated through the use of short-term and temporary task forces.

In a centralized, hospital-wide department, as shown in Figure 12–2, the "operations" component involves unit-level staff development in each separate department. The operations for the nursing department could consist of nursing educational consultants for each unit, with 24-hour responsibility. These consultants could answer to both the director of education and the vice-president for nursing. On the unit, the unit coordinator and nursing personnel would share the responsibility for continued staff development with the nurse-consultant, who assists and facilitates the educational process. Nurse-consultants could also form a committee to assess, plan, implement, and evaluate staff development processes for all nursing units. Rather than report to a staff development coordinator for nursing (and also to their director of education and vice-president for nursing), the committee could be the decision-making arm for decentralized learning. The multidisciplinary committee could oversee the hospital-wide educational processes and provide input for planning and decision making, while the nursing committee focused on operational levels.

Figure 12–3 shows a staff development department located under the nursing department. The director of nursing staff development is shown on a equal level with the other directors of nursing, and answerable to the vice-president for nursing. The committee approach should be used. This committee could be part of the nursing planning committee, quality assurance, or a separate committee for nursing education. It can be advisory for program assessment, planning, implementation, and evaluation. Temporary task forces could be formed for special needs, such as prioritizing programs, and include various representatives from the nursing department.

Nursing staff development is divided into four components: organizational development, operations, community relations, and research. Organizational development may focus on the *nursing* organization, but could include overall organizational plans, culture development, interdepartmental relations, and other aspects to be discussed shortly. The operations component would naturally consist of only nursing operations (versus departmental operations under the hospital-wide system). Unit-level staff development would occur through a similar mechanism, using nursing consultants in cooperation with unit coordinators.

In general, these examples have many similarities. Each consists of a department head who involves other employees and department heads in education through committee and task force interaction. The director is responsible for the four components of staff development. Organizational development, community relations, and research are organized centrally, and the operations component is totally decentralized under the director's authority. (Keep in mind that the vice-president for nursing is accountable for the performance of the nursing department, and is very much responsible for education and development.) The operations component is also involved in other staff development components, such as community relations and research. Each component must interact. Both of the models described, centralized and decentralized, can be effective; both designs implement the necessary components of staff development.

Some vice-presidents for nursing prefer the entire staff development process under their jurisdiction. Actually, this should not be the issue. Staff development should be organized according to the size, resources, qualifications of educators, type of employees, philosophy, and needs of the organization. The effectiveness of education will ultimately depend on administrative support and commitment, expertise of educators, interaction and involvement of employees, and specific educational strategies and methodology. There must be a cooperative and interactive relationship between practice and learning in order to see the results in improved functioning and patient care. Effective staff development depends on the proper climate and conditions, not upon specific organizational structure.

However the staff development department is organized, it must be headed by a director who can integrate its components into all aspects of organizational life. This director must not only be a learning specialist and educator; he or she must be an expert administrator over the department.[2] The director must be a consultant and a change agent, who works hand in hand with administration,[3] and must recruit, select, and develop top-notch educators who are closely integrated into resource planning and management. They must be able to focus on current, practical problems but keep an eye to the future. They must work to bridge theory and practice, and must maintain a broad view of the environment and organizational goals. They should serve as educational consultants for all levels of employees, from top administration to the staff level, and provide important input into management processes concerning human needs and development. Staff development personnel must be well read and knowledgeable resource people, experts in their specialty area, role models, and futurists. They should possess skills in interpersonal relations, management, and leadership, as well as in education. They must work cooperatively and collaboratively with management; they must be visible and accessible. Lastly, and most importantly, they must hold a high regard for the worth of human beings and an optimistic view and approach to life in general. The motivation to learn is usually preceded by the belief that something will change or improve, or some benefit will result. Educators must be optimistic about change and improvement before they can expect others to adopt an openness toward learning and new experiences.

THE COMPONENTS OF STAFF DEVELOPMENT

The components of staff development will be the focus of the following text. Together, each component comprises the process of staff development. This holds true regardless of the organizational design. Staff development can be hospital-wide with a variety of instructors and support systems, or a one-person nursing in-service division under the nursing department. Depending upon the budget, support, and resources available, the components will be developed and used in various degrees. In some facilities, community relations may consist of extensive community health education and patient education services. In other facilities, practically all time and resources will be devoted to operations. But even in the smallest departments with scarce resources, plans can include community relations or research. The following discussion will explore a wide range of activities and considerations in each component. These provide examples from which to choose, and when put together form an "ideal" staff development model.

The Organizational Development Component

Staff development ultimately is geared to organizational development. Plans must be made not only to integrate organizational and personal goals, but to develop a culture and climate for openness, communication, and lifelong learning. In addition, this component may involve providing integrated, hospital-wide, and repetitive educational experiences, as well as developing and maintaining materials and resources. Under the direction of the director of staff development, several or all of the following strategies can be planned and implemented for organizational development. These are just a few examples of what might be included in this component.

Planning. This involves the establishment of long-term educational strategies, objectives, and operational plans that serve to implement organizational plans. Staff development personnel must be involved in planning systems in order to ensure congruency.

Culture Development. This involves several ongoing processes including:

1. Ensuring administrative commitment to learning and the welfare of individuals by philosophy, standards, job descriptions, and performance evaluations that reflect this commitment. Policies and reward systems must reinforce continued learning. Administration and staff development personnel must demonstrate this commitment by role modeling, supporting ongoing learning, and providing needed time and resources. Staff development must assess the above and relate deficits to the planning committee and to administration.
2. Assessing the outcome of personnel processes to determine strengths and weaknesses in the organization. For instance, high turnover can reflect problems in selection, orientation, or retention efforts and stifle organizational development (OD) efforts. Staff development personnel must work with management to evaluate

the outcome of personnel processes and determine and correct problems. Staff development should be included in all aspects of the administrative function in order to provide important consultative input.

3. Continually identifying the individual employee's role in organizational success and communicating this in learning actitivies. It must explain how a specific learning objective relates to overall organizational goals and how the employee contributes to the whole.
4. Ensuring that the individual can effect change and control over the work environment. It must assess communication, employee support systems, openness to new ideas, and degree of autonomy on the work unit. It must work with management personnel and top administration to establish systems and procedures that will support creativity, innovations, and openness to learning.
5. Using principles of job satisfaction and motivation to stimulate the desire to achieve (see Chapter 11), and providing challenging opportunities and recognition for achievement.
6. Using formal and informal learning experiences to demonstrate high expectations, respect, and genuine concern for the growth and development of employees.
7. Providing ongoing intellectual and creative stimulation, and using strategies for creativity as discussed in Chapter 5 to promote the creative attitude and a climate for learning.

Human Resource Management Development. Ongoing management-leadership development should be provided to current and potential management personnel. In addition to skills such as decision making, communication, planning, or interviewing, management's role in human resource development and organizational development must be explored. Management expertise is critical to culture development, interdepartmental relationships, and achievement of organizational plans. Staff development cannot be effectively implemented without the proper environment, and this environment is dependent upon expert management practices.

Interdepartmental Relations. Creativity training, open forums, group discussions, and problem-solving task forces consisting of employees from different departments will serve to build sound interdepartmental relations. Opening communication and breaking down barriers among departments leads to a more receptive and unified organization. Staff development activities should include measures to enhance interdepartmental relations for total organizational growth.

Educational Resources for Growth and Development. Library materials or learning resource center and audiovisual equipment and materials should be available and accessible for continued learning. Although specific learning modules may be developed on each clinical unit, resources should be provided for independent, self-directed learning, group learning, and discussions, as well as classroom instruction.

Repetitive Instruction. Ongoing content required by the Joint Commission on Accreditation for Hospitals, such as safety, fire and disaster, and other similar required topics may be covered in a centralized manner. General hospital orientation, CPR, intravenous therapy certification, and other repetitive subjects may also be grouped under organizational development. Methodology for learning experiences may involve partial or total self-directed learning, such as viewing films and test-taking. Application of learning in many cases is evaluated on the clinical unit. Content remaining fairly standardized and applied to a large number of employees may be implemented in a more cost-effective manner through a centralized approach.

Organizational development is ultimately the responsibility of top administration. By placing the process under staff development, organizational development is linked, as it should be, to continued renewal and learning. Since organizational development involves progressing, evolving, and growing, it certainly will depend upon the continual growth and development of its human resources. Thus, staff development is the link to organizational development.

The Operations Component

The operations component of staff development consists of clinically oriented education on the unit level. Expert nurse-clinicians and educators serve as consultants to facilitate the ongoing competency and development of the nursing staff. Depending on the needs and resources of the facility, these nurses can be clinical nurse specialists or hospital-certified nurse-clinicians who cover specific units and shifts to ensure 24-hour educational coverage. In a small facility with limited staff development resources, this component can be implemented in several ways. The staff development director can devote time on units and each shift for problem-oriented, hands-on teaching. Preceptors and specialty nurses can be certified through staff development as specialists and take part in unit educational activities. Management personnel should receive continuing education in adult learning, consulting, and staff development processes, in order to take part in unit-level educational activities.

In any setting, unit-level staff development must be a responsibility that is shared by unit coordinators and the nurse-consultants. In addition, staff development must be included in nurses' performance evaluations and as part of career development, to enhance the nurses' accountability for self-directed learning and continued growth and development. In these rapidly changing times, a nurse-educator cannot possibly provide all learning experiences, nor can a nurse-educator make someone learn. Staff nurses must be motivated, independent learners; this requires effective personnel processes that result in professional, productive nurses, facilities and resources to support and help independent learning, and management development to ensure an environment conducive to learning and continual growth.

Nurse-consultants facilitate unit level education, but also take part in other components of staff development. They may become involved in a community relations project or research, and should be continually working toward organizational development and fostering a culture for learning. Other functions, such as patient education, are implemented on the unit level and would involve these educators. No one component is independent or distinct from another—each enhances the others' effectiveness, and together they determine the effectiveness of the staff development process. Nurse-consultants must understand how they all interrelate and take part in developing the whole process.

Operations involve unit-level orientation, achievement and maintenance of competency as well as individual assistance toward creativity and innovation, and fulfillment of potentials. Orientation processes and competency-based education were discussed in Chapter 8. The following is an example for implementing unit-level staff development and was derived from *Nursing Decentralization: The El Camino Experience.*[4]

Clinical staff development can be achieved through the use of nurse-consultants who support educational activites, and can be a means for independent learning and skills validation. Trained preceptors and nurse-specialists, as well as nurse-managers, can assist in evaluating on-the-job learning, competencies, and application of new knowledge. Carefully designed checklists and evaluation tools can be designed for objective assessments. Learning can be self-paced and enhanced through the development of educational modules, a learning resource center, and a core curriculum.

Educational modules consist of an individual educational activity or program, from learning objectives and pretest, to posttest following completion of content. Often a clinical evaluation is then conducted on the unit by a nurse-consultant or manager. These modules can contain material for anything from orientation (intravenous therapy or nursing care planning) to continuing education and advanced learning. They can be completed at any time, done at any pace, and be repeated by the individual nurse until he or she feels ready for the evaluation. Once the modules are prepared, instructor time in conducting and repeating classes is saved. The learning becomes self-paced and individualized—nurses choose the content according to their learning needs. Staff nurses can contract with nurse-consultants or management personnel to attain new skills and knowledge. These contracts can spring from performance evaluation (self-objectives) to career development programs. The contracts define staff development responsibilities, such as demonstrations, provision of resources, special assistance, and the staff nurse responsibilities, such as completion of learning modules and demonstration of certain behaviors. Modules designed for continuing education and advanced skills may be optional and completed on an employee's own time. Although the information is readily available, it is up to the individual nurse to use it, just as advancement on a clinical ladder is optional. Demonstration of new skills and knowledge on the unit must be rewarded and included in the performance evaluation system.

The learning resource center can be established to provide a place to complete modules and self-paced learning. It can consist of library materials, or be located next to the library. Lists of educational programs should be available with instructions for completion. Audiovisual equipment such as videocassettes, slides, and filmstrips should be provided, with a designated space for individual as well as small group learning.

A core curriculum can be developed, containing competency requirements for each particular unit. Each competency would have a subcompetency, delineating the exact criteria for evaluation. Learning modules then are designed to facilitate achievement of each subcompetency. This core curriculum is developed specifically for each unit, and consists of skills, processes, and behaviors necessary for minimum-level functioning on that unit. During orientation or transfer to a new unit, a skills inventory would be completed to assess the learning needs. Deficient areas would dictate the need for certain competencies and would direct the learner to appropriate learning activities, such as reviewing an article, completing an educational module, or viewing a film. The core curriculum groups all minimum-level competencies together with the corresponding learning experiences and evaluation methods. It must be updated and expanded as skills, knowledge, or behaviors change. Core curriculum can also be developed for advanced skills, such as for career development for a certain unit or specialty area. It would outline required competencies and related learning experiences, such as educational modules or certain clinical experience (see Chapter 8 appendices for ICU competencies, subcompetencies, skills inventory, and learning module).

The focus of unit-level staff development is demonstration of learning and competencies, or competency-based education using self-directed learning. A nurse may learn in any manner, or read a number of articles independently, or may forego a learning module and take the test or evaluation. Self-paced, independent learning leaves the learning experience up to the learner. Development of resources and modules provides the assistance, but it is demonstration of learning that counts. The core curriculum outlines needed competencies and related learning experiences. A nurse may demonstrate these competencies without completing the specific learning experiences. With this method, time and expense are not wasted teaching nurses what they already know. The adult learner is able to learn independently and is treated as a capable, responsible person.

Nurse-consultants work with unit coordinators and staff nurses to develop and revise core curriculum and educational modules. They counsel, coach, and validate skills and learning, and continually evaluate unit operations and functions to determine effectiveness of staff development. Teaching is done at the bedside, as well as in groups and classes, in addition to self-paced learning. While most learning experiences are problem-oriented and situational, future-oriented and conceptual content is offered for stimulation and creativity. With the development of self-paced modules and sharing responsibilities for skills validation and competency evaluation, consultants have more time to provide individualized, patient-centered teaching, as well as additional growth and development experiences.

In conclusion, unit-level operations focus on problem-oriented, situational learning and maintenance of ongoing competence. They also integrate nurses' performance and roles with other aspects of staff development, such as organizational development, community relations, and research. Through career ladders, performance evaluations, individual contracting, bonus systems, or other reward systems, management encourages nursing participation in activities outside of the clinical unit, and promotes nurses' growth and development. Staff development works with management to promote opportunities and guidance in this growth and development—to achieve progress towards creativity and innovation. By involving the staff in the planning and development of learning modules, brainstorming for ideas for teaching strategies, participating in classes, evaluating patient outcomes or assisting with community workshops and prevention programs, they can also achieve personal fulfillment and a sense of "making a difference." When staff members believe they count and do make a difference in the organization, they will strive to become better and more fulfilled and continue to grow. This is the goal of staff development, and it begins and ends with the staff nurse on the unit level.

The Community Relations Component

With growing competition in health care and the increasing number of options and choices for health care services by consumers, community relations has become an important aspect of organizational growth and development. Marketing and public relations are a significant part of the nurse-administrator's function, and maintaining the competitive edge in the marketplace is essential for organizational success. Staff development can greatly contribute to achieving this competitive edge through the component of community relations. By assessment of public perceptions and needs and continuous interaction with the community, a positive corporate image can be promoted. Ongoing community services, workshops, and activities must be integral to staff development planning and consistent with overall organizational goals. Not only must staff development help meet the community's health education needs, but it must promote the organization as consisting of progressive, expert, and caring clinicians. If the philosophy and goals involve research, high technology, or "down-home" personal care, this image should be promoted and transmitted to the community. Staff development can facilitate this process in conjunction with administrative marketing and public relations plans.

Community relations activities can be very simple or involve several full-time personnel in ongoing programs. A small, one-person staff development department can plan and coordinate a blood pressure screening, childbirth classes, or a diabetic class. A newspaper ad, flyers in local businesses and restaurants, or a spot on the local radio can inexpensively promote the activity. Some type of community relations activity should be included in staff development plans throughout the year. The number and type of activities will depend on the resources and available personnel. While in some cases community relations is organized as a separate department, it is still an essential component of the staff development process. The following are examples of the types of activities that can be included in this component.

Community Health Education. Ongoing classes can be offered for various problems and illnesses common in the community. A community hotline number can be promoted, offering brief teaching and assistance for health-related problems. Outpatient individual and group classes can be arranged following discharge, with audiovisual and material resources. Preventative classes can be offered regularly, such as childbirth, hypertension screening and clinics, stress reduction, coronary heart disease risk factors, and other topics of interest to the public. Health education and screening can also be provided to industries and businesses in the community on a regular basis.

In-house Patient Education. This may be organized as part of community relations. Although patient teaching occurs on the unit level, planning and coordination of in-house patient education classes, resources, and special assistance can be organized centrally. A patient education nurse-consultant can be available to assist unit-level consultants and staff nurses with discharge planning and teaching, and to provide materials, consultation, and assistance for patients with complex problems. This way, community health education plans and resources can be linked to in-house patient education services.

Community Communications. These can also be a part of this component. Physicians' office staff, home health agencies, and other related organizations can be oriented to admitting, discharge, and diagnostic procedures, or other policies and activities in the organization that can facilitate relations and interactions. Classes can be held to discuss problems, new technology, or other information necessary to maintain smooth transfer of patients or for continuity. Classes of this sort also serve to improve the image of the organization.

Corporate Image. Internal staff development on corporate image is another important part of this component. Employees should be knowledgeable of their role in public relations and how they can promote the image of the organization. They must be aware of the goals and philosophy of their organization, and the part they play in achieving the competitive edge in the community. Employees must understand that they make the organization and are a part of its success. This belief should be communicated through all staff development processes.

Community Services. The staff development department may want to take part in community services such as cancer drives, marathons for cystic fibrosis, or other related activities. The hospital should sponsor civic-related fund raisers or drives and take part in programs to improve the community. Staff development must be attuned to community needs and project a helping image.

Ongoing Assessment. Hospital marketing and long-range planning systems involve environment scanning and external assessment. Staff development personnel must also be involved in this assessment. They must have access to these data, and continually collect information during all community activities. Consumer satisfaction, perceptions of organizational image, and special needs and interests can be obtained during classes, screening clinics, and interactions. Ongoing evaluation must be integrated into all community relations activities.

Volunteer Orientation and Education. If there is not a separate department for volunteer services, staff development personnel may take responsibility for volunteer preparation and orientation and continual education. Staff development may still assist with this education even if a separate volunteer service department does exist. The treatment, guidance, and support provided to volunteers greatly affects their performance in the organization, as well as community relations. Volunteers communicate their attitude and perceptions of the hospital to others in the community, and this contributes to the corporate image.

Professional Workshops. Some staff development departments provide educational conferences and workshops for professionals in the community. This helps meet continuing education needs, as well as promoting the image of the hospital. Needed programs and conferences may also be sponsored by the hospitals in conjunction with a specialty association or group of professionals.

In conclusion, community relations are critical to an organization's continued growth and viability, and are an important part of the staff development process. The community relations component provides needed educational and health services in the community, promotes recruitment and retention of professionals, and helps meet the public's needs. This in turn helps improve the status of the organization in the community.

The Research Component

This component of the staff development process could be entitled quality assurance, educational research and development, or any number of names. It concerns a broad range of activities, from evaluation of the effect of staff development on services to clinical research. It may not always involve education *per se,* but it fosters creativity and innovation, development of ideas, improvement in systems and services, and evaluation of health care, all of which concern the development of human resources in some respect. Although quality assurance is the ultimate responsibility of administration, evaluation studies and processes may be coordinated and implemented through the staff development department. Any activity involving improvement, experimentation, and innovation could be considered part of this component. While a small facility would not have the capabilities for a separate division of research, efforts can still be made to evaluate services, test new ideas, and review patient outcomes.

This component should be under the direction of a person who is an open thinker with expertise in research. This person will serve as a consultant in designing, implementing, and evaluating research, as well as being an advocate for change and creativity. Although creativity and innovation are principles integrated into each personnel process, this component can serve as the "center for creativity and innovation." Not only can it train for creativity, brainstorming, and intuitive thinking; it can also provide an avenue to receive ideas and a guide for testing these ideas. It must be the avant-garde area of the organization.

In addition to promoting and guiding research, providing creativity training, and serving as the center for receiving new ideas and suggestions, this component can assist with evaluating the process and outcome of patient care, monitoring employee competency, monitoring efficiency and effectiveness of operations, identifying and solving problems, and implementing planned change, among other functions. Although these functions may be implemented by task force, committee action, through administration, or on the clinical unit, the staff development department coordinates, assists, and counsels during these processes. The research specialist can evaluate reliability and validity of methods and tools, provide resources and direction in planning, and see that plans are followed through to completion. Staff development personnel also promote and assist employees in publishing their research findings.

The evaluation process of staff development also comes under this component. While evaluation of clinical competency occurs on the unit level, educational program evaluations and evaluation for each component of staff development can be coordinated here. Data collection, assessment of findings, and follow-up action can be determined with assistance from the research component. The research component can serve as the "specialist" in evaluation, problem solving, and research, and provide direction and assistance in these matters.

The research component of staff development works to facilitate inquiry, discovery, and creativity, and to stimulate growth and development in all areas of the organization. By being involved in administrative planning and in committees, research can be integrated through the organization. It can become an important means for organizational development and for achieving excellence in patient care.

A MODEL FOR PROGRAM DEVELOPMENT

The first part of this chapter has dealt with staff development in a broad sense—how it relates to human resource management and the organization and components of the staff development process. This section will look at staff development on the unit level. It will present a model for planning and implementing an educational program or learning experience, from assessment through evaluation. This model is not the "only way," but a guide to ensure that staff development programs are appropriate, cost-effective, and improve services or patient care. The remainder of this discussion will explore the various components of this model, which are presented in Figure 12–4.

Identify and Analyze Problems and Needs

Needs assessment is a critical first step to program development. In these times of limited resources and economic constraints, no staff development activities can (or should) be offered without a justified need. But identifying a need is not enough. This need must be of sufficient magnitude to justify intervention and be amendable through staff development processes. Needs assessment can be accomplished through three steps: data collection, data analysis, and prioritization of needs and problems.

Data Collection. Problems and needs can be identified through a number of sources. A formal needs assessment should be conducted at least yearly, with continual additions and adjustments to data being made throughout the year. The following are some of the many sources of information to be used in developing educational activities.

Philosophy, Organizational Goals, Nursing Plans, and Human Resource Management Plans and Inventories. These provide current and future directions for growth and development and help identify learning needs when compared to other data such as performance evaluations.

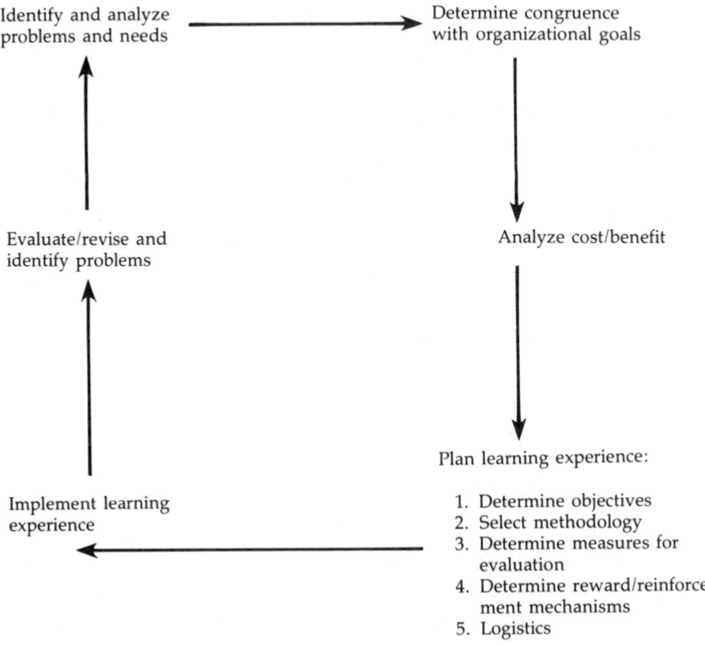

Figure 12–4. A model for program development.

Questionnaires and Surveys. These provide information concerning the staffs' perceived needs and interests.

Interviews with Experts or Review of Literature. This provides information concerning new developments in specialty areas, current trends and issues, and required skills for expert practice. In-house as well as outside clinical experts can provide input in this area.

Review of Charts, Incident Reports, Personnel Reports such as Turnover and Absenteeism, and Reports from Hospital Committees. These provide data relating to provision of services and performance, as well as productivity.

Patient Evaluations and Interviews. These provide information about level of satisfaction and perceived needs for improvement from the patient's perspective.

Performance Evaluations. These measure the quality of performance according to standards, and identify need for improvement. They also provide information about the application of learning.

Staff Interviews and Observation. These are performed formally or informally; information is collected for determining needs and problems.

Productivity Reports. Information regarding efficiency and effectiveness of services is used in determining performance needs.

Required Competencies. While standards and job description requirements are included in the performance evaluation results, identification of minimum-level competencies is necessary to needs assessment. Assessment of required competencies for practice is essential in analyzing and prioritizing learning needs.

Self-assessment by Skills Checklists, Self-evaluation of Performance, and Individual Contracting for Specific Learning Goals. These individual assessments can be used to identify group needs and dictate development of course content and staff development programs.

Management Input. This is critical to a needs assessment and should be performed continually on a formal and informal basis. Managers should identify operational problems, obstacles to achieving their unit objectives, critical and noncritical training needs for achieving objectives, and performance deficiencies.[5] Close working relations and open communication must be established between staff development and management personnel. This is greatly facilitated in a decentralized structure such as this organizational model where the manager, nurse, and nurse-consultant share the responsibility for competency and continued learning.

Data Analysis. Once data have been collected, they must be analyzed to determine the cause of the problem and whether it is appropriate for staff development intervention. Educators should use scientific problem solving when analyzing data and determining solutions. This includes defining the problem, examining all data related to a solution, evaluating and determining all alternatives, then selecting and implementing the most effective solution. Outcomes must be monitored and evaluated.[6] Sovie states that once identified, problems must be analyzed and grouped according to staff development, management, or a combination of the two for resolution. She defines problems appropriate to staff development according to the following criteria:

1. Evidence that a deficiency exists in skill or knowledge
2. Verification that support services and other departments are performing properly
3. Evidence of adequate policies and procedures
4. A problem is resolved when procedures are implemented by skilled or knowledgeable personnel[6]

Management problems can be identified when

1. Support services are inadequate
2. Supplies and equipment are inadequate

3. Policies and procedures are unclear or incomplete
4. There are unclear performance expectations by nursing and other health care providers
5. Policies, procedures, and practices require revision[6]

Sovie states that many needs and problems require the joint efforts of management with staff development for effective resolution. As mentioned earlier, staff development activities must receive total administrative support in order to be effective.

Prioritization of Needs and Problems. Once problems are identified as being amenable to staff development or a combination of staff development and management interventions, they must be prioritized. Minimum-level competency needs take top priority, because these needs have the greatest impact on patient care. Because various personnel will have various levels of expertise, learning activities will be planned to meet advanced growth and development needs as well as competency needs. But as problems arise, and when resources must be divided and allocated, competency or essential skills take priority.

After competency needs are met, prioritization will depend upon the philosophy and goals of the organization. Clinical, patient-oriented problems and needs should be high priorities, along with competency needs. But management and staff perceptions and evaluations should be included in needs assessment and prioritization. Interdepartmental concerns, communication, interpersonal relations, culture development, and creativity should also be included in staff development programs. Although essential and required skills and knowledge come first, there must also be a blend of "higher-order needs satisfaction" to produce a stimulated and more well-rounded staff. The degree to which the organization can help meet these needs will depend upon its staff development personnel and its resources. However, some attempt to facilitate growth and development can be made even with minimum efforts such as providing reading materials and audiovisuals, and supporting formal continuing education by nurses through time off or tuition reimbursement. Staff development educators should search for creative mechanisms for stimulating curiosity and learning in all aspects of work life. For example, the need to understand and test a progressive nursing methodology may be perceived by a unit's nursing staff as being important to their goal of innovative and progressive nursing care. Although the majority of time and resources may be allocated to meeting minimum-level standards, a study group can be formed to meet for 15 minutes each day and share information. The nurse-consultant could guide and facilitate learning and provide reading materials and other resources from a search of the literature. Then discussion of the new methodology could be part of the team conference or integrated into patient care planning, to be applied to actual practice—or be "put to use." Knowledge must not be "for knowledge's sake," but be tied to application or need. Knowledge of issues and trends, creativity, philosophy, or whatever is considered a growth and development need can always be linked to application. It is important that nurse-educators identify the usefulness and effect of educational programs on patient and organizational outcomes. The link between education, need and problem resolution, and effect on organizational outcomes will determine the priority of a given staff development program.

Determine Congruence with Organizational Goals

Closely related to and in addition to prioritization is the need for determining the congruence of an identified need with overall organizational goals. A need must first be identified and analyzed as being amenable to staff development. In prioritizing needs and problems, it must be determined to have an impact on organizational outcomes and patient care. In leading up to cost–benefit analysis and planning objectives, it then must be delineated how the solution to this problem or need will help achieve nursing and organizational goals. A solution's effect or outcome must be connected to organizational plans and goals. The following provides an example: The nurses on a medical–surgical floor want to learn to read 12-lead ECGs. While nurses in the intensive care units are required to have this knowledge, medical–surgical competencies require only identification of the basics, such as sinus rhythm, tachycardias, bradycardias, ventricular rhythms, etc. As the request is investigated, it is determined that more acutely ill patients are being placed on the medical–surgical units, requiring more extensive knowledge of physical assessment and cardiac arrhythmias. Knowledge of 12-lead ECG interpretation would facilitate telephone communications with the physicians and help prevent cardiac complications. Although staff development personnel can identify the need as being amenable to education and as directly affecting patient care, they are not presently prepared to put a large number of staff nurses through the ECG course. In addition to cost–benefit analysis, they must relate this need to achievement of organizational goals. In this case the organization's goals include promoting the institution as consisting of progressive and expert health care providers. In conjunction, the nursing goals include developing a program for certifying advanced nurse-clinicians. An educational program for training medical–surgical nurses in ECG interpretation could become part of this certification and contribute to developing a staff of expert clinicians. Marketing tactics could include "staff nurses certified in cardiac assessment and ECG interpretation." In addition and most importantly, this knowledge could contribute to the ultimate goal of quality patient care.

All needs do not fit so perfectly into organizational plans, and even if they do, they may not be cost-effective (discussed later). But it is important to relate all desired outcomes to nursing and organizational plans to ensure that all energies are headed in the same direction. It is also important for the employee to understand why required attendance and performance of new competencies is necessary. When the employee can see how learning and application of new skills or knowledge will contribute to achievement of hospital goals, he or she can understand the importance of learning and the employee's role in organizational success. Every educational activity should include an organizational purpose along with its behavioral objectives. For instance, nurses required to attend an in-service program on a new patient teaching and discharge planning procedure would receive behavioral objectives with the following purpose: "It is the goal of this institution to serve as a leader in the promotion of health and prevention of illness in the community. Patient education and discharge planning are critical to continuity of care from hospital to home, and are a vital link to achieving this goal. Understanding and implementing this procedure will ensure effective patient education and discharge planning." This is not a cure-all, but it is an important first step in helping nurses to see the need to learn and the importance of their performance to organizational success.

Analyze Cost–Benefit

While cost effectiveness and cost versus benefit are part of the evaluation process, it is helpful to project anticipated expenses for educational programs and compare this to predicted benefits from the outcome of the program. Whenever a new program is proposed, requiring staff development time and expense, it must be justified. Cost–benefit analysis looks at the benefits to be derived from the program compared to the costs. When benefits cannot be quantified according to dollars and cents, they are usually analyzed by quality or effectiveness of the outcome. This analysis not only helps in decision making, but facilitates developing clear goals concerning the outcome of the educational program.

Cost–benefit analysis is also important when considering repeating a previous program, or choosing among other alternatives. In the evaluation process the costs versus benefits or effectiveness should reveal important information concerning revising, repeating, or deleting the program. This analysis should be done at the completion of every program to determine actual costs and outcomes.

Cost–benefit analysis projects any costs incurred through planning, developing, conducting, and evaluating a program, versus the results, such as improved job performance, improved attitudes, job satisfaction, or improved patient outcomes. Costs might include materials, media, personnel time away from patients, salaries of instructors, time involved in developing and evaluating content, equipment, and facilities, among other things. Benefits might include achievement of goals and objectives, improved safety, increased efficiency, increased patient satisfaction, improved job proficiency, among other things. The goal is to evaluate costs versus effectiveness or benefits, and balance the two to produce the same or improved outcomes with decreased costs, or improved outcomes with

TABLE 12–1. QUESTIONS TO ANSWER THROUGH COST–BENEFIT ANALYSIS

1. Is staff development the best solution to this problem?
2. Is the cost worth the outcome or benefit? (Is the problem worth it?)
3. What is the likelihood of solving the problem?
4. What is the cost of the solution in relation to available resources and other priorities?

the same costs. Evaluation of costs and benefits involves deciding what is affordable, what are the payoffs, and what are the most effective approaches or strategies to achieving the results.[7]

Cost–benefit analysis is an important step in justifying a program offering as well as in planning for teaching methodologies and strategies. It causes the educator to examine various solutions to a learning deficit and to identify the most cost-effective one. Cost-effectiveness is evaluated at various stages of program development and implementation, from planning specific content to evaluating achievement of objectives. It is important that the educator predict costs versus benefits prior to devoting time, energy, and resources to a specific solution, only to evaluate after the fact that the solution was either ineffective or more costly than the original problem. A problem or need must be identified as being amenable to staff development. It must be prioritized as important enough to warrant intervention. It must be related to the achievement of nursing and organizational goals. Then the cost of the solution must be weighed against the need or problem, and compared to available resources and other priorities. Cost–benefit analysis consolidates the processes in the first three steps of program development (see Figure 12–4), and ensures within reason that the solution *will solve* the problem or need in the most cost-effective manner (Table 12–1).

Plan the Learning Experience

This step deals with the specifics of the educational program. It has already been determined that a staff development need exists, that it is a high priority and worth the expenditure of time and resources. Now the actual planning of the learning experience must take place. This includes five major concerns: determining objectives, selecting methodology, determining means for evaluation, determining reward mechanisms, and logistics.

Determining Objectives. Since the problem or need and the purpose or relation to organizational goals have been determined, specific objectives or behavioral outcomes must be identified to achieve the purpose and resolve the problem. These must delineate who will learn what, how, when, under what conditions, and the means or criteria by which this learning will be demonstrated or evident. The behavioral objectives should be developed with input from management and the learners involved, and will dictate the content of the program.

Selecting Methodology. The strategy or method for achieving the behavioral objectives and purpose will vary according to the resources, time available, needs of the staff, expertise of the educators, and the educational content. A variety of methods will help keep interest in learning high and provide a more stimulating learning environment. Cost–benefit analysis also is used in selecting methodology—a self-paced learning module for certain basic and repetitive skills training would prove to be more cost-effective than an ongoing lecture format. Also included in selecting methodology is the use of audiovisual material as a medium for teaching. Principles of adult learning theory should be utilized in selecting methodology. Participation of learners, varying learning styles, and varying experiences and needs are a few of the many factors influencing adult learning.

Determining Measures for Evaluation. Program evaluation should be planned prior to implementation, and will be based on the behavioral objectives and program content. It is important that evaluation become an integral part of staff development, and not a paper-and-pencil exercise. If a program cannot be justified as cost-effective and shown to achieve the desired outcomes, it cannot be continued. Measures for determining learning and its application in the work setting must be planned. Evaluation should include achievement of behavioral objectives, application of learning, and learner satisfaction with educational content and methodology. Plans should also include a means to follow up evaluation and control results. Plans for return demonstrations, written tests, follow-up observations on the unit, and other evaluation mechanisms must be developed prior to program implementation. These evaluation tools must be pretested for validity and reliability.

Determining Reward or Reinforcement Mechanisms. As discussed in Chapter 11, people are more motivated to achieve when they are rewarded for their efforts. Systems must be developed to promote learning and improvement and reward achievement. Performance evaluations with merit systems, bonuses for special projects and contributions, promotions and salary increases for clinical advancement or expertise, and career ladders are a few ways established by administration to reinforce continued learning. Special recognition and awards, praise and positive feedback, and other psychic rewards are also invaluable. Program planners should identify specific reward systems for educational activities and work with management to reinforce and reward the application of learning to the work setting. It is essential that management support and understand the learning objectives and provide the reinforcement necessary for transfer of learning to the unit operations. Reward and reinforcement efforts should be planned to result in behavioral changes and improved performance. An intermittent spot check by managers for correct use of a new technique, with approval and praise, may be all that is necessary. Simple and effective reward measures can be built into each program.

Logistics. Any educator knows that program planning involves a number of details for effective implementation. Times, dates, advertising in advance, facilities, materials and resources, and many other factors enter into program planning. Time schedules for program development, flow charts for project completion, and other logistics are necessary to prepare and implement an educational program.

Implement the Learning Experience

Once planning is completed, the learning experience is implemented. If it is independent or self-directed, arrangements are made with management for staff time to complete modules or use the learning resource center. Directions, resources, and completion dates will have been identified so the nurses can work individually at their own pace. Implementation should be a matter of simply carrying out plans.

Evaluate or Revise and Identify Problems

Following implementation, data are collected using preplanned evaluation tools and compared to objectives to determine achievement or nonachievement. The process of the program, as well as the outcome, should be evaluated to determine needed revisions and new needs and problems, which will feed into Step 1, needs assessment and analysis. Evaluation should involve management and the learner, and should include self-evaluation by participants and their reaction or satisfaction with the program. The chief concerns of staff development evaluation are: Did learning occur? Is the learning being transferred to the work setting? Are there improvements in systems, operations, patient satisfaction, or patient outcomes? Was the program cost-effective? The following discussion will address these concerns.

Did Learning Occur? The answer to this question should be found by evaluating achievement of behavioral objectives. Can the learner perform the competencies delineated in the objectives? If clear-cut objectives were developed with measurable criteria, this should be relatively straightforward. The learner scores 90 percent on a written posttest, demonstrates the procedures on a checklist, verbalizes appropriate responses as indicated in the criteria, etc. Of course, all educators know that evaluation is not that simple. Evaluation tools must be objective, valid, and reliable. Testing and ensuring accurate evaluation methods and tools are carried out in the planning stage. With valid and reliable evaluation tools, achievement of objectives should indicate learning did occur.

When objectives are *not* achieved, a determination should be made as to the reason. Questions that should be asked are

1. Were the evaluation tools accurate?
2. Were the objectives realistic and attainable?
3. Were the instructors capable and effective?

4. Was the content appropriate for the learners' preparation and knowledge level?
5. Were the teaching methods and pace for learning appropriate to the learning styles and abilities of the participants?
6. Was practice time provided?
7. Were resources, equipment, and facilities adequate?
8. Were feedback, support, and reinforcement of learning provided?
9. Were there appropriate reward systems?

These and other questions should be asked to determine the reason for failure. If learning is not acquired at this stage, it cannot be transferred to the work setting, and the program will not be cost-effective. All efforts must be made to correct errors and obstacles and to achieve objectives. Special guidance may be needed for slow learners or those in need of additional help.

Is the Learning Being Transferred to the Work Setting? Determining the answer to this question would involve evaluating immediate and long-term effects of the educational program and involves the management team. Preplanning should have included follow-up tools to observe performance according to objectives, or require demonstrations on the unit. By being involved in program planning, management works closely with staff development to achieve mutual objectives. Educational programs geared to achieve organizational goals are part of the performance evaluation and included in the reward system or merit raise system. Not only are employees expected to apply, and assisted in applying, new knowledge; they are evaluated on this application. Management may also complete special evaluation forms for the staff development department, identifying and evaluating the performance of new skills and maintenance of new competencies. Because management is greatly involved in the staff development process, management works hard to reinforce new learning and achieve successful outcomes. Evaluation may occur at invervals—immediately, after 3 to 6 months, and after a year. Again, this is preplanned prior to implementation.

Transfer of learning to the work setting is one of the most important concerns for staff development educators. Although acquiring knowledge is an important first step, this knowledge must be used in order to be effective. The results of staff development are evaluated according to improvement in the nurses' performance. Transfer of learning must take place and result in this improvement. Belinda Puetz[8] described the elements necessary for transfer of learning to practice. These are:

1. The learning experience is based on a learning need identified by both planners and participants, and it can be resolved through education.
2. The closer the relation of a learning need to patient care, the more likely learning will be transferred into practice.

3. The learning experience is planned for a specific audience who have the prerequisite skills and knowledge on which to build.
4. The learner has participated in needs assessment and program planning.
5. Learning objectives are stated behaviorally and the exact desired outcome is clear to the learner.
6. Objectives are realistic and attainable.
7. Program content and learning methodology are appropriate and based on participants' learning styles.
8. Learning experiences actively involve participants, versus passive attendance.
9. Practice and clinical experience are provided in a situation similar to the work environment.
10. Baseline performance is established prior to learning, then follow-up evaluation of objectives is systematic.
11. Newly acquired skills and behaviors are reinforced by peers and management, and rewarded.

Are There Improvements in Systems, Operations, Patient Satisfaction, or Patient Outcomes? The ultimate determinant of successful staff development is its link to organizational success and improvements and patient outcomes. While every educational program will not involve developing extension methods for determining these types of outcomes, it is essential to tie these ultimate outcomes to staff development in some manner.

Baseline data can be established by patient surveys and interviews, time studies, productivity measures, patient turnover and complications, and a vast amount of other sources. Research can be instituted to show the relationship between learning and systems improvement. Although research of this sort is still in its infancy in the clinical setting, educators can take steps to establish "before-and-after" data useful in evaluating progress in the organization. Elaborate methodologies are not required. For example, a simple and clear-cut study showing a relationship between catheter care and decreased urinary infections could be translated to dollars and cents for the organization. While management support and reinforcement is involved in application and transfer of this learning—thus affecting the results—the focus is still on how learning has improved patient outcomes. Staff development educators will become more proficient in this area of evaluation as they are required to become more accountable for results and usefulness of their programs. This accountability is a growing trend.

Was the Program Cost-Effective? Once the evaluation results are determined, these can be compared to the cost of providing the program. Outcomes and costs can be compared to the predicted cost–benefit and cost-effectiveness analysis to help identify problems and improve future predictions and analyses. Summaries of evaluation findings with total costs can be recorded and used for an annual evaluation of staff development costs versus effectiveness, and for future planning. Or program results or "quality" of outcomes can be rated by some numerical scale for determining ratios to cost and for evaluating the cost-effectiveness of the program. In some cases, program outcomes can be quantified into dollars and cents and compared to the cost of assessing, planning, implementation, and evaluating the program. The actual program costs and outcome "earnings or savings" can be compared to determine the cost–benefit ratios. This is helpful in deciding about program revisions and future plans. According to Del Bueno,[9] such comparisons can assist in determining the need to change methodology and strategies, revise plans and objectives, retest evaluation tools for validity and reliability, continue the program, or use different resources and time schedules.

It must be noted that the process of comparing costs to outcomes can in itself be an expensive undertaking. Staff development directors must assess the cost of evaluation and compare it to the actual use of the evaluation results, and decide whether it is worth it. This decision will depend upon the director's expertise, resources, time, needs, and support services. In addition, there are a variety of approaches to assessing cost-effectiveness in staff development, and different approaches may be necessary for different purposes. No one approach is perfect or appropriate for all situations. Directors should determine what information they need and their goals. Evaluation must be realistic and, ideally, fit into existing hospital-wide evaluation systems. The evaluation methodology must be efficient, and results must be usable. The goal is to determine whether the program has achieved its objectives in the most cost-effective manner.[10] Actual program costs can be computed by assessing costs for labor, materials, and overhead.[10] Or costs can be determined for each stage of the program, from assessment to evaluation. Planning costs would include salaries and fringe benefits, travel and meal expenses, and any marketing costs for developing and mailing materials. Implementation costs would include faculty and secretarial salaries for preparations, materials used, supplies, meals and breaks, overhead costs, teaching materials and classroom use. Learner salaries and benefits would also be included with the cost of replacing learners on the unit. Then the cost for evaluating the activity, in terms of time, materials, and secretarial support, would be figured. The total costs can then be divided by the number of participant hours, to determine the cost per participant hour for the program.[9]

If the benefit or outcome can be calculated in terms of dollars, this total dollar amount could be divided by the program cost to result in a ratio. Ratios are useful for comparing and choosing among alternatives.[10]

When program benefits cannot be quantified monetarily, the quality of the results should be measured for comparison to cost. Outcomes can be "qualified" by a variety of mechanisms. Del Bueno suggests using a sliding, numerical scale. Each level on the scale would be assigned a number, which is then used in a ratio with the cost of the offering. The scale could be one to five, and include: *1*, attendance only; *2*, evidence of acquisition of knowledge and skills; *3*, application of knowledge in a simulated setting; *4*, application in a real setting; *5*, maintenance of behaviors. Hard data must support these determinations, using valid and reliable tools.[9]

Cost-benefit and cost-effectiveness ratios can be derived by dividing the *value* of the benefit by the *value* of the costs. These values may be determined by formulas, sliding scales such as the one mentioned, or exact costs, if possible. The value of the cost of the program can also be subtracted from the value of the benefit. A positive or negative result can aid decision making. Or the two values can be compared, using ratios. Projects can be ranked in order of decreasing ratios, to facilitate prioritizing programs and choosing among alternatives. Of course the values must be stated in equal terms, such as using the same numerical rating scale for both program costs and outcomes, or using dollars.

All results cannot be reduced to mathematical formulas. And other factors will enter into outcomes, such as deviations from unit to unit, due to managerial support.[11] But these types of analyses and ratios can result in improved data collection and documentation, and validation of learning and performance. It can ensure that evaluation is not based solely on attendance or participant evaluation ratings.[9] Determination of investments versus outcomes can enhance the total staff development process and enable staff to reach more accurate evaluation results.

CONCLUSION

Human resource development is critical to the successful functioning and overall development of the organization. The most precise and accurate planning systems require human resources who are able to put them into operation effectively. A politically active and progressive marketing team is immobilized if the staff cannot provide competent care and services for the patients. The development of able, proficient, and self-renewing human resources affects the success of every system and process within the organization. Staff development is an integral link to effective human resource management, and ultimately to organizational progress and viability.

This chapter has barely scratched the surface of the staff development process. Rather than focus on specifics of the teaching and learning process, or theories of adult learning, it has concentrated on the components of the process as a whole, and on developing an educational program. A volume could be written on each subject introduced. It is hoped that the nurse-administrator has grasped a perspective of staff development's relationship to human resource management and will provide the needed guidance, support, and direction so vital to staff development personnel. In this world of continual change, commitment to learning and renewal is no longer an option, but a responsibility.

The subject of our last chapter is labor relations. In coordination with the other personnel processes, staff development serves to foster effective employee–employer relations, by building a competent, innovative, and satisfied work force. These relations are enhanced through open communication, trust, and mutual respect. But achievement and maintenance of effective labor relations requires other important strategies, and is a process within itself. These strategies are not only essential to the effectiveness of labor relations, but can affect the outcome of all operations and functions in the organization, and each personnel process. Therefore, the process of maintaining effective, sound employee–employer relations must be closely integrated into human resource management practices. This process is another important determinant of a successful administrative function, and ultimately of organizational progress and viability. And now for the last personnel process: labor relations.

REFERENCES

1. Rowland, H. S., & Rowland, B. L. *Nursing administration handbook.* Rockville, Md.: Aspen, 1980, pp. 160–189.
2. Nadler, L. *Corporate human resources development: A management tool.* New York: Van Nostrand Reinhold, 1980, pp. 26–40.
3. Tobin, H. M., Yoder Wise, P. S., & Hull, P. K. *The process of staff development: Components for change.* St. Louis: C. V. Mosby, 1979, pp. 46–49.
4. Althaus, J. N., Hardyck, N. M., Pierce, P. B., & Rodgers, M. S. *Nursing decentralization: The El Camino experience.* Rockville, Md.: Aspen, 1981, pp. 103–129.
5. Bucalo, J. P. An operational approach to training needs analysis. *Training and Development Journal,* 1984, *38*(12), 80–84.
6. Sovie, M. D. Investigate before you educate. *JONA,* 1981, *11*(4), 16, 17–20.
7. Kearsley, G. *Costs, benefits, and productivity in training systems.* Reading, Mass.: Addison-Wesley, 1982, pp. 2–26.
8. Puetz, B. Evaluation in staff development. Audio-Tape #NEC-167, from *Nursing Resources Spring 1982 Conference.* Chicago: Teach-em, 1982.
9. Del Bueno, D. J., & Kelly, K. J. How cost effective is your staff development program? *JONA,* 1980, *10*(4), 31–36.
10. Puetz, B. *Evaluation in nursing staff development: Methods and models.* Rockville, Md.: Aspen, 1985, pp. 153–161.
11. Stevens, B. *The nurse executive* (2nd ed.). Wakefield, Mass.: Nursing Resources, Inc., 1980, pp. 340–342.

SUGGESTED READING

Adams, S. Self-study for independent learning. *Journal of Continuing Education in Nursing,* 1971, *2*(3), 27–31.

Alexander, C. P. A hidden benefit of quality circles. *Personnel Journal,* 1984, *63*(2), 54–58.

Bell, C. Building a reputation for training effectiveness. *Training and Development Journal*, 1984, *38*(5), 50–54.

Bell, D. F. Assessing learning needs: Advantages and disadvantages of eighteen techniques. *Nurse Educator*, 1979, *3*(5), 15–21.

Bennett, B., & Griswold, D. F. Proving our worth: The training value model. *Training and Development Journal*, 1984, *38*(10), 81–83.

Betz, C. L. Methods utilized in nursing continuing education programs. *Journal of Continuing Education in Nursing*, 1984, *15*(2), 39–44.

Bille, D. A. *Staff development: A systems approach.* Thorofare, New Jersey: Charles B. Slack, Inc., 1982.

Borich, G. D. (Ed.). *Evaluating educational programs and products.* Englewood Cliffs, N.J.: New Jersey Educational Technology Pub., 1974.

Boyle, P. B. *Planning better programs.* New York: McGraw-Hill, 1981.

Bratt, E. M. & Vocrell, E. Concept mastery in nursing staff development. *JNSP*, 1986, *2*(4), 162–164.

Brown, B. (Ed.). Continuing education—Who cares? *Nursing Administration Quarterly*, 1978, *2*(2).

Calkin, J. D. Let's rethink staff development programs. *JONA*, 1979, *9*(6), 16–19.

Cantor, M. M. Staff development: What are the qualifications? In Journal of Nursing Administration, *Staff development. Volume II. A contemporary nursing resource book.* Wakefield, Mass.: Contemporary Publishers, Inc., 1977, pp. 5–7.

Coffey, L. *Modules for independent-individual learning in nursing.* Philadelphia: F. A. Davis, 1975.

Dailey, N. Adult learning and organizations. *Training and Development Journal*, 1984, *38*(12), 64–68.

Davies, L. K. Fitting the media key into instruction. *Training and Development Journal*, 1984, *38*(12), 23–27.

Del Bueno, D. J. Continuing education, spinach and other good things. *JONA*, 1977, *7*(4), 32–34.

Del Bueno, D. J. Need to know versus nice to know. In Journal of Nursing Administration, *Staff development. Volume II. A contemporary nursing resource book.* Wakefield, Mass.: Contemporary Publishers, Inc., 1977, pp. 46–47.

Fay, P. Contracting: A collaborative approach. *JNSP*, 1986, *2*(4), 157–162.

Flanagan, J. C. The critical incident technique. *Psychological Bulletin*, 1954, *51*, 327–358.

Fojtasek, G. A model for evaluating a staff development program. *Journal of Continuing Education in Nursing*, 1985, *16*(2), 58–62.

Frederiksen, N. Proficiency tests for training evaluation. In R. Glaser (Ed.), *Training research and education.* Pittsburgh: University of Pittsburgh Press, 1962.

Gardner, D. E. Five evaluation frameworks: Implications for decision making in higher education. *Journal of Higher Education*, 1977, *48*(5), 571–593.

Gardner, J. *Self-renewal: The individual and the innovative society.* New York: Harper & Row, 1964.

Garen, M. E., & Daniel, J. Construct a training quality control system. *Personnel Administrator*, 1983, *28*(11), 33–79.

Georgenson, D., & Del Gaizo, E. Maximize the return on your training investment through needs analysis. *Training and Development Journal*, 1984, *38*(8), 42–47.

Gessner, B. Second thoughts on needs assessment. *Journal of Continuing Education*, 1982, *13*(3), 46–49.

Gladwin, L. A. The impact of artificial intelligence on training. *Training and Development Journal*, 1984, *38*(12), 46–47.

Goodykoontz, L. Evaluating a continuing education program. *Journal of Continuing Education in Nursing*, 1980, *11*(4), 25–28.

Gosnell, D. Evaluating continuing nursing education. *Journal of Continuing Education in Nursing*, 1984, *15*(1), 9–11.

Greaves, P. E., & Loquist, R. S. Impact evaluation: A competency-based approach. In B. Brown (Ed.), Quality assurance update. *Nursing Administration Quarterly*, 1983, *7*(3), 81–86.

Haggard, A. Decentralized staff development. *Journal of Continuing Education in Nursing*, 1984, *15*(3), 90–92.

Hillelsohn, M. J. How to think about CBT. *Training and Development Journal*, 1984, *38*(12), 42–44.

Hoffman, F. O. A responsive training department cuts costs. *Personnel Journal*, 1984, *63*(2), 48–53.

Jazwiec, R. M. Learning needs assessment: A complex process. *JNSD*, 1985, *1*, 91–96.

Johnson, J. A. Cost, value and productivity: The bottom line in education. *JNSD*, 1986, *2*(1), 28–32.

Kelley, A. I., Orgel, R. F., & Baer, D. M. Evaluation: The bottom line is closer than you think. *Training and Development Journal*, 1984, *38*(8), 32–37.

Kirkpatrick, D. L. Four steps to measuring training effectiveness. *Personnel Administrator*, 1983, *28*(11), 19–25.

Knowles, M. *Self-directed learning: A guide for learners and teachers*. New York: Association Press, 1975, pp. 34–37.

Laird, D., & Belcher, F. How master trainers get that way. *Training and Development Journal*, 1984, *38*(5), pp. 73–75.

MacDonald, D. R., & Stewart, M. R. An increasingly promising training and development alternative to streamline training efforts. *Personnel Journal*, 1983, *62*, 821–825.

Metzger, N. J. Revisiting the preceptor concept: Cross training nursing staff. *JNSP*, 1986, *2*(2), 70–76.

Mitchell, W. S. Wanted: Professional management training needs analysis. *Training and Development Journal*, 1984, *38*(10), 68–70.

Mouton, J. S., & Blake, R. R. Principles and designs for enhancing learning. *Training and Development Journal*, 1984, *38*(12), 60–63.

Munro, B. H. A useful model for program evaluation. *JONA*, 1983, *13*(3), 23–26.

Popiel, E. S. Long-range evaluation of a continuing education course. *Journal of Continuing Education in Nursing*, 1973, *4*(4), 15–17.

Puetz, B. E., & Peters, F. L. Assessing needs and planning learning activities. In *Continuing education for nurses: A complete guide to effective programs*. Rockville, Md.: Aspen, 1981.

Puetz, B., & Rytting, M. B. Evaluation of the effect of continuing education in nursing on health care. *Journal of Continuing Education in Nursing*, 1979, *10*(2), 22–25.

Rothwell, W. J. Curriculum design in training: An overview. *Personnel Administrator*, 1983, *28*(11), 53–57.

Scherer, J. J. How people learn: Assumptions for design. *Training and Development Journal*, 1984, *38*(1), 64–66.

Schileger, P. R. A guide for people who use your video program. *Training and Development Journal*, 1984, *38*(12), 32–34.

Sims, H. P., & Manz, C. C. Modeling influences on employee behavior. *Personnel Journal*, 1982, *61*, 58–65.

Smith, C. E. Planning, implementing, and evaluating learning experiences for adults. *Nurse Educator*, 1977, *3*(6), 31–36.

Smith, C. M. Learning on your own for credit. *AJN*, 1980, *80*(11), 2013–2015.

Steele, S. *Educational Evaluation in Nursing*. Thorofare, New Jersey: Charles B. Slack, 1978.

Stein, L. Adult learning principles: The individual curriculum. *Journal of Continuing Education in Nursing*, 1971, *2*(6), 7–13.

Stufflebeam, D. L., & Webster, W. J. An analysis of alternative approaches to education. *Educational Evaluation and Policy Analysis*, 1980, *2*(3), 5–20.

Thomas, W., & Thomas, C. The payoffs and pitfalls of video-based training. *Training and Development Journal*, 1984, *38*(12), 28–29.

Thompson, M. A. A systematic approach to module development. *Journal of Nursing Education*, 1978, *17*(8), 21.

Tobin, H. Quality staff development: A must for change and survival. In Journal of Nursing Administration, *Staff development. Volume II. A contemporary nursing resource book*. Wakefield, Mass.: Contemporary Pub., Inc., 1977, pp. 40–43.

Vinton, K., Clark, A. O., & Seybolt, J. W. Assessment of training needs for supervisors. *Personnel Administrator*, 1983, *28*(11), 45–51.

Wilson, J. D. Factors influencing results. *Journal of Continuing Education In Nursing*, 1984, *15*(2), 59–62.

13 The Process of Labor Relations

Labor relations are usually thought of in terms of the employer–union relationship. Actually, they should be viewed in a broader context. With the increasing complexities of work life and the rapid rate of change, labor relations are now a concern of all nurse-administrators in any setting. For our purposes, they can be thought of as synonymous with employee relations, and can be defined as the interactions, dealings, or relationship between management and those being managed in a unionized or non-unionized setting.

Labor relations are not a typical personnel process, as are those previously presented. Rather, they constitute a state of being that is continuous and dependent upon various processes. One does not *implement* labor relations, as one can select a new employee or counsel the underachiever. Instead, one must apply knowledge of human resource management in conjunction with an understanding of change to plan and develop strong and productive labor relations. Various processes must come into play to reach the state of effective labor relations. This is the ultimate goal: achieving mutually cooperative employer–employee interactions based on respect, shared values, and unified purposes. Attaining this goal requires effective application of each of the personnel processes, monitoring and controlling of day-to-day employee relations, and an understanding of the collective bargaining process.

EFFECTIVE APPLICATION OF EACH OF THE PERSONNEL PROCESSES

Each personnel process is designed to maximize human potential and talent for both personal and organizational growth. Each process has a specific purpose contributing to organizational viability, such as retaining productive workers or fostering growth and development. These purposes help to produce a competent, innovative, and satisfied workforce committed to organizational success. There is also a by-product from each personnel process that is of great importance. This is the process's contribution to sound, effective employee relations. When effectively implementing each process, a trusting employer–employee relationship evolves. Strategies such as participative management or the use of task forces work to strengthen the link between managers and the managed, and build mutually supportive relations. Although each process has its specific purpose, each process works to build sound and effective employee relations. That is why the status of labor relations greatly depends upon the effective implementation of each personnel process. Table 13–1 reviews some specific aspects of each process that contribute to effective labor relations.

TABLE 13–1. REVIEW OF PERSONNEL PROCESSES AS RELATES TO LABOR RELATIONS

Recruitment

Factors in the recruitment process that directly enhance labor relations include giving priority to internal recruitment, providing equal employment opportunities, job posting, employee participation in the recruitment process, and developing current employees to fill future positions. Fostering a supportive and communicative environment, providing competitive salaries and benefits, and using strategies such as career ladders aid recruitment, retention, and labor relations.

Selection

Strategies in the selection process that enhance labor relations include ensuring equal employment opportunities in selection processes, fairness in all procedures, staff involvement in selection of candidates, and selecting the most qualified person who can grow in the job.

Orientation

Orientation serves to foster the cultural fit and begin the growth and development process, as well as to assist employees to attain minimal level competencies and adjust to the new job. Effective orientation promotes well-being, security, and satisfaction with the job. It creates good feelings about the organization, clarifies roles and expectations, and helps develop a trusting, communicative relationship. All of this contributes to the development of effective employer–employee relations.

Performance evaluation

Performance evaluation contributes to effective employer–employee relations by providing individual guidance for ways to improve; providing feedback concerning performance; increasing and opening communication; being applied fairly, consistently, and objectively; being

TABLE 13–1. (cont.)

based on valid indicators of performance; communicating caring and concern for individual well-being and growth; focusing on ways to improve skills, knowledge, and talents for self-satisfaction; being based on clear expectations and criteria, and providing resources, support, and direction for continued growth and development. Also, the use of self-evaluation, self-objectives, and peer review of standards and quality of care contribute to effective labor relations.

Counseling and coaching

Counseling and coaching enhances labor relations by assisting employees with problems and in need of counseling; offering peer assistance programs; assisting in overcoming performance problems; developing trust and open communication; providing justified progressive discipline procedures based on due process and just cause, and offering appeals and grievance mechanisms that are fair and accepted by employees.

Retention and productivity

An effective retention and productivity process directly enhances labor relations. This process serves to promote and maintain job satisfaction by meeting employee needs for good working conditions; competitive salaries and benefits; a trusting, communicative, and caring environment; a sense of competency; and satisfying group interactions. It promotes individual motivations congruent with organizational needs by offering attainable opportunities to succeed and advance; psychic income; incentives linked to performance and rewarded objectively and fairly; and individual freedom to exercise controls over work. This process serves to develop satisfied employees who will stay and grow with the organization. It promotes a mutually satisfying employer–employee relationship.

Staff development

This process enhances effective labor relations by offering continual growth and development experiences that satisfy personal achievement and competency needs. It promotes individual accountability through contracting, self-objectives, and self-directed learning. This meets needs for control, independence, and individuality. Staff development programs are based on needs analysis completed and compiled by employees, as well as involve employees in planning, implementation, and evaluation. Programs include all hospital employees and are geared to break down barriers among departments and open communication. Staff development programs not only assist with gaining new skills and knowledge needed for the job, but include outside trends, future plans, issues concerning health care workers, and physical and mental health programs for employees. Staff development trains for creative thinking and offers a means for self-expression through participation. It opens communication and offers a means to channel ideas and suggestions and test new ideas. This all promotes effective labor relations.

MONITORING AND CONTROLLING EMPLOYEE RELATIONS

Although each personnel process has a mechanism to evaluate its effectiveness, special attention must be given to the overall monitoring, improvement, and controlling of day-to-day labor relations in all aspects of human resource management. Steps must be taken to resolve issues, conflicts, and disequilibrium that can stress these relations. Measures to identify and solve problems have been previously discussed, such as employee surveys, employee evaluation of managers, exit interviews, one-to-one communication, and problem-solving task forces. There are a multitude of approaches to eliciting employees' attitudes and concerns and involving them in problem solving. All efforts must be made to ensure fair, uniform application of policies and procedures in a supportive, communicative way. These measure and practices must be instituted *before* an organizing drive occurs. Employees must be given continual feedback, and open communication must be maintained. Management actions must be taken to detect problems early and ensure immediate corrections.

One very important means for monitoring, improving, and controlling labor relations, as well as resolving conflicts, is through an appeals or grievance system. These procedures provide a means for identifying inequities, issues, and perceived unfair management practices, and for allowing fair resolution of grievances. Not only can disputes between management and employees be resolved, but steps can be taken to correct and improve poor conditions or relationships. Grievance procedures will only be briefly discussed in this chapter, as they were explored in Chapters 9 and 10.

THE COLLECTIVE BARGAINING PROCESS

The goal of achieving sound, effective labor relations also depends on a broad understanding of unions and collective bargaining. If a nurse-administrator is functioning under a union contract, he or she must possess an intricate knowledge of the roles, responsibilities, and legal requirements of employers and employees under this contract. The entire management team must understand the principles and conditions for effective collective bargaining and maintenance of sound employee relations throughout the day-to-day administration of the contract. An administrator faced with an organizing effort must possess knowledge of legalities and forces involved in organizing, from recognition to negotiations.

If a nurse-administrator is in a nonunionized setting, the entire management team must understand these principles and concepts to better adapt, predict, and respond to the forces of change. Understanding trends, issues, and facts about unionization can improve awareness of needs in the organization. From an understanding of negotiations and codetermination of decisions, issues and conditions contributing to dissatisfaction can be resolved and a more satisfying, participative organizational climate established.

The process of building effective labor relations does not begin when an organizing drive is within the organization. The process begins voluntarily by an enlightened administration that realizes the need for good employee relations. Ensuring effective implementation of personnel processes, providing mechanisms to correct conflicts, and using knowledge of collective bargaining are all necessary to provide a mutually satisfying, productive climate. An administrator working currently in an organized setting who undertakes these efforts will foster effective, productive relations. An administrator in a nonunionized setting who voluntarily undertakes these efforts will rarely be faced with an organizing effort. In either case, building effective labor relations is an important part of human resource management.

Because much of this book has been devoted to discussions concerning effective personnel processes and building sound employee relations, this chapter will focus mainly on the collective bargaining process. An overview of the literature on important aspects of collective bargaining will be presented. This overview is meant to serve as an introduction and framework for further study. It will proceed from trends and changes, through legislation affecting unionization, to negotiations and contract administration.

COLLECTIVE BARGAINING AND THE FORCES OF CHANGE

Basically, collective bargaining is a process in which employee representatives meet with hospital representatives to negotiate a contract defining the terms of employment for a certain period of time. This process goes through various stages but, according to Berkeley, concerns promise making, or contract negotiation and promise checking or contract administration.[1] Collective bargaining does not just happen. Many conditions and factors set the stage for an employee move to organize or form a union for the purpose of collective bargaining. The forces of change have affected nurses' perceptions of unionization, need to take control over the conditions and terms of their work, and willingness to resort to collective bargaining. The following discussion will provide an overview of some of these changes.

According to Cohen,[2] registered nurses' participation in unionization has drastically increased over the past 20 years. She cites the following factors as contributing to this increased activism:

1. Legislation allowing and regulating employees in private, nonprofit hospitals the right to strike
2. The inattention by employers to individual employee needs and working conditions, unless organized into a collective group
3. Observance of semiskilled employees' growth in earnings and rights due to their organization
4. The observance of other professional groups', like teachers', involvement in unionization
5. Frustration with the "handmaiden" role and poor image

6. Eroding power in unions and their need for increased membership and strength, causing them to turn to health care employees
7. The experience, resources, and support unions are offering to nurses to organize and negotiate

Flanagan[3] cites the factors contributing to increased unionization of health care employees as being: (1) growth in larger, multisystem hospitals; (2) highly technical, specialized, and depersonalized work environments; (3) legislation favoring employee rights to unionize; (4) poor working environment and conditions; (5) increased assertiveness and activism by professional nurses; and (6) the need for unions to increase their membership.

A report by the National Labor Relations Board (NLRB) representatives predicted an increase in strained relations between employers and organized labor resulting from mounting financial pressures. Hospitals are cutting staff and shifting responsbility, causing growing disputes between labor and management.[4]

Flanagan[3] describes eight major factors that are affecting nurses' propensity toward collective bargaining. These include:

1. Widened scope of nursing practice and responsibilities resulting in need for appropriate autonomy and authority consistent with this heightened responsibility
2. Collective bargaining activities of other professionals such as physicians, teachers, and social workers, making it appear less "unprofessional"
3. Effects of the feminist movement to improve pay and women's rights and to correct inequities in the work environment
4. The consistently low salaries of nurses
5. Dissatisfaction with administrative attitudes towards professional nurses, nonnursing tasks, lack of inclusion in work-related decision making, poor staffing, and other working conditions
6. Growth of the concept of "professional collectivism," which justifies collective bargaining. This concept is based on the belief that nurses are responsible for ensuring quality patient care, but this quality is dependent upon maintaining work satisfaction and appropriate working conditions
7. Growth of the number of labor unions intent on soliciting registered nurses
8. Increased negotiations concerning standards of practice, nursing roles, establishment of practice committees, and other professional concerns

The forces of change have affected the worker, the work, and the work environment in ways that contribute to increased collective bargaining. As discussed in Chapter 11, nurses are staying in the work force longer, are more aware of their rights, and are more politically active. As a whole, they have become more assertive and seek professional respect, job satisfaction, and control over their practice. Concurrently, the work has become increasingly complex and demanding. Decreases in length of stay, cutting costs, increased patient acuity, and high technology have contributed to this complexity and demand. The hospital environment has also changed. Growth in the size of hospitals can increase the complexity and distance between administration and employees. The emphasis on cost control and competition can lead to lack of concerns for employee satisfaction. All of these changes can set the stage for employee organizing. A frustrated, overworked work force that is cut off from top administration and feels abused will turn to collective bargaining. To them, it is the only way to be heard or be involved.

Issues of concern to nurses that are motivators toward collective bargaining include control over nursing practice and redistribution of power in the organizational setting;[5] comparable economic conditions among similar employees in other local hospitals and within the facility; lack of job security resulting from ineffective grievance systems; favoritism in applying policies and in staffing; lack of support for continuing education; and lack of orientation for assignment to various units.[6] Lack of reward and recognition, lack of communication, mounting work pressures and paperwork, lack of advancement opportunities, and lack of input into patient care were also identified as concerns of nurses. The stress of understaffing along with conflicting physician–nurse relationships add to this dissatisfaction and interest in unions as an alternative. Many nurses realize that unions do not solve all problems, but it is the perception that hospitals do not care and will not work to alleviate these problems that is the impetus for unionizing.[6] Nurses want to voice their concerns, be heard, and be involved in working out solutions. These concerns and issues should sound familiar, as they have been explored through this text, and affect the status of labor relations. Basically, when nurses lack a satisfying, motivating environment and have poor employer–employee relations, they seek solutions. In more and more cases, collective bargaining is this solution.

While activity in unionization has increased, many nurses are just beginning to view collective bargaining as a means for resolving problems. They are concerned with injuring their professional image with the public. Some nurses fear losing individual decision making and autonomy to group and collective decision making. Others fear an autocratic union leader or the effects of a strike on patient care. Stern[7] states that these concerns stem from misconceptions and lack of understanding of the collective bargaining process. Proponents state that strikes can gain nurses needed security, economic rewards, and working conditions so they can provide quality patient care. Ample notice is given for preparation and coverage during the walkout. When job satisfaction is restored, energies can be directed toward providing patient care.[8] Collective bargaining contracts can contain provisions for nursing practice councils and sharing of governance, provisions for individual accountability, and peer evaluation or review, defining the professional nurse's role, and maintaining standards of care. The contract can be used to hold both the nurses and administration accountable for quality service to the public.[9] The trend away from pure economic interests to issues of governance, accountability, and standards of care has helped the collective bargaining movement in nursing.

LEGISLATIVE CHANGE

Legislative change has also affected the rise of union activity in the health care setting. In 1935 the National Labor Relations Act (NLRA) was passed, legalizing unionization by private sector employees in order to negotiate wages and working conditions. This act exempted public employees from collective bargaining under the provisions of the act, but not employees of private, nonprofit hospitals. The employees of profit-making or nonprofit private hospitals were protected by the NLRA.[10] Passed during the Depression, the NLRA was designed to help restore stability and ease tensions among the nation's work force, and by improving purchasing power, to increase spending and employment.

The NLRA created the National Labor Relations Board (NLRB) to administer the NLRA. The functions of the NLRB are to determine the appropriate bargaining unit for collective bargaining, to conduct elections concerning employee representation, and to investigate and prevent unfair labor practices. The determination of the appropriate bargaining unit involves questions of which employees should be included in a bargaining unit, as well as what is considered an appropriate unit. The needs of each occupation must be considered without creating an unnecessary proliferation of bargaining units in one facility.[11]

In 1947 the Labor-Management Relations Act, or the Taft-Hartley Act, was passed, amending the NLRA. These amendments served to balance many prounion practices by further defining and restraining unfair labor practices. The Federal Mediation and Conciliation Service (FMCS) was established as an independent agency under the federal government to provide third-party assistance in labor disputes. Also, and most importantly for nurses, the NLRA was amended to exempt private, nonprofit hospital employees from NLRA coverage and made them subject to varying state laws. This Tydings Amendment served to restore the charitable image of the nonprofit hospital, and was passed with the support of the American Hospital Association.[10]

Between 1947 and 1974 several other significant acts were passed. The Landrum-Griffin Act, or the Labor-Management Reporting and Disclosure Act, was passed in 1959. This was a means to monitor union and employer financial transactions, internal union practices, and require disclosure of operations in order to prevent abuses and improve individual union members' rights. Then Executive Orders 10988 and 11491 established procedures, guidelines, and regulations for collective bargaining in the federal sector.[10]

After the Taft-Hartley Act in 1947, nonprofit hospitals were exempt from the requirement to negotiate with their employees. Hospital administrators could *voluntarily* elect to recognize a unit and negotiate, but employees were not protected or regulated by the NLRB. Although this exemption was amended in 1974, Arndt and Huckabay state that nurses experienced major setbacks due to the Taft-Hartley amendment. The lack of protection for employees in private, nonprofit hospitals between 1947 and 1974 caused an effect on nursing that is still present today. This effect includes:

1. The continued opposition by hospital administrators to recognition and meaningful bargaining with nurses
2. A lack of knowledge and general apathy by nurses towards collective bargaining
3. A lack of economic strength to support collective bargaining[12]

With the increase in union activity in federal and public sectors and the large number of recognition strikes by employees exempt from NLRB certification procedures, the Taft-Hartley Act was finally amended.[13] In 1974, as we have seen, Congress removed the exclusion of private, nonprofit hospitals and provided their employees coverage under the National Labor Relations Act. (Privately owned proprietary hospitals came under NLRB jurisdiction in 1967.) Now any nongovernment-operated hospital was subject to NLRB regulations. In order to avoid disruption of patient care, certain special requirements were established for the field of health care. These requirements concerned giving a ten-day strike notice, notice of contract expiration, and mediation through the Federal Mediation and Conciliation Service in the potential event of interruption of services. Those not complying with NLRB regulations were committing unfair labor practices.[14]

NLRB and Appropriate Bargaining Units

When the NLRB was established, it was given responsibility for administering the Labor Relations Act, along with the congressional instruction that it not contribute to the proliferation of the number of units in a single facility. Congress did not want a multitude of small bargaining units to exist within one hospital. Prior to an election, the NLRB determined which employees could constitute a bargaining unit, based on the following factors: common interests among the employees, common skills and supervision, degree of contact with other employees, degree of integration of functions among employees, and previous bargaining practices and patterns. The appropriate employee bargaining units determined by the Board were set as:

1. R.N.s
2. Physicians employed by a hospital
3. All other professionals
4. Service and maintenance workers
5. Technical employees
6. Office clericals
7. Maintenance and boiler operators with special interests

Despite this decision, there remains much controversy over the number of appropriate units, and there is conflict between NLRB and the courts. Employers can refuse to accept an NLRB decision and take it to the courts. In some cases the courts are overturning NLRB rulings. Decisions by NLRB are being made now on a case-by-case basis.[2]

To complicate the matter, the NLRA stipulates that supervisors may not be included among others in a unit, nor may professional employees be included with nonprofessional employees in a unit unless the professionals voted for this inclusion. The NLRB determines who are supervisors and who are professionals when determining an appropriate bargaining unit. This decision is made according to the individual employee's function and the congressional statutes.[15] According to the statutory definition, a supervisor is someone with the authority to hire, discharge, suspend, lay off, transfer, promote, recall, discipline, reward, assign, adjust grievances, direct other employees, and exercise independent judgment. This definition makes it difficult to distinguish between a nurse-supervisor and a nurse who is supervising other employees as part of the nurse's professional role in patient care.[11] Several employers argue against representation by the state nursing associations because supervisory nurses are members and pay dues to the association. Past NLRB rulings have stated that no clear conflict of interest is present that impedes the collective bargaining process with professional organizations. But employers can contest this representation, stating domination by supervisors in the association, and tie up organizing efforts for years. To avoid this, some state associations are establishing separate economic and general welfare functions as an independent organization.[16] In addition, state associations are concerned about a drop in membership due to collective bargaining functions. Separation of the economic and general welfare component from the other aspects of these associations has become a big issue among the membership—especially among supervisory nurses. This issue is further contributing to the establishment of separate economic and general welfare functions within many state associations.

Where the NLRB has been determining appropriate bargaining units according to the community of interests cited, a 1984 circuit court ruling rejected this and recommended determination based on *broad groups with diverse interests*. Sharper differences would have to be shown among employees' working conditions, functions, and hours.[17] In different regions the NLRB is issuing conflicting rulings concerning the appropriateness of the all-R.N. unit. Due to this change in interpretation, in one region the Maryland Nurses' Association is now representing the first all-professional unit of R.N.s, pharmacists, medical laboratory technicians, counselors, nurse-anesthetists, and physician assistants.[18] Much conflict can be expected to exist over the special needs of R.N.s and the appropriateness of an all-R.N. bargaining unit.

Federal Mediation and Conciliation Service

As stated earlier, the Taft-Hartley Act created the Federal Mediation and Conciliation Service. The FMCS is a government agency that helps prevent labor disputes. According to the 1974 amendments to the NLRA, newly organized bargaining units must notify the FMCS 30 days prior to contract negotiations, and with an existing unit, 60 days prior to the expiration of the contract when an agreement has not been made. Of course, an additional ten-day strike notice is also required. Once notice is received, the FMCS assigns a mediator to contact both parties and investigate the entire situation and status of negotiations. The mediator will report to the FMCS, who then determines the need for appointing an impartial board of inquiry (BOI). This BOI undertakes fact-finding, which is a neutral investigation with recommendations that the parties can accept, reject, or use in negotiations. The mediator from the FMCS continues to meet with both parties. He or she simply acts as a resource and neutral person to aid the bargaining process.[19]

EMPLOYEE ELECTIONS

The National Labor Review Board monitors and determines unfair labor practices and conducts elections for employees deciding about their representation. The following discussion will briefly review these functions.

A union becomes the exclusive bargaining agent for a group of employess in two ways. The union can present authorization cards signed by a majority of employees in that group, and make a formal demand to the employer to be recognized. Or the union can file a petition to NLRB for an election and present authorization cards by 30 percent of the employees in that group. If no agreement is reached by the employer and the proposed union for a consent election, a hearing officer from the NLRB will conduct a hearing of the facts and evidence and present a report to the regional director, who in turn either dismisses the petition or directs an election. A date is then set and an election held, usually on the premises of the employer.[20]

Elections are supervised by the NLRB regional office. Employees vote in favor of or against unionization, and if more than one union is on the ballot, the winner gets exclusive representation rights for the group. The winner is determined by majority vote, *not* by the majority number of employees. Therefore, the outcome is determined by how many employees cast a vote. Either party can contest the verdict on grounds of unfair labor practices, such as intimidation of employees by employer or unions, interference of the election process, or misrepresentation by either party.[20]

UNFAIR LABOR PRACTICES

Heylman states that unfair labor practices are committed by both management and employees and are defined by law.[21] The following lists some examples of unfair practices on both parts.

Unfair Labor Practices by Employers

1. Threatening employees who vote or join a union
2. Questioning employees concerning their union activities
3. Awarding salary increases to prevent employees from joining or voting for a union
4. Firing an employee for participating in organizing drives or joining a union
5. Firing employees who engage in lawful strikes, following appropriate notice of intent to strike
6. Firing an employee who testifies at an NLRB hearing
7. Changing salaries or benefits without collaborating with union representatives
8. Threatening to shut down the hospital if employees join a union
9. Spying on union meetings
10. Discriminating against a qualified applicant due to union membership

Unfair Labor Practices by Unions

1. Picketing tactics that prevent nonunion employees from working
2. Picketing for extended periods (over 30 days) without petitioning for a union election
3. Excessively raising union member fees when members have a union–shop agreement, or must become members of the union
4. Threatening to picket the employer due to a business association with another business the union sees as "unfair"
5. Refusing to negotiate with designated employer representatives

6. Terminating a contract and engaging in a strike without proper notice to the employer and FMCS, or state agency
7. Threatening employees with job loss if they do not support the union
8. Engaging in violence during picketing or strikes
9. Pressuring employers without union–shop agreements to hire only employees who belong to the union[21]

An unfair labor charge is filed with the NLRB by an individual, union, or the employer. A hearing is conducted by an administrative law judge and reviewed by the board, who issues a decision. If a decision states that unfair labor practices have occurred, a corrective action is ordered, which could include reinstatement with back pay, an order to supply certain information, an order to bargain, or other orders.[22]

UNION SOLICITATION

Employees' rights to participate in union activities, attempt organization, and to strike, as well as employer rights to make views known on unionization, are defined by law, along with the unfair labor practices.[20] Additional legal specifications have been added for hospitals in regard to strike notification (as previously mentioned) and union solicitation. In general, a hospital can forbid union activity, such as distributing prounion literature in patient-care areas. Conversely, union solicitation cannot be forbidden in areas where it would not disrupt patient care, such as in cafeterias, main lobbies, and lounges. Court rulings and NLRB decisions have been conflicting on this issue. Court rulings have been in favor of solicitation in gift shops, cafeterias, and nonpatient lounges, as not to interfere with the organizing rights. The burden seems now to be on the hospital to show that solicitation would be detrimental to patient care or disturb patients.[10]

UNIONS REPRESENTING NURSES

Before delving further into the collective bargaining process, mention should be made of the various unions representing registered nurses. Once nurses decide to organize, they must determine who will represent them. Flanagan[3] describes the following unions as representing the majority of health care employees:

American Nurses' Association

This is a professional association that assists and supports its state level associations in organizing and collective bargaining. Each state develops its own policies and procedures in regard to the bargaining process, and some are very active, while others do not participate in any collective bargaining activities. Most employees represented are registered nurses, but licensed practical nurses or other professional employees are represented by some state associations. The American Nurses' Association sets standards, position statements, and recommendations. In addition to economic issues, state nurses' associations are negotiating issues concerning professional standards, practice-related committees, roles and responsibilities of nurses, as well as staffing and assignments, staff development, performance evaluation procedures, and mechanisms for peer review of quality of nursing care.

Service Employees International Union (SEIU)

This union is the oldest union in the health care industry and has the largest membership. Organized under the American Federation of Labor in 1921, it began representing hospital employees in the 1930s. It represents employees in public, nonprofit, and private facilities, and is composed of professionals, paraprofessionals, and technicians. Negotiating teams consist of elected members and an officer, and must ratify all negotiations with the affected members.

National Union of Hospital and Health Care Employees

This union began in 1932 as the bargaining agent for pharmacists in New York City. It began representing hospital employees in the 1950s. Known as Local 1199, this union is part of the Retail, Wholesale, and Department Store Union of the CIO and has four main divisions: registered nurses; hospital employees; professional, technical, and office employees; and the drug division. A specific unit in one facility would be a part of the appropriate division, but make decisions based on individual bargaining unit needs.

The American Federation of Teachers (AFL-CIO)

This is a teachers' union that developed a division for nurses—the American Federation of Nurses. It is now engaged in actively organizing health care employees and nurses.

The American Federation of Government Employees

The largest federal union, it consists of a professional and nonprofessional bargaining unit in Veterans Administration facilities.

American Federation of State, County, and Municipal Employees

Primarily a union representing public employees, it has begun organizing in the private sector. With a drop in membership and government cutbacks, it is beginning to focus on the health care industry.[3]

Summary

The above discussion has focused on changes, trends, and general background information in unions and collective bargaining. It has only provided a condensed overview, and should be supplemented with further study and reading. It is important that nurse-administrators on all levels understand the history and developments of collective bargaining in health care, whether practicing in a unionized or nonunionized facility. This information can serve as a knowledge base in maintaining effective employer–employee relations, effectively administering an existing contract, or negotiating a new contract.

NEGOTIATIONS

Once nurses have organized, held elections, and been recognized as a bargaining unit, employment issues must be settled. The final results of the settlement between employer and union depend on the relative bargaining power of each party and the negotiating skills of the bargainers. Bargaining power is the ability to secure a settlement on one's own terms, and involves the relative cost of disagreeing versus the cost of agreeing with the other bargainer's demands. Although the cost of agreeing versus disagreeing is manipulated and altered during the negotiations, there are definite factors that affect the motivation to accept or reject demands.[23]

Cost of Disagreeing

The union's ultimate bargaining power is its ability to hurt the employer by imposing a strike. The *cost of disagreeing,* resulting from a strike, will depend on the union's ability to increase a strike's effectiveness, and an employer's ability to minimize its effect on operations. A union's bargaining power in imposing costs on the employer through a strike is affected by

1. Internal unity, which increases with the proportion of members who will strike and remain on strike
2. Strike funds, collected through dues and other financial support, which can minimize the adverse economic effects of strikes on members and prolong the ability to remain on strike
3. Other financial support systems to members, such as information about food stamps, financial aid, and extended credit from local banks and merchants during strikes. Financial counseling for ways to prepare for strikes by saving portions of paychecks will also help workers to survive while on strike
4. Another union's willingness to honor the strike and not cross picket lines can prevent employers from operating and increase costs from the strike[23]

An employer's ability to minimize the cost of a strike and to increase bargaining power is affected by several factors, some of which include:

1. Preparation in advance for a strike and buildup of needed inventories so as not to totally disrupt operations

2. Preparing trained supervisors to operate the facility
3. Preparing the financial position of the facility in case of a strike through special savings, short-term loans, or special insurance for strikes

Both unions' and employers' cost of disagreeing are affected by other factors, such as unemployment (which would increase the employer's ability to replace workers during a strike) and nature of the workers involved in the strike (strikers in key positions can disrupt the entire operation of the facility).[23]

Cost of Agreeing

The other main determiner of bargaining power is the *cost of agreeing* with the other bargainer's demands. The cost of agreeing falls into three areas: direct costs, secondary costs, and nonmarket costs. Direct costs concern the specific cost of demands such as wage increases, extended vacation time and holidays, and the expected duration of the provisions. Secondary costs of agreement include the associated costs for increased benefits to other employees in another bargaining unit or nonunion workers. Nonmarket costs involve union provisions that interfere with decision making of administration and the freedom of workers. These are noneconomic costs that subjectively influence willingness to agree to the other's demands. Bargaining power in relation to the cost of agreement depends on what is being bargained. A union's bargaining power will be decreased if the cost of agreement is too high for management to agree to its demands. The cost of agreeing and disagreeing is further determined and clarified through the negotiation process.[23]

Preparing for Negotiations

Even if the nurse-administrator does not sit at the bargaining table, he or she is involved in directing the negotiators in decisions regarding nursing service. The nurse-administrator must live with the contract on a day-to-day basis, and therefore must be active in its development. The following are some guidelines for preparing to work in an organized work force and for negotiations.

1. Understand the content of the laws applicable to your institution, such as the Labor Management Relations Act, or Executive Order 11491
2. Review the original NLRB certification to understand which employees are legally recognized as a bargaining unit
3. Enroll in a course in labor relations to gain an understanding of the collective bargaining process
4. Educate supervisors about labor relations *prior to* a drive
5. Know the rights of management personnel as well as employee rights

6. Contact and use labor relations experts and consultants
7. Anticipate union demands by reviewing previous issues, problems, and grievances of employees
8. Continually review labor relations literature and periodicals for updates and trends
9. Learn the vocabulary of labor relations and negotiations
10. Keep in mind that employees have the right to organize and are protected by law. Their representative must try to obtain the best contract possible for the members. You, as the nurse-administrator, are responsible for the level of nursing care and for managing that nursing care
11. Also, consider the possibility of a strike and prepare for this possibility
12. Review existing contracts and anticipate changes
13. Study the current salaries and benefits in the immediate geographic area and determine your facilities' position on this scale
14. Understand that issues concerning wages, hours, and conditions of employment must be negotiated in good faith. Understand what constitutes unfair labor practices[24]

Claus[25] states that successful negotiations depend upon the composition of the bargaining team, the timing of negotiations, and the content of negotiations, as well as the negotiation site. He states that management's bargaining team should consist of an expert in labor relations or personnel, finance, administration, and nursing. Team members should at least equal the number on the union's team. The nursing director, hospital administrator, and board members should not sit at the bargaining table, but should meet with the bargaining team to direct decision making. Each team selects a spokesperson. The union's team usually consists of selected employees with influence and a representative from the labor organization.

Negotiations begin 90 days before an existing contract expires, and shortly after a new bargaining unit's legal recognition and certification. Areas to be negotiated are defined by law, and although they must be discussed, an agreement or concession is not mandatory. The site for negotiations must be agreed upon, and should be in a neutral setting without interference.[25]

In preparing for bargaining, inside negotiators who remain in the organization throughout the day-to-day contract administration are favored. While an outside negotiator can maintain objectivity, he or she will leave the contract administration to others. It is possible that an outside negotiator could also seek spectacular results as a means to enhance his or her own reputation and future prospects. Preparations should include gathering all possible information about the employee team; obtaining guidelines and parameters from top administration and the board; anticipating and evaluating union demands; gathering internal and external financial information; gathering demographic data on the employees; and developing an employer's negotiation position.[26]

Additional suggestions for preparing negotiations include[27]:

1. Keep both negotiating teams small enough to be productive
2. Agree to the length of time for each bargaining session
3. Proposals should be exchanged prior to negotiations
4. Negotiators need the authority to make a commitment during the bargaining process
5. Negotiations should be preceded by an agenda and list of relevant economic data (developed through a prenegotiation conference)
6. Less controversial issues should be resolved and put in writing prior to approaching more difficult issues
7. Economic and noneconomic issues should be separated for negotiations
8. A decision must be reached concerning negotiating economic issues separately or as a total economic package

Negotiating Techniques

Successful bargaining agreements depend upon skill in negotiating. Although it is not possible to provide comprehensive information on negotiating strategies and techniques in this text, a summary of points and tips can be provided. These serve as an overview of the negotiating process and provide insight into the need for extensive training and expert knowledge prior to bargaining.

Some ground rules for negotiators should first be understood. These include[28]:

- Do not agree to a press blackout, because the employer may decide to take some issues to the public in the event of an impasse (inability to mutually resolve an issue)
- The employer should see the union's demands prior to submitting its proposals—do not submit a joint proposal
- Prohibit tape recorders during the negotiations, as they inhibit the flow of communication
- Refuse to allow settlements to become retroactive

Some techniques for negotiating contracts include[28]:

1. Attempt to agree on some items early in order to build the climate for negotiations
2. Try to deal in packages, combining union demands into one package
3. Agree on ideas first, then clarify with specific language

4. When an issue cannot be resolved, pass over it for the time being rather than becoming bogged down
5. Try to trade a significant union item for a "not so significant" employer issue
6. Put agreements in writing as they are reached
7. Show good-faith bargaining when not agreeing to a proposal by explaining rationale and offering counterproposals as a compromise
8. Use subcommittees to help resolve complex items
9. Use the word "no" very carefully, and do not imply flexibility on a issue the board will never agree to change
10. Use "sidebar" conversations between chief negotiators to discuss issues confidentially in private
11. Use contract language that does not require an oral explanation; refrain from phrases such as "every effort," "if possible," and use absolute terms
12. Negotiators should keep their sense of humor to relieve tensions and keep communications open
13. The chief negotiator should call a caucus of his or her team to help plan strategies, share information, break tensions, and refresh members, allow time to think, and give the impression of difficulty
14. Ensure that the union can claim some type of victory in order to sell the settlement to its members

Deadlocks

When issues cannot be resolved, certain steps can be taken to help reach an agreement—mediation, fact-finding, arbitration, and strike. Mediation and fact-finding were discussed earlier under the section concerning the Federal Mediation and Conciliation Service. Neither of these can dictate the terms of a settlement, but only provide assistance in resolving issues.[25]

Arbitration is a nonjudicial means for resolving a dispute, and results in a binding decision for both parties. *Interest arbitration* concerns a binding decision by the arbitrator for a new contract, and is usually used where a no-strike agreement is in effect or required by law. *Rights or grievance arbitration* is used more often, and is the means for resolving an issue under an existing contract. A contract will define the steps in a grievance procedure, where arbitration is the final step (refer to Chapter 9 and 10 concerning grievance procedures). The arbitrator's verdict is binding and rarely taken to court (if so, it may meet with little success). Arbitrators are selected by both parties and must be neutral. Usually they are selected from a list provided by the American Arbitration Association (AAA) or the FMCS.[1]

Strike Contingency Plans

If both parties fail to reach an agreement through negotiations, mediation, and fact-finding, the result can be the collective stopping of work by employees—a strike. Because a strike is always a possibility, advanced planning or a strike contingency plan is a must to minimize the adverse effects of the strike as well as to promote positive employee relations once the strike is over. The negotiating process and the strike will eventually be over, and employers and employees will be left to work together under the contract. All interactions and communications occuring through these processes will affect the long-term relationships of management and union members, so must be undertaken with an attitude of mutual respect and cooperation.

The first step before developing a strike contingency plan is to examine the circumstances surrounding the potential strike. The employer should ask himself or herself the following questions:

1. Is the strike avoidable? Are there other avenues left that could help settle the dispute?
2. Have prestrike nogotiations been constructive, or is the dispute not significant enough to justify a strike?
3. What are the chances of winning for both sides?
4. Can the facility hold out indefinitely, and what personnel will be used?
5. Does the employer believe that his position is morally right?
6. What does the union really want, and what promises has it made to members?
7. What position is the union in to compromise?
8. What are the financial resources available to members on strike?
9. How many employees can be expected to strike, and how many employees can be expected not to cross picket lines?[29]

In preparing for a strike, it is important to understand what *kind* of strike is occurring—unfair labor practice strike, economic strike, or unprotected strike.

A strike occurring due to an *unfair labor practice* is when the employer violates the Labor Act in some way, such as by firing an employee for union activities, and the employees strike over this issue. If this charge is later substantiated, these employees are entitled to reinstatement to their previous positions upon request.

The *economic strike* occurs over issues such as salaries and benefits, or even work schedules. These strikers may be permanently replaced, as long as during the strike the employer does not commit unfair labor practices.

The third type of strike is the *unprotected strike,* where employees lose protection under the Labor Act and give up rights to reinstatement. This would occur if employees did not give the required ten-day notice and could be discharged.[29]

In preparation of a strike contingency plan, a committee should first be formed representing the hospital departments. Everyone should be kept informed of contract expiration and the status of negotiations. A plan for a shutdown with layoffs of nonstriking employees or for operating during the strike should be developed. Preparations for hiring strike replacements, possible mass picketing and potential violence, prevention of unfair labor practices, and preparation for disseminating information to the public should be included in the plan.[29] Contingency measures should include stockpiling of necessary supplies; arranging patients into three categories: those who can be discharged, those who *may* be discharged if absolutely necessary, and those who will still require care; and assigning the strikers' work to supervisors, volunteers, and nonstriking professionals.[30]

In developing a strike contingency plan, the employer must consider the long-term effects of a strike and attempt to balance the needs of the organization with a concern for good employee relations. A coordinator of the strike plan should be appointed who can support management personnel and also communicate that employees have the right to free speech and to strike. He or she must provide the leadership to maintain cooperative relationships with striking employees and set the stage for a smooth transition once the strike is over.[31] Supervisors must be coached in interpersonal techniques to restore harmony and prevent or reduce hostilities once employees are back at work.

CONTRACT ADMINISTRATION

Once a contract has been ratified, the negotiating process does not end. Throughout the life of the contract, cooperative and productive labor relations must be maintained. Open and ongoing communications and meetings between the employer and union representatives are necessary for a sound relationship. The contract must be interpreted and implemented, and a means for settling differences in this interpretation must be developed. Mechanisms for handling violations of the contract must also be specified. These are the concerns of contract administration.

A crucial part of contract administration is the grievance procedure. When issues arise concerning employer–employee relations and the administration of the contract, a grievance system is intact for handling and resolving these issues. The definition of a grievance, as well as the exact procedure, is specified in the contract. Discussion of grievance procedures was presented in Chapters 9 and 10. The only real difference is that in unionized settings a union representative assists the employee throughout the process, and arbitration is typically the last step.

The purpose of a grievance procedure is to work out differences in interpretation of the contract and provide a means for controlling conflict. It allows employees a means to complain without fearing retribution and provides a means for continuous negotiations throughout the day-to-day life of the contract. It allows identification of problems and a way to correct these problems, building stronger labor relations. It ensures the uniform application of personnel policies and can open communications between employees and management.[23]

Union grievances usually fall into the categories of job security of an individual employee, such as discipline and discharge issues, or group grievances surrounding job assignments, work standards, and working conditions. Disciplinary actions often cause employees to file grievances charging arbitrariness in applying disciplinary procedures or lack of due process. A system must be fair, uniformly applied, and based on just cause and due process.

Incentive systems for merit pay can also contribute to grievances when employees feel the system is used unfairly. Specific procedures and objective criteria must be used in performance evaluations and in awarding salary increases based on performance.

A change in past practices, though not written into a contract, is seen by the union as a management obligation. Sudden changes in past practices often cause employee grievances. Issues over which job classification should perform certain new tasks or responsibilities, individual transfers, promotions, assignments, and layoffs also give rise to grievances. Many contracts require that seniority and merit or experience be a factor in assignments. Shift preference, overtime, and health and safety issues also cause employee grievances. Steps must be taken to handle grievances effectively at the first-line management level, in order to decrease time and complications resulting from lengthy dispute resolution and arbitration. The following are causes for lengthy and ineffective grievance procedures:

1. Lack of screening by union of significant grievances
2. A union seeking trouble and filing any and all grievances
3. A union not unified, so fearing that refusal to arbitrate weak grievances might result in a loss of power
4. Lack of union investigation and training in grievance handling
5. First-line managers with lack of authority to handle and resolve grievances, and lack of training in grievance resolution
6. A hard-line approach by management on all grievances
7. An employer who maintains an uncooperative and antiunion attitude and makes little attempt to build sound relations
8. Mutual hostilities resulting from a bitter strike
9. Unclear or ambiguous contract language and performance evaluation systems[32]

While contract administration is a responsibility placed largely on the employer, it is a mutual process requiring continual, cooperative negotiations. First-line managers are instrumental in effective contract administrations and grievance resolutions. They must be aware of the provisions of the contract and be well trained in personnel management and leadership styles. A caring manager who is concerned for the employee as an individual will receive fewer grievances.[23]

CONCLUSION

The term "labor relations" brings to mind unions and collective bargaining. Effective management of collective bargaining from the initial organizing stage through contract administration is an essential part of labor relations, and has been the main topic of discussion in this chapter. But the *process* of building effective labor relations involves much more. It concerns the interactions, dealings, or relationship between management and employees in a unionized or nonunionized setting. A sound relationship based upon mutual cooperation, respect, shared values, and unified purposes is the ultimate goal. Although there is no such thing as a "perfect state," and relations must be continually renewed and maintained, certain steps can be taken to build toward this goal. That has been a theme throughout this book—that building sound employee relations serves to maximize individual gratification and build commitment to organizational success.

The process of building and maintaining effective labor relations must involve all aspects of human resource management. To achieve its goal, it must first ensure sound and effective personnel practices. It must continually monitor, improve, and control employee relations throughout the personnel processes and ensure the resolution of issues, conflicts, and disequilibrium that can stress employee relations. Lastly, it must effectively manage the collective bargaining process, including day-to-day contract administration.

As with all personnel processes, the status of labor relations depends upon developing an organizational climate that fosters individual satisfaction and effective employee relations. Practicing a philosophy that embraces the value of each human resource, along with an enlightened leadership team, can create such a climate. That has been the purpose of this book—to provide such a philosophy and integrate it into expert management practices, for maximum growth of the individual and the organization.

REFERENCES

1. Berkeley, A. E. Arbitration: The process and the participants. In I. M. Shepard, & A. E. Doudera (Eds.), *Health care labor law*. Ann Arbor, Mich.: University of Michigan Health Administration Press School of Public Health, 1981, p. 166.
2. Cohen, A. G. Labor relations in the health care industry. *Hospital Topics*, Nov./Dec. 1982, p. 34.

3. Flanagan, L. *Collective bargaining and the nursing profession.* Kansas City, Missouri: American Nurses' Association, 1983, p. 7.
4. American Hospital Association. *Washington Memo.* Chicago:AHA, November 2, 1984, #525, p. 4.
5. McClelland, J. Q. Professionalism and collective bargaining: A new reality for nurses and management. *JONA,* 1983, *13*(11), 36–38.
6. Elliot, C. L. Hospitals must face heavy unionization drives in '80s. Part 2. *Hospitals,* 1981, *55*(14), 99–102.
7. Stern, E. M. Collective bargaining: A means of conflict resolution. *Nursing Administration Quarterly,* 1982, *6*(2), 9–28.
8. Luttman, P. A. Collective bargaining and professionalism: Incompatible ideologies? In B. J. Brown (Ed.), *Nursing Administration Quarterly,* 1982, *6*(2), 25.
9. Cleland, V. S. Taft-Hartley amended: Implications for nursing—The professional model. *JONA,* 1981, *11*(7), 17–21.
10. Taylor, B. J., & Witney, F. *Labor relations law* (4th ed.). Englewood Cliffs, N.J.: Prentice-Hall, 1983, pp. 735–744.
11. Emerson, W. L. Appropriate bargaining units for health care professional employees. *JONA,* 1978, 10–11.
12. Arndt, C., & Huckabay, L. M. *Nursing administration: Theory for practice with a systems approach.* St. Louis: Mosby, 1980, pp. 308–309.
13. Horvitz, W. L., & Moffett, K. E. The FMCS and the peaceful resolution of disputes. In I. M. Shepard & A. E. Doudera (Eds.), *Health care labor law.* Ann Arbor, Mich.: University of Michigan Health Administration Press School of Public Health, 1981, p. 147.
14. Zimmerman, D. A. Trends in National Labor Relations Board Health Care Industry Decisions. In I. M. Shepard & A. E. Doudera (Eds.), *Health care labor law.* Ann Arbor, Mich.: University of Michigan Health Administration Press School of Public Health, 1981, pp. 6, 7.
15. Alexander, E. L. *Nursing administration in the hospital health care system* (2nd ed.). St. Louis: Mosby, 1978, pp. 51–56.
16. *The American Nurse.* Labor law hasn't met nurses' expectations. 1984, *16*(3), 1, 6, 10.
17. *AJN.* NLRB reversal threatens all-RN bargaining units, says ANA. *AJN,* 1984, *84*(10), 1303, 1312, 1324.
18. *The American Nurse,* Rulings differ on appropriate unit issue. 1985, *17*(3), 6.
19. Graczyk, B., & Castrey, R. T. Mediation—What it is, what it does. *JONA,* 1980, *1*(11), 24–28.
20. Rowland, H. S., & Rowland, B. L. *Nursing administration handbook.* Rockville, Md.: Aspen, 1980, pp. 141–143.
21. Heylman, P. M. Employee relations in an unorganized facility: How to preserve the status quo. In I. M. Shepard & A. E. Doudera (Eds.), *Health care labor law.* Ann Arbor, Mich.: University of Michigan Health Administration Press School of Public Health, 1981, pp. 122–131.
22. Miller, R. L. Anticipate questions, seek answers for adept labor relations efforts. *Hospitals,* 1976, *50*(13), 50–54.
23. Allen, R. E., & Keaveny, T. J. *Contemporary labor relations.* Reading, Mass.: Addison-Wesley Pub. Co., 1983, pp. 241–249.
24. Fralic, M. F. The nursing director prepares for labor negotiations. In C. Lockhart & W. E. Werther (Eds.), *Labor relations in nursing: The management anthology*

series. Theme five: Organizational security and longevity. Wakefield, Mass.: Nursing Resources, 1980, pp. 81–85.

25. Claus, R. C. The ins and outs of collective bargaining. *JONA*, 1980, *10*(9), 18, 19.
26. Gonder, P. O., & American Association of School Administrators. *Collective bargaining: Problems and solutions.* Sacramento, Calif.: Education News Service, 1981.
27. Elkin, R. D. Negotiating and administering a union contract. In C. Lockhart & W. B. Werther (Eds.), *Labor relations in nursing: The management anthology series. Theme five: Organizational security and longevity.* Wakefield, Mass.: Nursing Resources, 1980, pp. 75, 76.
28. National Education Association and RCH Systems. *Verbal skills and negotiations.* Westwood, N. J.: National Education Association.
29. Heylman, P. M. Developing a Strike Contingency Plan. In I. M. Shepard & A. E. Doudera (Eds.), *Health care labor law.* University of Michigan: Health Administration Press School of Public Health, 1981, pp. 137–139.
30. Brody, P. E., & Stamm, J. B. Strike two: Hospitals down but not out. *Health Care Management Review,* 1978, *3*(3), 53–61.
31. Anderson, C., & Van Norman, D. How to handle a strike. *Hospitals,* 1985, *59*(2), 109–112.
32. Fossum, J. A. *Labor relations: Development, structure, process* (2nd ed.). Plano, Tex.: Business Publications, Inc., 1982, pp. 361–383.

SUGGESTED READING

Addison, J. T. Are unions good for productivity? *Journal of Labor Research,* 1982, *3*(2), 125–138.

Arbeiter, J. S. Strike! When nurses walk out. *RN,* Oct. 1984, pp. 50–58.

Ashton, D. (Ed.). Developments in employee relations. *Management Decision,* 1982, *20*(5 & 6), 2–67.

Azoff, E. S. Sensitized supervisors—A key to preserving nonunion status. *Hospital Progress,* 1979, *60*(1), 57–59.

Barash, J. Trade Unionism from Roosevelt to Reagan. *The Annals of the American Academy of Political and Social Science,* 1984, *473,* 11–22.

Batstone, E., Ferner, A., & Terry, M. Unions on the board. *Employee relations (West Yorkshire),* 1983, *5*(5), 2–4.

Behrens, C. K., & Sollenberger, J. R. The National Labor Relations Act: A potential legal constraint upon quality circles and other employer-sponsored employee committee. *Labor Law Journal,* 1983, *34,* 776–780.

Beletz, E. E. Nurses participation in bargaining units. *Nursing Management, 13*(10), 48–58.

Bernstein, A. H. Hospitals under federal labor law. *Hospitals,* 1980, *54*(15), 30–34.

Blair, D. H., & Crawford, D. L. Labor union objectives and collective bargaining. *Quarterly Journal of Economics,* 1984, *99*(3), 547–566.

Botan, C. H., & Frey, L. R. Do workers trust labor unions and their messages? *Communication Monographs,* 1984, *50*(3), 233–244.

Boyce, M. T. Protected activities of nonunion employees. *Employee Relations Law,* 1983, *9*(2), 292–307.

Bright, D. Industrial relations of recession. *Industrial Relations Journal*, 1983, *14*(3), 24–33.

Burton, D. F., & Hewlett, S. A. Labor-management relations and productivity: A framework for success. *National Productivity Review*, 1983, *2*(2), 185–194.

Carson, C. B. Unionism revisited. *The Freeman*, 1984, *34*(4), 209–218.

Casey, J. R. Reorganizing in the eighties: An internal participatory model. *Public Administration Review*, 1982, *42*(6), 576–583.

Champagne, P. J. Using labor management committees to improve productivity. *Human Resources Management*, 1982, *21*(2), 67–73.

Cole, R. E. QC warning voiced by U.S. expert on Japanese circles. *World of Work Report*, 6 July 1981, pp. 49–51.

Coney, A. C., & Barmish, A. What to do when organized labor comes calling. *Hospitals*, Dec. 16, 1979, pp. 85–90.

Coombe, J. D. Peer review: The emerging successful application. *Employee Relations Law Journal*, 1984, *9*(4), 659–671.

Dannemiller, K. After the nurses' strike: A healing project. *Group and Organization Studies*, 1982, *7*(2), 193–206.

Dimse, C. A. Can unions get you what you want? The case against: Nurses and management share common goals. *Nursing Careers*, 1982, *3*(5), 8.

Dumphy, D. C., & Dick, R. *Organizational change by choice*. Roseville East, Australia: McGraw-Hill, 1981.

Dunlap, J. T. *Dispute resolution: Negotiation and consensus building*. Dover, Mass.: Auburn House, 1984.

Farish, P. Improved output. *Personnel Administrator*, 1982, *27*, 18.

Freeman, R. B., & Medoff, J. L. Trade unions and productivity: Some new evidence on an old issue. *Annals of the American Academy of Political and Social Science*, 1984, *473*, 149–164.

Friedheim, K. K. Negotiating a union contract. *MLO*, 1982, *14*(12), 58–64.

Gordon, M. E., & Johnson, W. A. Seniority: A review of its legal and scientific standing. *Personnel Psychology*, 1982, *35*(2), 255–280.

Gordon, T. Organizing efforts of public employees thwarted: "Millions" spent on anti-union tactics. *American Teacher*, 1981, *65*(7), 1.

Harrison, E. L. The discipline of hospital professional employees. *Hospital Topics*, 1979, *57*(4), 6–9.

Horvitz, W. L. On the labor front: A rough 1984. *Dun's Business Month*, 1983, *122*, 61–62.

Hospitals. Nonunion staff has right to representation. 1983, *57*(8), 48.

Kassalow, E. M. The future of American unionism: A comparative perspective. *Annals of the American Academy of Political and Social Science*, 1984 *473*, 52–63.

Levitan, S. A., & Johnson, C. M. Labor and management: The illusion of cooperation. *Harvard Business Review*, 1983, *61*(5), 8–10.

Lopez, M. The pros and cons of managing union and nonunion labs. *MLO*, 1982, *14*(12), 69–71.

Metzger, M. Labor relations demand special attention in multihospital systems. *Hospitals*, 1981, *55*(1), 57–59.

Metzger, N. Hospital labor scene marked by union issues. *Hospitals*, 1980, *54*(7), 105–112.

Metzger, N., & Ferentino, J. M. Labor relations: How to administer the grievance procedure. *Hospitals*, May 1, 1982, pp. 89–92.

Oswald, R. New directions for American unionism. *Annals of the American Academy of Political and Social Science*, 1984, *473*, 141–148.

Parker, H. J., & Gilmore, H. L. The unfair labor practice caseload: An analysis of selected remedies. *Labor Law Journal*, 1983, *34*, 172–179.

Regan, W. A. Freedom of speech for employer in hospital labor controversy. *Hospital Progress*, 1979, *60*(5), 84–86.

Rehmas, C. M. Writing the opinion. In A. M. Zack (Ed.), *Arbitration in practice*. Ithaca, N.Y.:ILR Press/Cornell, 1984.

RN Magazine. State association won't bargain anymore, *RN*, March 1983, p. 14.

Salkever, D. S. Hospital unionization trends. *Journal of Health and Human Resources Administration*, 1983, *6*(2), 267–285.

Sargis, N. M. Will nursing director's attitudes affect future collective bargaining? *JONA*, 1979, *8*(12), 21–26.

Schwartz, S. J. The National Labor Relations Board and the duty of fair representation. *Labor Law Journal*, 1983, *34*, 781–789.

Shanin, D. B. NRB versus Baptist Hospital, Inc.: Union solicitation in health care institutions. *American Journal of Law Medicine*, 1980, *6*(1), 105–123.

Spelman, J. Can unions get you what you want? The case for: Unions in your own image. *Nursing Careers*, 1982, *3*(5), 8.

Stepp, J. R. Helping labor and management see and solve problems. *Monthly Labor Review*, 1982, *105*, 15–20.

Union-busting today: Assault with a deadly briefcase. *Allied Industrial Worker*, 1982, *25*, 8.

Unions' View of Industrial Relations. *Worklife/IR Research Reports*, 1983, *3*(4), 12–13.

Van Houten, D. R. Bibliography: Industrial and economic democracy. *Economic and Industrial Democracy*, 1982, *3*(3), 366–379.

Veninga, K. S., & Veninga, R. L. The PATCO problem and nursing: A comparative analysis. *Nursing Outlook*, Apr. 1982, pp. 265–267.

Winpisinger, W. W. The "Japanese miracle." *Labor Today*, 1983, *22*, 6.

Zippo, M. Labor-management relations in the 80s. *Personnel*, 1982, *59*(5), 45–46.

Index

Page numbers followed by f or t refer to figures or tables.